C.J.P. Thijn J.T. Steensma

Tuberculosis of the Skeleton

Focus on Radiology

Foreword by E.G. Theros

With 126 Figures in 344 Separate Illustrations

Springer-Verlag Berlin Heidelberg New York
London Paris Tokyo Hong Kong

Professor Dr. Cornelis J.P. Thijn
Department of Radiology
University Hospital Groningen
Oostersingel 59, 9700 Groningen
The Netherlands

Dr. Jieldouw T. Steensma
Department of Tuberculosis
Beatrixoord Hospital
Haren/Groningen
The Netherlands

Radiographs prepared by Harry van der Zwaag

ISBN-13:978-3-642-74667-3 e-ISBN-13:978-3-642-74665-9
DOI: 10.1007/978-3-642-74665-9

Library of Congress Cataloging-in-Publication Data. Thijn, Cornelis Jacob Pieter, 1933– Tuberculosis of the skeleton: focus on radiology / C.J.P. Thijn, J.T. Steensma; foreword by E.G. Theros. p. cm. Bibliography:p.Includes index.ISBN-13:978-3-642-74667-3(U.S.:alk. paper)1.Human skeleton–Tuberculosis. 2. Human skeleton–Radiography. I. Steensma, J.T. (Jieldouw T.), 1942– . II. Title. [DNLM: 1. Tuberculosis, Osteoarticular. 2. Tuberculosis, Osteoarticular–radiography. WE 253 T439t] RC312.5.B6T45: 1989 616.9'9571–dc20 DNLM/DLC for Library of Congress 89-11484 CIP

Softcover reprint of the hardcover 1st edition 1990

2121/3130-543210 – Printed on acid-free paper

Foreword

Tuberculosis is on an accelerated march again, not only in third-world nations where it has always been endemic but also in more advanced nations with vast technological resources. This worldwide increase in tuberculosis has been due in part to two major factors: first, the widespread use of immunosuppressive drugs and, secondly, the rising incidence of immunodeficiency diseases, particularly exemplified by AIDS. These are in addition to the increased incidence caused by the recent unprecedented population migrations.

Against this background, the authors have provided us with a timely contribution which will be of value for understanding and diagnosing the manifestations of tuberculosis in the musculoskeletal system. Although musculoskeletal involvement is much more frequent in third-world countries, it is increasing in more advanced nations because of the flow of immigrant populations and the severely immunosuppressed states of many patients encountered in practice. This book should be a must for all those involved in the practice of radiology in the third world and will be of great value for radiologists everywhere because it is so topical. Also, it assembles in one place a veritable panorama of the multifaceted features that can occur in bone and joint tuberculosis.

The authors have very effectively organized their material so that easy reference can be made to specific anatomic areas. Appropriately, they begin with an epidemiological overview of anatomic sites of involvement, and then proceed to evaluate each site in sections of the text, beginning with the most common and proceeding to the more unusual ones. The whole is preceded by a good summarizing discussion of the pathogenesis, clinical background, and methods of investigation and diagnosis. The largest portion of the textual material is devoted to tuberculous spondylitis since the spine is by far the most common site. Numerous illustrations have been carefully selected to give the reader a thorough survey of the possible manifestations of tuberculosis of the spine. This is followed by a discussion of tuberculous arthritis since involvement of the hip and knee joints is second in frequency only to that of spondylitis. Thereafter, the authors deal with other parts of the skeleton with typical examples of radiographic findings. Because of the importance of understanding and differentiating intramedullary bone involvement from synovial involvement, the authors have devoted a special section to osteomyelitis. The book ends with a clear summary of the principles of management of musculoskeletal tuberculosis.

One of the strengths of this work is the authors' dedication to relating the radiologic images to the underlying pathology and the clinical background. The degree to which the authors develop this makes this text unique amongst others that have been written on the same subject. Thus, the reader not only has a source of easy reference because of the way the book is organized, but will gain further understanding of the pathogenesis of this remarkably persistent disease.

ELIAS G. THEROS, M.D.
I. Meschan Distinguished Professor
of Radiology
Wake Forest University
Bowman Gray School of Medicine
Winston-Salem, North Carolina, USA

Preface

The incidence of tuberculosis has declined dramatically in the more industrialized countries over recent decades, but the disease is still present. In the Netherlands, new manifestations of tuberculosis are found in about 1400 patients every year. Some 70 of these are in the skeletal system. Immigrants from Mediterranean countries and the Tropics account for 25% of the tuberculosis population in the Netherlands [23]. Clinicians and radiologists must remain aware of the disease and consider the possibility of tuberculosis in their patients. Pulmonary tuberculosis is a very common disease in countries in which living conditions are poor due to malnutrition, inadequate housing, and lack of health education. The manifestations of skeletal tuberculosis may present a clinical and radiologic picture there that is different from that in western countries: the course of the disease tends to be more acute and to involve severe destruction, resembling a nontuberculous osteomyelitis or arthritis.

This book is based on material from the Beatrixoord Hospital. This Hospital was originally founded in 1909 as a sanatorium for the treatment of patients with tuberculosis, when the disease was still common in the Netherlands. Since the 1950s it has served as a hospital for a broader range of diseases. The Tuberculosis Department today is one of the few remaining in this country, where patients with all forms of tuberculosis can be treated. Since 1955 the clinical data on each patient have been carefully noted and the radiographs archived. For many years Dr. E.H.J. Warns was closely involved in the treatment of patients with skeletal manifestations of tuberculosis in the Hospital. His meticulous description of the radiologic findings testify to his great enthusiasm and to his extensive knowledge of this disease. His contributions have been of great help.

The clinical and radiologic material on 460 manifestations of skeletal tuberculosis in 370 patients were studied (over the period 1955–1987). The spine, hip, and knee joint proved to be the most commonly affected sites. A number of radiographs presenting rare sites of osseous tuberculosis were also kindly placed at our disposal, mainly by radiologists practicing in other countries. The authors wish gratefully to thank them for their help.

Books that are oriented particularly to the radiologic aspects of skeletal tuberculosis are hardly available today. In addition to the radiologic focus of the present work, chapters are devoted to the pathogenesis, clinical findings, diagnostic methods, and therapy of skeletal tuberculosis. In our opinion, this book will be worth while both for the treatment of patients with tuberculosis of the skeletal system and as a reference work for clinicians and radiologists who want to be informed about skeletal manifestations of tuberculosis.

The radiographic material in this book was carefully prepared by HARRY VAN DER ZWAAG. The authors gratefully appreciate his work. We also wish to thank the clerical staff of the Beatrixoord Hospital (Mrs. A. DE BOER) and the University Hospital of Groningen (Mrs. G. WELTEVREDE, Mrs. A. BUITENDIJK) for their efforts. The authors owe a great debt to Dr. R.J. MULDER and Dr. M.T. MULDER-DE JONG for their comments on parts of the manuscript and for their suggestions as to improvements.

Groningen and Haren
Autumn 1989

C.J.P. THIJN
J.T. STEENSMA

Contents

1 Pathogenesis

Tuberculosis is a generalized disease with local manifestations. VILLEMIN (1865) was the first to prove in animal experiments that tuberculosis is a contagious disease. KOCH (1882) discovered the tubercle bacillus and thereby brought about a revolution in medical science. Nevertheless, many mysteries are still to be solved.

1.1 Species and Types of Mycobacteria

The causative agents of tuberculosis are bacteria belonging to the so-called *Mycobacterium tuberculosis* complex. The main representatives are *M. tuberculosis, M. bovis, M. bovis* BCG and *M. africanum*. The Indian subcontinent has yet some other variants. *M. tuberculosis* is by far the most common cause of tuberculous involvement in bone and joints. Where cattle are free of tuberculosis, *M. bovis* has been eliminated as a source of infection through the consumption of raw milk. In England and Wales a decline was noticed in disease caused by *M. bovis* in tuberculous cervical lymph nodes from 57.5% in 1945 to 1% in 1984, while in bone and joint disease there was a decline from 10.6% to 4% over the same period. The difference in these two sets of figures is probably due to a different length of time between the moment of primary infection, on the one hand, and the occurrence of lymph node lesions or of bone or joint lesions, on the other, the latter often appearing only after many years [41]. Vaccination with BCG may result in the involvement of bone and joints; this, however, is exceptional [55, 123, 131, 148, 182]. *M. africanum* is a mycobacterium that bacteriologists place between *M. tuberculosis* and *M. bovis*. In the Western world it does not play a significant role.

Mycobacteriosis, caused by atypical mycobacteria, falls beyond the scope of this book. Mycobacteriosis in bone tissue is seldom described in individuals with a normal immune system [44, 108, 150, 155]. In immune-impaired patients, such as those with AIDS, disseminated disease caused by human or atypical mycobacteria with involvement of bone tissue is quite common [75].

Mycobacteria usually spread through the body by hematogenous or lymphogenous pathways. The micro-organisms may settle for years in tissue, as co-called dormant bacilli or persisters, before they cause disease. Disease in bone and joints, however, may also affect adjacent tissues. On the other hand, miliary disease, as a result of hematogenous spread of mycobacteria, may have its origin in a tuberculous bone lesion.

1.2 Genetic Influences: HLA-DR

It has long been known that tuberculosis is more common in some families than in others. But even within one family the individual members may react differently. Most risk factors for developing tuberculosis are believed to be acquired. Yet the susceptibility for tuberculosis may also be under genetic control, because only a small fraction of all infected persons eventually develop tuberculosis.

There is a difference both in qualitative and in quantitative immune response, regulated by immune response genes. The human leukocyte antigen (HLA) system is a powerful genetic marker. HLA-DR antigens regulate host responses to infections through cell-mediated immunity. HLA determinants cause only relative, not absolute, differences in sensitivity to the disease. Other factors, including exposure, concurrent disease, immune competency of the host, and antigen composition, also play a role in expression of the disease and may mask the association of tuberculosis with HLA phenotypes [76, 132].

Much research has been carried out to gain a better understanding of the pathogenesis of tuberculosis. An interesting finding is that mycobacteria and rheumatoid arthritis seem to share corresponding antigens [74]. At the end of the last century Poncet [135] suggested a link between tuberculosis and inflammatory rheumatoid arthritis. Other investigators also came to this conclusion, and some were interested in the role of immunity to tuberculous antigens [58, 62, 133, 178], while others doubted the existence of any such link [77]. A recent hypothesis has been that HLA-DR4 is able to present an antigen of synovium or cartilage which possibly also occurs in infectious micro-organisms [49]. More research is needed to gain further insight in these complex mechanisms.

1.3 Development of Cellular Immunity and Hypersensitivity Reaction to Mycobacterial Antigens

After the first contact with mycobacteria (primary infection) there is only a mild local and systemic reaction, because of the lack of a specific immune response. The lungs are usually the first site of such infection. Most mycobacteria ingested by macrophages are killed after phagocytosis, and disease does not occur. The bacteria may, however, survive intracellularly and multiply. Release of mycobacteria after lysis of these macrophages causes dissemination by hematogenous and/or lymphogenous pathways, and the bacteria may settle in any organ in these first weeks, before specific immunity is provoked [37]. Local circumstances such as oxygenation, pH, and the development of specific cell-mediated immune response (4–6 weeks after infection) determine whether the bacteria in these seondary stations are killed or remain alive and lead later to postprimary disease (secondary tuberculosis).

Mycobacteria can survive in a dormant state as so-called persisters. These hardly metabolize, seldom multiply, and may survive thus for a period or months or even many decades. When, for some reason, host resistance is diminished, and the cellular immune response becomes insufficient, dormant bacteria may "wake up", start to multiply, and cause disease.

There is a difference in susceptibility of various organs to tuberculosis. Genetic as well as local factors play a role, however little is known about this.

Mycobacterial antigens evoke both a specific cell-mediated immunity and a cellular hypersensitivity reaction (delayed, type IV).

The balance between immune reaction and hypersensitivity reaction determines the histological findings and the clinical symptoms.

1.3.1 Cell-Mediated Immunity

Macrophages and T-lymphocytes in combination with the antigen load are responsible for what happens. The macrophage has an essential role as effector cell, while the T-lymphocyte is mainly the immune responsive cell [37]. Cell-mediated immunity is mainly a local phenomenon. Macrophages are activated by lymphocytes and their lymphokines at the site of infection. This results in the formation of granulomas (tubercles). After activation, macrophages differentiate functionally. Some activated macrophages may kill the tubercle bacilli.

1.3.2 Hypersensitivity Reaction

After contact with tubercle bacilli the host develops a hypersensitivity to the mycobacterial antigen(s). Genetic factors play a role in the degree of hypersensitivity [4, 9, 101]. The hypersensitivity reaction to a low amount of bacillary antigen(s) causes an accelerated tubercle formation and often the destruction of the bacilli (see Sect. 1.3.1). In the presence of a high amount of antigen(s) the hypersensitivity reaction itself causes cell death and tissue destruction; this is known as caseation.

Liquification (formation of pus) is the most harmful response in secondary tuberculosis and is also linked to delayed-type hypersensitivity. During the liquification process the tubercle bacilli also multiply extracellularly. With excess bacillary antigen the formerly beneficial reaction, which is responsible for the cell-mediated immunity of tuberculosis, is then responsible for almost all tissue damage present in tuberculosis, specifically that in caseation and liquification [143].

1.3.3 Progression or Healing

Progression of the disease is dependent on the ability of the macrophage to kill or inhibit the growth of the mycobacteria in its cytoplasm. In bone and joint disease the hypersensitivity reaction plays an important role. The number of bacilli in the pus is usually low because the local circumstances (lack of oxygen and low pH) are not beneficial to bacterial growth. During the healing process, fibrosis walls off the caseous foci, and at the edges increasing osteosclerosis is seen. In the end, remineralization and (re)calcification may occur. Destruction and healing can thus be seen at the same time.

1.4 Endogenous Reactivation

Tuberculosis of bone and joints is a postprimary manifestation of tuberculosis. The clinical disease may begin either soon after primary infection or even many years later, when a specific cellular immune response exists. The balance between the interaction of cellular immunity and (persistent) mycobacteria may be disturbed by certain medicines (cytostatics, corticosteroids), radiation, intercurrent infections (measles, HIV infection), and other circumstances that diminish resistance to infectious disease, such as diabetes, malignancy, and stress [33, 50]. Local traumata may also result in endogenous reactivation of a tuberculous infection and cause symptoms after a latent period of 1–6 months [80, 160, 176]. The mechanism which causes this disturbance in cellular immune response and results in multiplication of dormant bacilli is still unknown.

2 Clinical Findings

Pulmonary tuberculosis can be seen as a composite of many local processes: some lesions heal, others progress, some stabilize, and others reactivate – at the same time [37]. The same is true in bone and joint disease: active disease and healing can be seen together with old inactive processes in the same patient, close together or at different locations.

In earlier times, when many patients died of tuberculosis, it was possible to study the various stages which tuberculosis in bone and joint may present. It is tempting to follow the old masters, such as CALVÉ and MENARD, in their description of pathology in connection with clinical findings in the patient [25, 117]. One should realize, however, that the stages that are described may overlap with each other. Depending on the time at which treatment is started, antituberculous drugs may influence the course of the disease.

In tuberculosis of bone and joints three clinical stages can be distinguished [137, 141].

Stage I: *Early Onset ("phase d'ensemencement").* In the beginning the patient has only intermittent pain, and there is a slight disability. At rest, the pain subsides, although after a while pain may become more prominent and may occur even at night, due to loss of the normal muscle spasms that protect against pain in the daytime [45]. In joint disease, movement of the involved joint is avoided, which results in slight contractures and muscle atrophy. The patient quickly feels tired and is sometimes with fever up to $\pm 38.5°$ C. Because the pain is not permanent, it may take weeks and even months before the patient seeks medical advice. In joint disease the complaints resemble those of chronic monoarthritis. There may be a local increase in temperature and sometimes signs of intra-articular hydrops. A slight resistance may be felt upon palpation, caused by periarticular edema. Circumscribed tenderness may be elicited by local pressure. Regional lymph nodes may be enlarged [121].

Physiotherapy is of no help in this stage; on the contrary, it often aggravates the pain. The patient is then often accused of being neurotic and feels misunderstood. Progression is often slow, especially in patients who are otherwise in good physical condition. However, rapid progression is also possible, as in malignant disease.

Radiologic blurring of contours and demineralization are the most prominent findings in this early stage.

Stage II: *Active Disease ("phase d'état" or "phase de focalisation").* Gradually the destruction proceeds, resulting in an abscess. The pain is no longer intermittent and becomes more severe upon weight bearing and even slight movements. Abscess formation may exert pressure on surrounding tissue. This is especially dangerous in vertebral involvement with extension of lesions towards the spinal canal. Contractures and muscle atrophy become more prominent. Muscle tonus diminishes. The patient may have bouts of fever of up to 39°–40° C, highest in the late afternoon and often with a normal temperature in the morning. But body temperature may also be normal. Local swelling and a draining sinus are relatively late signs, but these may be the first alarming symptoms for the patient. When an abscess extends to the skin, a local swelling can be felt – round and at first hard but later more fluctuant.

The so-called "cold" (tuberculous) abscess differs from a pyogenic abscess in that it is less warm and red, relatively less painful on pressure, and shows slow progression. A cold abscess may descent between, and also through, muscle sheets a long way downward, e.g., from lumbar vertebrae along the psoas muscle down to the upper leg and there perforate at last. The overlying skin discolors to a typical purple-red. In the end, a draining sinus may occur. A cold abscess may contain pus of variable consistency; thin in the upper layers and thicker, more or less curdled in the lower layers. In the course of the disease it may also vary in consistency. The pus is often greenish in color and may even contain small sequestra. After perforation of the abscess the pain becomes less severe, and if the patient had fever, the temperature usually drops, although not always, to normal. Return of pain and/or temperature is often due to secondary pyogenic infection.

In this second stage the patient not only suffers pain on pressure, both direct and indirect (axial compression elicits pain in the involved vertebrae), but there is also circumscribed percussion pain. A gibbus may be seen, caused by collapsed adjacent vertebrae. In knee and hip involvement, drawing in the longitudinal axis is often painful. Since pain is conducted by nerves, the pain is often felt distal to its origin (e.g., pain medial in the knee caused by coxitis, in breast or abdomen in spondylitis, in the hand caused by omarthritis). Neurological symptoms such as pareses and alterations or loss of sensibility may occur, as well as incontinence of urine or feces, depending on the site of the lesion, caused by compression of the spinal cord.

Radiologic findings in this stage show considerable destruction, loss of normal anatomical contours in joint disease or collapse of vertebrae, but at the same time also gradually better demarcation between diseased and normal healthy tissue. Considerable swelling of soft tissue may be present because of abscess formation, which may be missed on ordinary radiographs when they are focused on the bones only. Especially in the lumbar region the psoas abscesses may be very wide, and a large film is needed in order not to overlook these cold abscesses.

Stage III: *Healing Stage ("phase de cicatrisation").* If nothing is done, the patient may die of complications: miliary spread of mycobacteria or secondary infection and subsequent septicemia. Many patients, however, have enough resistance to overcome the infection, even without surgical or medicamentous intervention. Although these patients recover, endogenous reactivation of tuberculosis is imminent as long as no bactericidal drug therapy is given. Without medical intervention, however, some patients, never reach the final stage but have chronic disease, with stage II and III seen together. The patient may suffer from a chronic draining sinus, which often is secondarily infected.

In this third stage of healing, fibrosis in the center and peripheral osteosclerosis are found. The pain subsides and disappears completely when a bony or fibrous ankylosis develops. The sinus heals from inside outward. This takes a long time, often with a long period of intermittent draining (*periode du désespoir*). In a definitely healed sinus the skin is retracted and pale.

3 Diagnostic Methods

Tuberculosis is often called the great imitator. Whereas tuberculosis once ranked high on the list of differential diagnoses, its frequency has since declined substantially. In countries with low prevalence it is often even forgotten as a possible diagnosis [30, 64, 100]. This may be disastrous for the patient and even lead to death – in a potentially curable disease. The patient may die of a presumed "cancer with metastasis to the bone," while at autopsy tuberculosis is found.

One should always bear in mind the reason why a person develops tuberculosis at this particular moment. In some way or other the host resistance has been undermined. The reason may be a simultaneous disease: viral or bacterial infections, a (newly detected) diabetes, malignancy, postnatal stress, undernourishment due to insufficient food or gastrectomy, treatment with drugs that cause immune suppression (e.g., corticosteroids and cytostatics) or radiotherapy [33]. A local trauma or psychological stress may also lead to reactivation of tuberculosis. We have found the combination of tuberculosis and other pyogenic infection at the same location only in the case of a sinus.

The only absolute proof of tuberculosis is a positive culture of mycobacteria, but especially in extrapulmonary disease this is often difficult to obtain. A combination of findings often leads to a "clinical" diagnosis [7, 121].

Suspicion is already half the way to diagnosis. Other diagnostic methods may be helpful, and these are reviewed briefly below.

3.1 Patient and Family History

A history of previously untreated or insufficiently treated tuberculosis may give a clue to the possibility of an endogenous reactivation. If the patient is under suspicion of having tuberculosis but shows no history of such, close contact with a contagious tuberculosis patient is important information, especially in children and adolescents. But often the origin of the disease in a contact person is not known, or this person dares not admit that he suffers from tuberculosis. Information about a sick and coughing member of the household, a grandparent, or a friend may arouse suspicion of tuberculosis. One might also ask whether some acquaintaince has died of an unknown pulmonary disease.

There is often an insidious onset, with complaints which, at first slight, were intermediate, but which grew slowly worse (see Chap. 2). Pyogenic infections are usually more acute. Other possibilities of disease must be considered in the differential diagnosis.

Tuberculosis is principally a systemic disease. One should not focus only on complaints at one location but also inquire as to other symptoms. Every complaint, however slight, must be taken seriously. In many patients tuberculous activity is found at more than one location in the body. Concomitant active pulmonary or renal tuberculosis is very common. More than half of adult patients have a history of pleuritis.

3.2 Symptoms and Signs

A total body examination of the nude patient, including a neurological screening is necessary in order not to overlook tuberculous involvement at more than one site or concomitant disease. (See Chap. 2).

Pain, possibly elicited by pressure or percussion, local rise in temperature, swelling, muscle atrophy, contractures, and impaired function are frequent findings. Normal walking rhythm is usually disturbed. In vertebral involvement neurological symptoms may be found. A draining sinus is suspicious for tuberculosis, especially in the case of a long-standing sinus with intermittent pus production. Long healed, retracted sinuses, also on other parts of the body, may help one find the proper diagnosis. An abscess or sinus in the thigh, for example, must lead to suspicion of spondylitis in the lumbar or sacral region. Enlarged lymph nodes are not always malignant. Today, even tuberculous involvement of regional lymph nodes in bone and joint disease is possible [121].

3.3 Laboratory Findings

Routine blood examination is of no help at all in the diagnosis of tuberculosis. One may find normal as well as elevated levels of erythrocyte sedimentation rate, leukocytes, enzymes, and γ-globulins, but none of these is pathognomonic for tuberculosis. More advanced techniques for ascertaining specific antigens or antibodies cannot yet discern between active and inactive tuberculosis.

3.4 Tuberculin Skin Test

The skin test with purified protein derivative (PPD) injected intradermally and read after 72 h is an inexpensive and helpful test. However, a positive test (≥ 10 mm induration) is no proof of active tuberculosis. A negative skin test with PPD, however, absolutely does not exclude tuberculosis! The combination of active tuberculosis and negative tuberculin skin test may be expected in the following cases: (a) in persons in bad general condition, and especially in old age; (b) after some infections (viral, including HIV, mononucleosis); and (c) with the use of corticosteroids and/or cytostatics. Many such cases may have a (temporarily) negative skin test [6]. A repeated skin test after 1 week may often show a positive reaction (boosting). A small number of patients (in the Netherlands $\pm 5\%$) are also anergic to other antigens and never show a positive skin test.

The size of the skin area affected by the skin test is not correlated to the severity of disease. It is only an expression of delayed-type hypersensitivity to certain surface antigens of mycobacteria. There is a cross-sensitivity with tuberculins of mycobacteria other than *M. tuberculosis* because of corresponding antigens. The homologous tuberculin usually produces the greatest reaction [16, 51]. The skin test is expressed in millimeters induration (not redness). One should avoid talking about positive or negative. A 5-mm PPD skin test, for example, in a sick child with a history of tuberculosis contact should not be considered negative or unimportant but should be taken seriously until another diagnosis is proven [28, 152].

3.5 Biopsy or Puncture

In many cases it is not clear what disease is responsible for the bone lesions found on radiographs. A puncture or biopsy is needed to confirm diagnosis [173]. Techniques such as ultrasonography, computed tomography (CT), and magnetic resonance imaging (MRI) may be helpful in localizing the extent of the abscess. We prefer open biopsy over puncture. If it is decided to perform a puncture of an abscess that may be of tuberculous origin, special precautions need to be taken (see Sect. 11.4.1.). Histological findings in the borderline may be confusing (many plasma cells and lymphocytes). Microscopic examination and cultures are needed to confirm the diagnosis, but results are often inconclusive. Such results do not exclude tuberculosis, and treatment should be given as long as another diagnosis is not confirmed.

3.6 Bacteriology

A positive culture is the only proof; a positive microscopic finding is very suspicious of tuberculosis. Mycobacteria stained according to the Ziehl-Neelsen method or with auramine can be seen microscopically. In bone and joint tuberculosis the number of bacteria is often low, and the micro-organisms are not always easy to find in pus or tissue specimens [54]. It cannot be stressed strongly enough that negative findings do not exclude tuberculosis. Cultures on specific media are rather sensitive, but the bacteria grow slowly, and only after 6–8 weeks may they be considered negative. Also, negative cultures do not exclude active tuberculosis.

Many surgeons do not think about routine examination of material for bacteriological examination by microscopy and culture, and tissue is often dropped in formalin in the operating theater solely for histological examination. This is most regrettable. When tissue or pus is obtained under sterile conditions, it should be cultured both for pyogenous bacteria and for mycotics and mycobacteria. For culture of mycobacteria pretreatment with an acid or base should be avoided in order not to kill the few mycobacteria that may be present. A mixed infection without a sinus is seldom encountered. An even more sensitive, but also time-consuming test is injection of patient material into a guinea pig.

3.7 Histology

Tuberculosis is a granulomatous disease. The granulomas or tubercles caused by mycobacteria often cannot be distinguished typically from other granulomatous lesions, unless mycobacteria can be seen, making diagnosis quite certain. Central necrosis and caseation cannot always be found. This means that histological examination can also be confusing and may give no proof.

A "typical" tubercle in active disease consists of numerous macrophages, including epithelioid cells and giant cells, surrounded by layers of lymphocytes, plasma cells, and fibroblasts. Capillaries, lymphatics, collagen and ground substance are also part of a fresh tubercle but vanish soon as the disease progresses. In the center there is often necrotic or caseous material, in which mycobacteria may be seen. Mycobacteria may be noticed both intra- and extracellularly [94]. The originally caseous material may liquify and form pus. If the abscess wall is insufficient, a sinus may result. Sometimes eroded vessel walls can be seen. Bone structures may be destroyed and collapsed, but there is also considerable demineralization.

During healing the fibrous tissue layers become thicker. Remineralization and osteosclerosis beginning at the edges mean that healing is proceeding. Although radiographs may show a bone cavern during the active disease, complete restoration is possible in the healing phase, if weight bearing is avoided long enough, by remineralization of the not completely destroyed bony tissue (Fig. 9).

Various stages of activity can be seen close together (Chap. 2).

3.8 Imaging Modalities

Conventional radiologic examinations and modern imaging modalities may be helpful, but these give only an indication as to the correct diagnosis, not proof. Tuberculosis, the great imitator, shows a wide variety of possibilities, from hardly visible or invisible lesions to extensive destruction and healing. This is dealt with in the following chapters.

In practice, it may take a long time before radiologic examination is considered. A delay of 2–3 years in bone and joint disease is not uncommon today in countries in which the disease shows low prevalence [100].

4 Epidemiology of Bone and Joint Tuberculosis

The incidence of skeletal tuberculosis differs between Europe and North America, on the one hand, and developing countries, on the other, it being higher in the latter [109, 128, 140]. In addition, the character of the disease is different: in tropical countries (India, tropical Africa, Asia, South America) and among immigrants from these countries, tuberculous skeletal involvement more often presents as an acute osteomyelitis or arthritis, has a toxic cause [43], and can be very destructive [18, 29, 128, 140, 166]. In these countries factors such as malnutrition, inadequate housing, poor medical services, and lack of health education contribute to the high incidence of bone and joint tuberculosis [140]. Interracial differences are also found as regards the age at onset of the tuberculous process – this being low among nonwhite populations [12, 29, 31, 40, 47, 64, 78, 109, 136, 140, 173]. In low-prevalence countries, skeletal manifestations usually present with less severe bone destruction. Although the clinical features may occur within a very short period, radiologic findings of the tuberculous process often suggest that the bone lesion has already been present for a considerable time. In low-prevalence coun-

Table 1. Sites of tuberculous bone involvement: reported relative distributions (percentages)

	Sanchis-Olmos 1948 [147]	Lafond 1958 [93]	Goldblatt and Cremin 1978 [64]	Silva 1980 [158]	Eckel and Düe 1985 [48]	Martini 1988 [109]	Thijn and Steensma 1988[a]
Spine	40.8	47.5	59.9	60.0	57.0	44.0	52.0
Knee	9.6	10.0	8.2	8.0	11.0	18.0	10.9
Hip	29.0	4.8	10.6	18.0	13.0	10.0	12.6
Wrist, finger joints	5.6	3.2	–	4.0[b]	6.0	2.0[b], 1.8[c]	3.3
Elbow	1.4	2.4	0.8	0.5	3.0	8.0	1.7
Shoulder	–	2.8	1.2	1.5	3.0	2.5	3.7
Ankle/foot	5.8	5.9	2.6	7.0	6.0	12.0	3.7
Sacroiliac joint	–	–	4.2[d]	0.5	–	0.5	2.6
Pubis, ischium, symphysis, ilium	0.8	–	–	–	1.0	0.5	1.2
Sternum/sternoclavicular joint	–	–	–	–	–	–	3.0
Cranium	–	–	–	–	–	–	0.7
Ribs	–	–	–	–	–	–	2.0
Greater trochanter	–	–	–	–	–	–	2.2
Long tubular bones	1.2	–	5.0	–	–	–	0.4
Multifocal lesions	16.0	–	8.2	–	–	–	11.3
Number of osseous manifestations	480	230	499	–	969	529	460

[a] Previously unpublished data from Beatrixoord Hospital, Haren/Groningen, The Netherlands.
[b] Only wrist.
[c] Only finger joints.
[d] Includes pelvis.

tries, the patient-and-doctor's delay may add up to 2–3 years; physicians, for example, have become unfamiliar with tuberculosis and sometimes wait until the origin of disease is proven [100]. Alas, this may be too late for some patients: at autopsy! The significance of a previous trauma as a cause of tuberculous bone involvement is suspected but not proven [22, 80, 160, 176].

Common sites of tuberculous bone involvement are the thoracic and lumbar spine, the hip, and the knee joint [166]. Unusual sites of infection are the limb bones, pelvis, ribs, sternum, and skull; not a single bone is safe from tuberculous involvement. Multifocal bone lesions are found both in white and in nonwhite patients and have been described at frequencies ranging from 7.6% to 20%, predominating in colored patients [64, 70, 93, 127, 128, 140, 147]. In our material on 370 patients, 460 manifestations of tuberculosis in bones and joints were studied (Table 1). In 42 patients (11.3%) multifocal lesions were encountered, 37 of whom presented with two, 4 patients with three, and a single patient with four foci of bone or joint tuberculosis.

5 Tuberculous Spondylitis

5.1 General Remarks

In about 1% of patients with tuberculous infections the skeleton is affected. The majority of tuberculous infections are caused by *M. tuberculosis*. Other mycobacteria, for example, *M. bovis*, are also found, but at much lower rate. BCG spondylitis has been described and is found mostly within 2 years after vaccination [13, 55, 123, 148, 182]. Tuberculous spondylitis is the most frequent form of osseous tuberculosis, being encountered in about half of these patients [40, 78, 109, 136, 140] (Table 1). In a large majority of cases the thoracic and lumbar spine is affected [129, 164, 175]. The atlas and the epistropheus seem to be the least common location of tuberculous spondylitis [109, 124]. In our material of 460 manifestations of osseous tuberculosis, 239 instances (52%) were localized in the spine: 13 cervical spine, 107 thoracic spine, 106 lumbar spine, and 13 sacrum. The number of affected men and women was about the same, and only few patients were children.

In Asia, tropical Africa, South America and among immigrants from these countries, the tuberculosis is more serious and results in much more destruction and more uncommon manifestations of osseous infection. In the tropics neurological involvement occurs in half of patients with tuberculosis of the spine; it varies from less severe features to paraplegia and even quadriplegia [140]. In patients from the tropics higher rates of involvement of the cervical spine, the vertebral arches, and the adjoining ribs may be found; also described are manifestations such as multiple noncontiguous vertebral lesions, osteosclerotic bone response, single vertebra affection, preservation of intervertebral discs, widening of intervertebral discs, florid paravertebral abscesses, but also absent paravertebral abscesses [8, 29, 92, 95, 97, 105, 113, 164, 169]. Probably because of the high prevalence of tuberculosis in the above-mentioned countries, tuberculous spondylitis is mainly a disease of childhood. In the first decade of life reported frequencies of 32% [129], 40% [175], 50% [64], 61% [164], and 70% [73] are found in the literature. Among whites tuberculous spondylitis is mostly a disease of adults. The mode of infection is thought to be hematogenous. Arterial as well as venous routes may be responsible for the spread of tuberculous bacilli to the spine. Arguments for the importance of a venous pathway are a similarity in the distribution of pyogenic infection of the spine following urologic procedures and the production of tuberculous infections of the spine experimentally by injecting bacilli into the abdominal or pelvic organs. Especially the paravertebral venous plexus seems to be responsible for tuberculous infection of the spine [15, 69, 73, 142, 177]. Besides the hematogenous and lymphohematogenous modes of infection, in some patients tuberculous lesions of vertebrae or paravertebral tuberculous lymph nodes may contaminate adjacent vertebrae; even spinal tuberculosis extended from the subarachnoid space is also described by some authors [24, 76].

5.2 Radiologic Modalities

In the latent period between the onset of tuberculous disease of a vertebral body and the appearance of abnormalities on radiographs, a radionuclide bone scan may be able to detect the initial focus as a "hot spot" (Fig. 21). In cases with destruction only of bony tissue, early bone scanning with technetium polyphosphate and gallium is usually negative [175, 177]. MRI is able to diagnose initial spondylitis because of the larger content of water in the focus. In the later stages of active disease and during the healing process conventional radiographs and tomograms are usually sufficiently reliable to follow the spondylitic process (Fig. 1). Abscess formation in the lumbar area may be missed on conventional radiographs when these are focused on the vertebrae only. The abscesses may be very extensive, and a large film is needed in order not to overlook these cold abscesses.

The use of ultrasonography, CT, and MRI improves the diagnosis of paravertebral abscesses, burrowing abscesses, destruction of the vertebral canal, soft tissue calcifications, affection of the vertebral arches, and encroachment in the vertebral canal [65, 69, 81, 92, 95, 107, 138, 175, 177]. CT features of retroperitoneal abscesses are low-density masses with peripheral rim enhancement adjacent to mild or extensive bone destruction. It is wise to use scintigraphy and CT in every nonwhite patient with unexplained and significant low back pain [177]. CT can also be helpful in needle localization during the procedure of abscess aspiration. Myelography is sometimes indicated in the patient with neurological features to determine the site(s) of canal encroachment (Fig. 21). Sinography and opacification of abscesses after punction and the injection of contrast medium may be indicated in selected cases.

5.3 Usual Presentation of Tuberculous Spondylitis

A latent period, lasting from several months to many decades following primary tuberculous infection, may be seen before clinical signs of spondylitis become manifest [1, 98, 142, 174]. The thoracolumbar region is most frequently affected [129]. Only below the age of 7 years is the intervertebral disc vascularized, and it may therefore be affected initially. In adults there is usually no initial infection of the disc [98]. In the majority of cases tuberculous infection of the vertebral bodies either by the arterial or venous pathways is primarily localized in the center of the vertebral body or in the large blood lacunae adjacent to the layer of hyaline cartilage which covers the subchondral bone plates and intervertebral discs. The initial foci are mostly located close to the anterior contour of the vertebral body (Figs. 1–4). Progressive extension of the lesion takes place in the direction of the intervertebral disc. The disc itself is only affected by the tuberculous process if the integrity of annulus fibrosus is disturbed, and the nucleus pulposus is infected. Otherwise, cartilage is very resistant to destruction by tuberculosis. In pyogenic infections, invasion of the intervertebral disc occurs more rapidly because proteolytic enzymes are present in this type of infection. Perifocal inflammation and penetration of both the bone plate and the hyaline cartilaginous end plate cause rupture of the annulus fibrosus, herniation, and subsequent contamination of the discal tissue. Infection of the adjacent vertebral body often occurs, as may the collapse of the two affected vertebrae. If so, sequestra are commonly present (Figs. 3, 6).

In many cases flattening of the intervertebral disc is the first sign of affection on a conventional radiograph of a single vertebra or of two adjacent vertebral bodies, whereas tomography at the same time already shows considerable vertebral involvement (Figs. 1, 3). Tuberculous affection of the spine may be confined to a single vertebra, and the adjacent intervertebral discs may be spared or only slightly affected (Fig. 5). A frequency of even 65% for single vertebral affection has been described [29, 39, 159]. Other unusual manifestations of tuberculous affection of the spine are mentioned later in this chapter. Multifocal foci of tuberculous spondylitis have been described in 4%–9% [147] and in 11% [175] of cases. The multifocal foci of tuberculous spondylitis in our material were found in nonwhite as well as in white patients (Figs. 6–9, 19). Depending on the anatomy and the localization of the tuberculous process, extension is possible in the anterolateral and posterior directions.

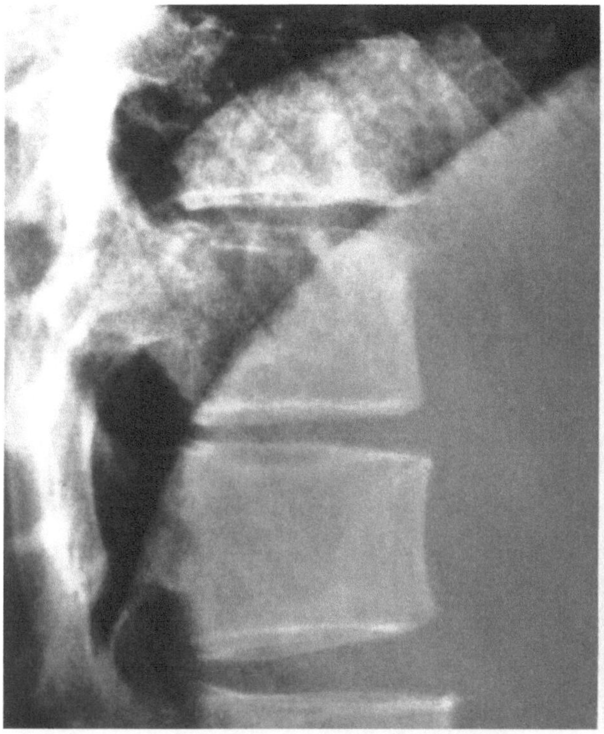
a

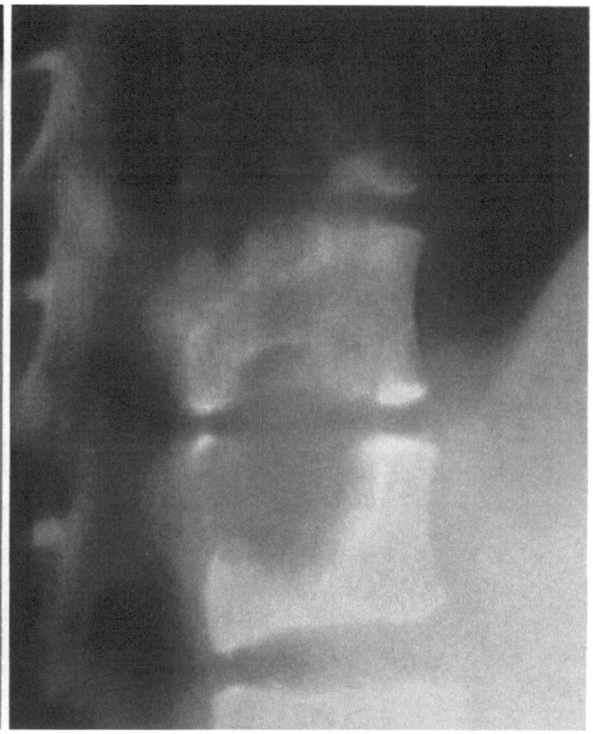
b

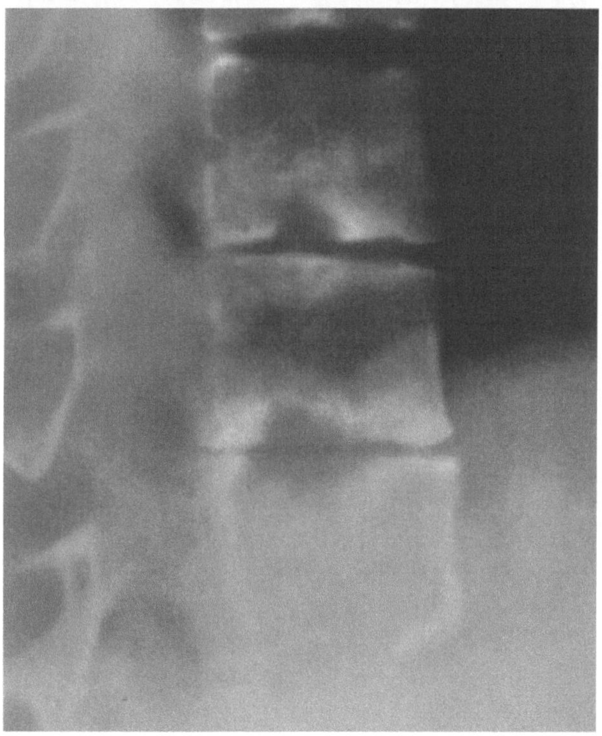
c

Fig. 1a–c. Tuberculous spondylitis. White sailor, 40 years old. Spondylitis at T-10–L-1, probably resulting in miliary tuberculosis after 1 year. Other spinal localization of tuberculosis at the level T-5–T-6 (Fig. 10). **a** The conventional radiograph presents only narrowing of the intervertebral disc. **b** Tomography at the same time shows three contiguous affected vertebral bodies. **c** Tomography after 1 year, immobilization, and chemotherapy: narrowing of the intervertebral discs, osseous defects diminished in size, restoration of bone structures and marginal osteosclerosis. Healing process

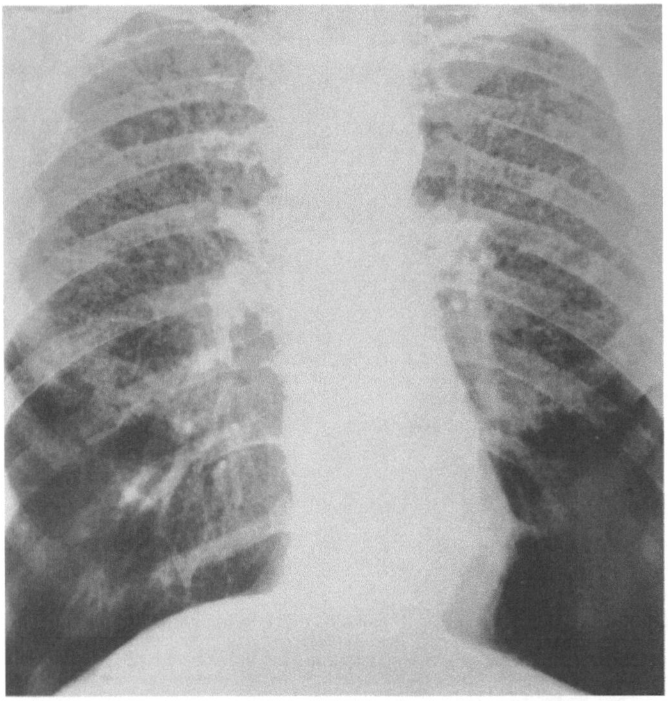

a

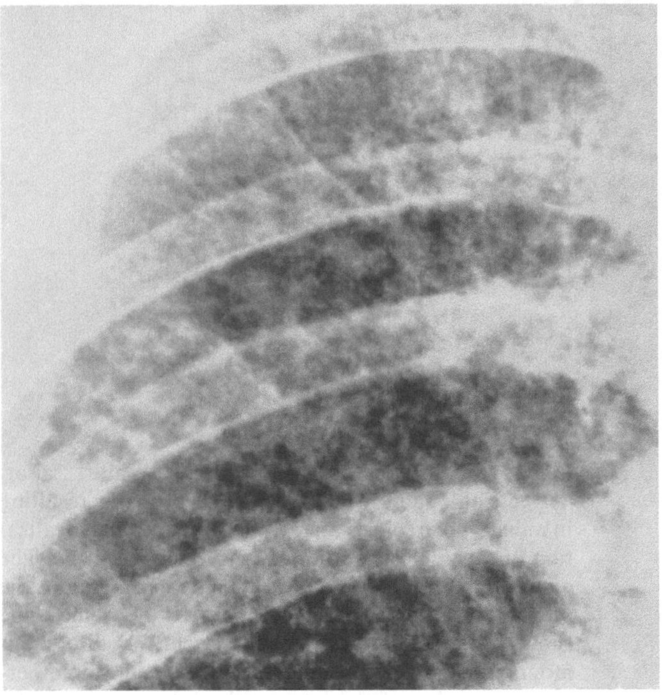

b

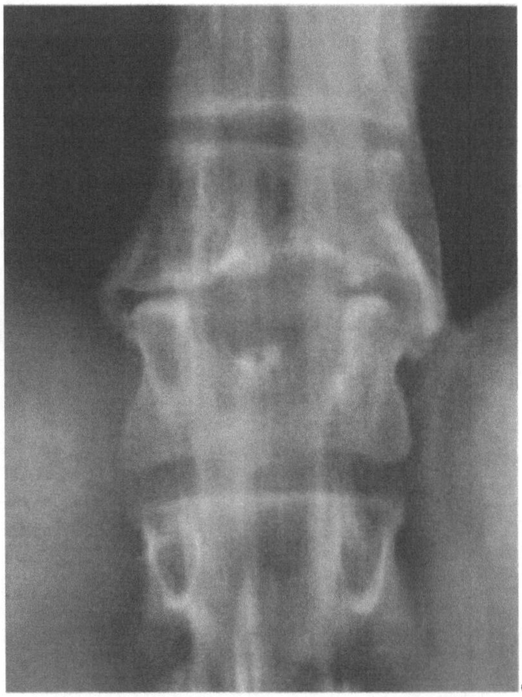

c

Fig. 2a–c. Tuberculous spondylitis. Man, 56 years old. Twenty years earlier, partial gastrectomy; 14 years later, total gastrectomy. On admission, old spondylitis with recent reactivation, miliary pulmonary tuberculosis, and tuberculous spondylitis. **a, b** Miliary pulmonary tuberculosis (*detail*, **b**). **c** Two affected vertebrae and affection of the intermediate disc. Marginal osteosclerosis and degenerative changes around the affected vertebrae as a consequence of the old tuberculous disease

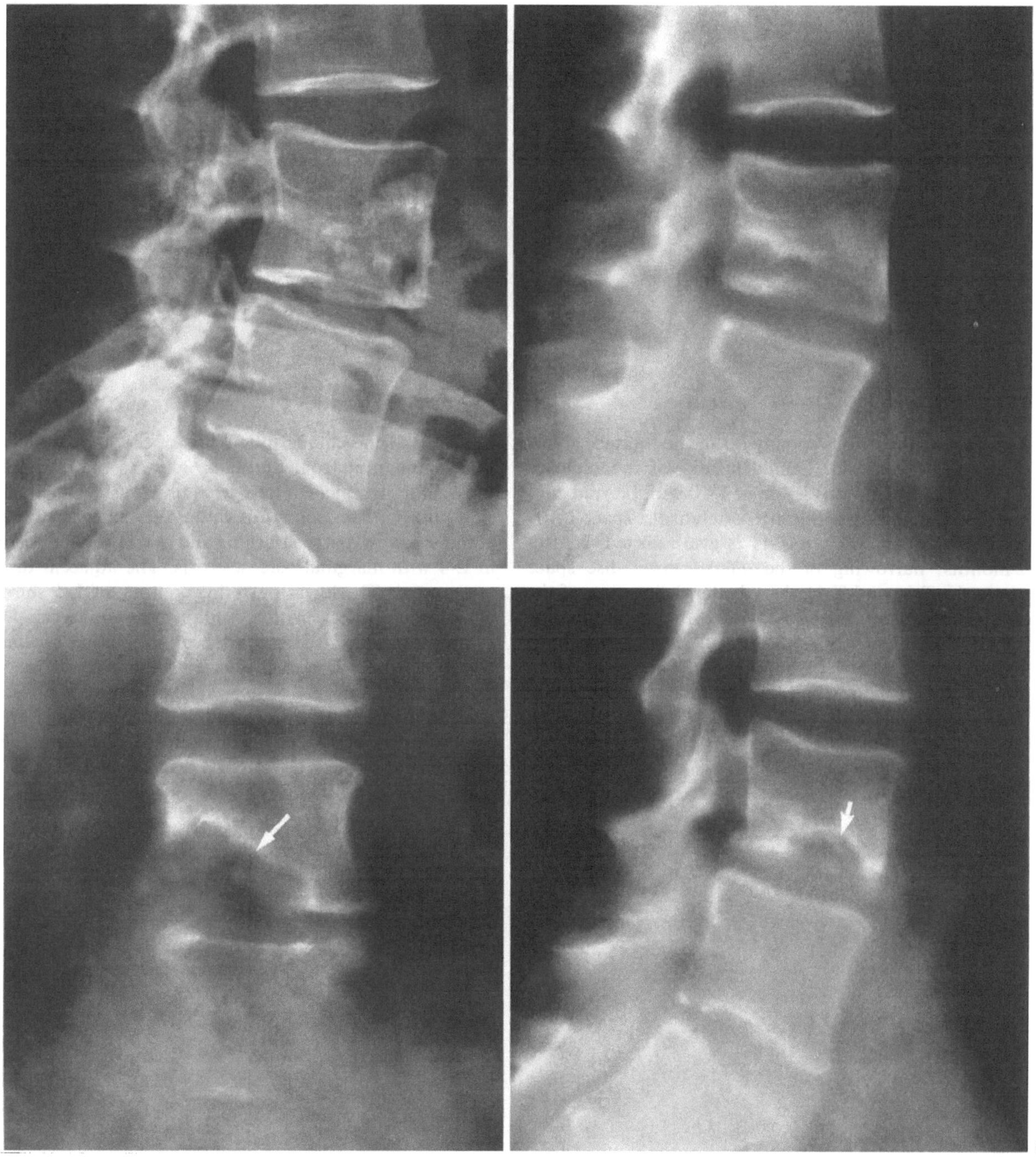

a b c d

Fig. 3a–d. Tuberculous spondylitis. At the age of 4 years, positive tuberculin skin test. At adult age, mixed connective tissue disease, Sjögren's disease and Raynaud's syndrome. After 3 months therapy with steroids, tuberculous spondylitis. **a–c** Conventional radiography and tomography: narrowing of the intervertebral disc L-4–L-5 and significant osseous defect in L-4. The conventional radiograph shows only intervertebral disc flattening and an irregular lower bone plate of L-4. **d** After 1 year, immobilization and chemotherapy: the osseous focus has decreased in size and marginal osteosclerosis is present. Healing process. *Arrows*, sequestrum

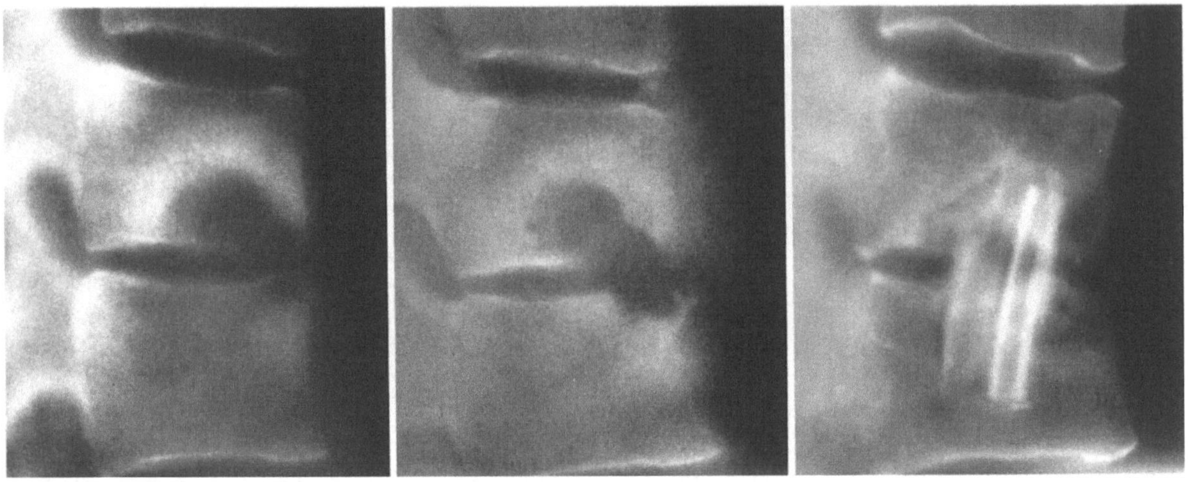

a–c

Fig. 4a–c. Tuberculous spondylitis of the thoracic spine. Woman, 46 years old. Family history of tuberculosis. **a** Tomography: osseous lesion in T-10 with blurred contours and narrowing of the intervertebral disc space T-10–T-11. Anterior border of T-11 is also affected. **b** After 2 months: narrowing of the intervertebral disc space proceeds. T-10 and T-11 show better delineation of the osseous defects. **c** One year after **b**, after chemotherapy spondylodesis anterior with excochleation of the bone lesions, implantation of bone grafts, and immobilization: slight kyphotic angle and no further compression of the vertebral bodies

Fig. 5a–d. Tuberculous spondylitis of the lumbar spine. ▶ Male immigrant from Surinam, 30 years old. Possibly tuberculous lymphadenitis 3 years previously. On admission, tuberculous spondylitis with a very extensive psoas abscess. **a, d** Soft tissue swelling and circumscribed lesion in L-4 with marginal osteosclerosis. The adjacent discs are normal! The lower posterior contour of L-5 shows an osseous defect with beginning osteosclerosis. **b, c** After 2 months: the prevertebral soft tissue swelling has diminished. Decrease in size of the osseous lesion and improved delineation as well as osteosclerosis. Ossification of the anterior longitudinal ligament and some osteosclerosis of L-5 as a consequence of tuberculous involvement of the intervertebral disc L-5–S-1

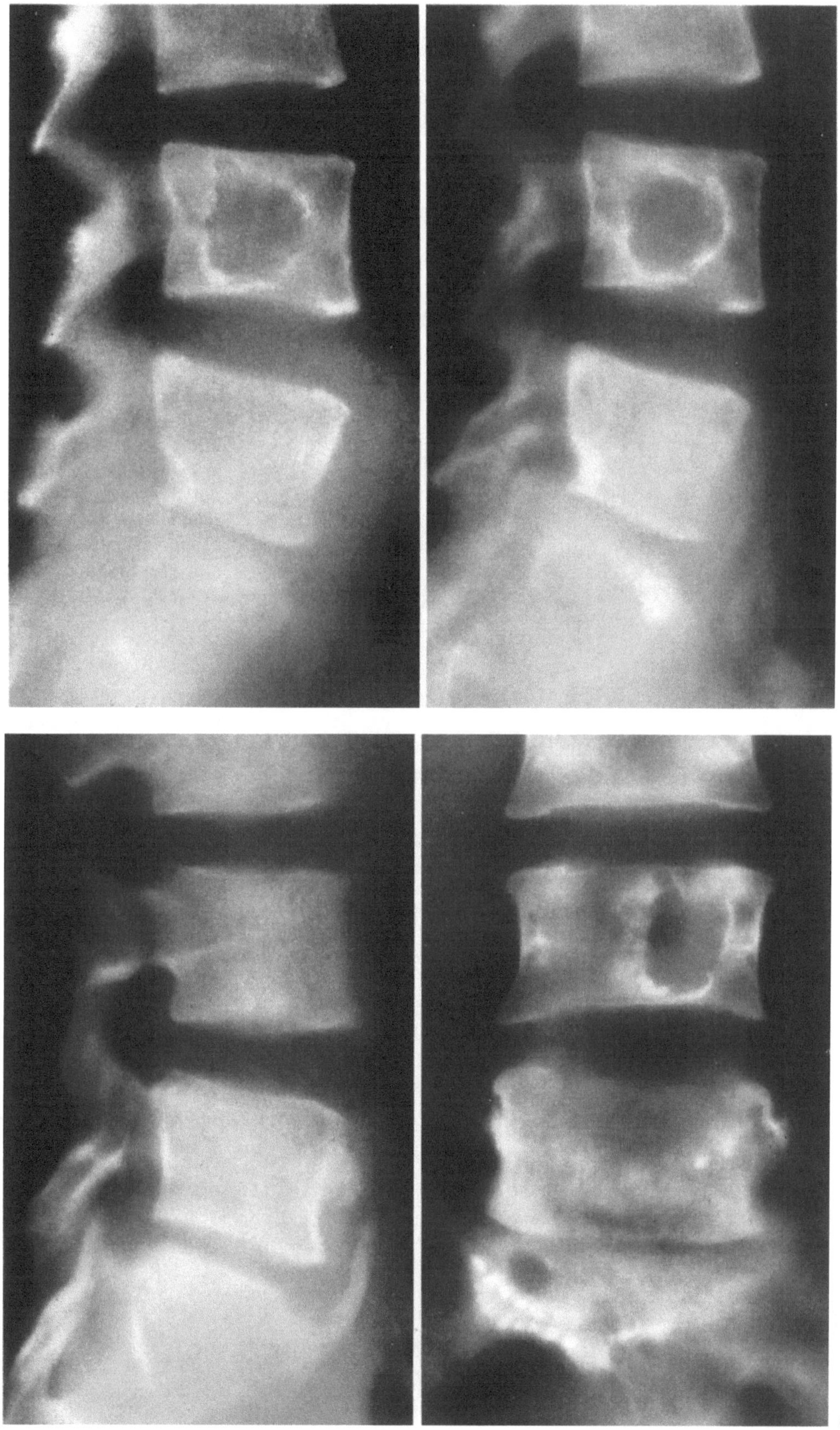

a b c d

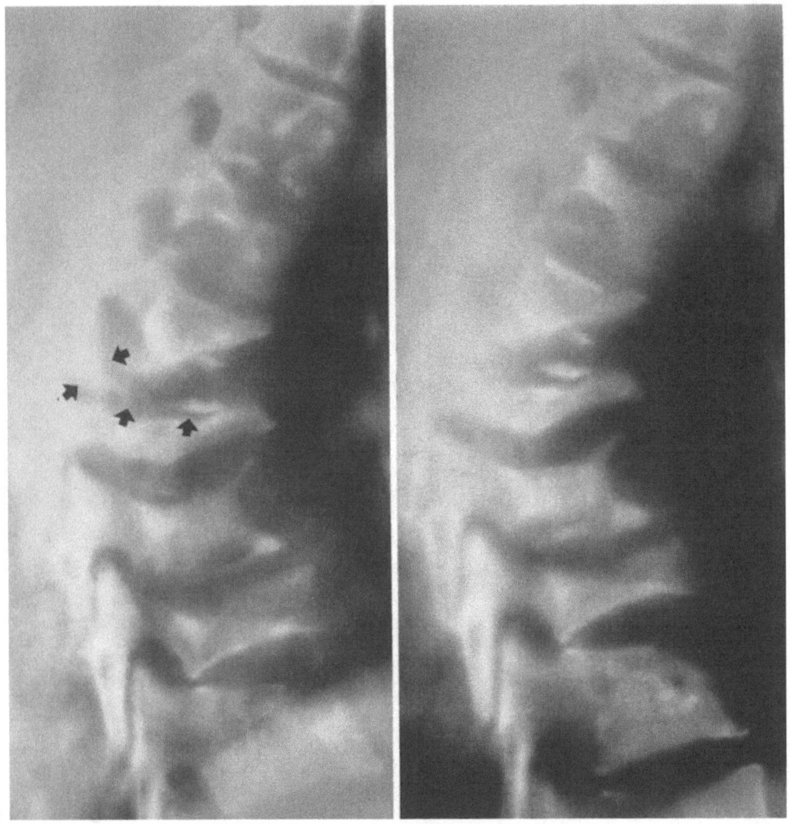

a, b

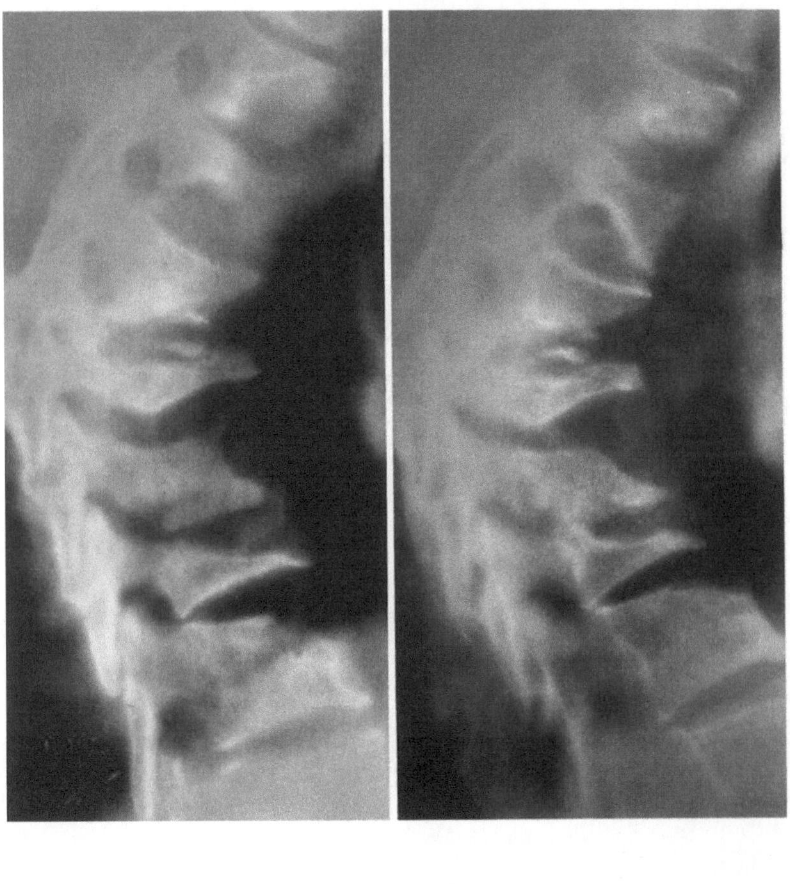

c, d

Fig. 6a–d. Tuberculous spondylitis in nine vertebrae! chinese woman, 41 years old. Paraparesis. After a doctor's delay of 3 years and progression from two involved vertebrae to nine, the diagnosis of tuberculous spondylitis was confirmed. Sequence of four radiologic examinations. **a** Nine thoracic vertebrae are involved, which could be checked by counting the vertebral arches. T-6 is almost completely vanished (*black arrows*); severe destruction with collapse, anterior gouge defects, and sequestra are present. During immobilization and chemotherapy, gradual improvement with fibrous ankylosis. The pain disappeared, but the spastic paraparesis remained. **b** Six months after **a**. **c** One year after **a**. **d** Two and a half years after **a**

Fig. 7a–d. Tuberculous spondylitis. ▶ Adopted boy from Korea at the age of 4 years. No history of tuberculosis available. On admission, 12 years old. **a** Five contiguous vertebral bodies are affected in the thoracolumbar spine. Two-thirds of the vertebral body of T-11 has disappeared. Kyphotic angle at T-11 – T-12, anterior gouge defects in the vertebral bodies T-9 and T-10. **b** Four months after **a**, after chemotherapy, spondylodesis anterior with bone grafts over four vertebrae and immobilization. **c** One year after **a**: healing with remarkable restoration of the vertebral bodies T-10 and T-12. Significant kyphotic angle. **d** Two years after **a**: Pott's gibbus after healed tuberculous spondylitis

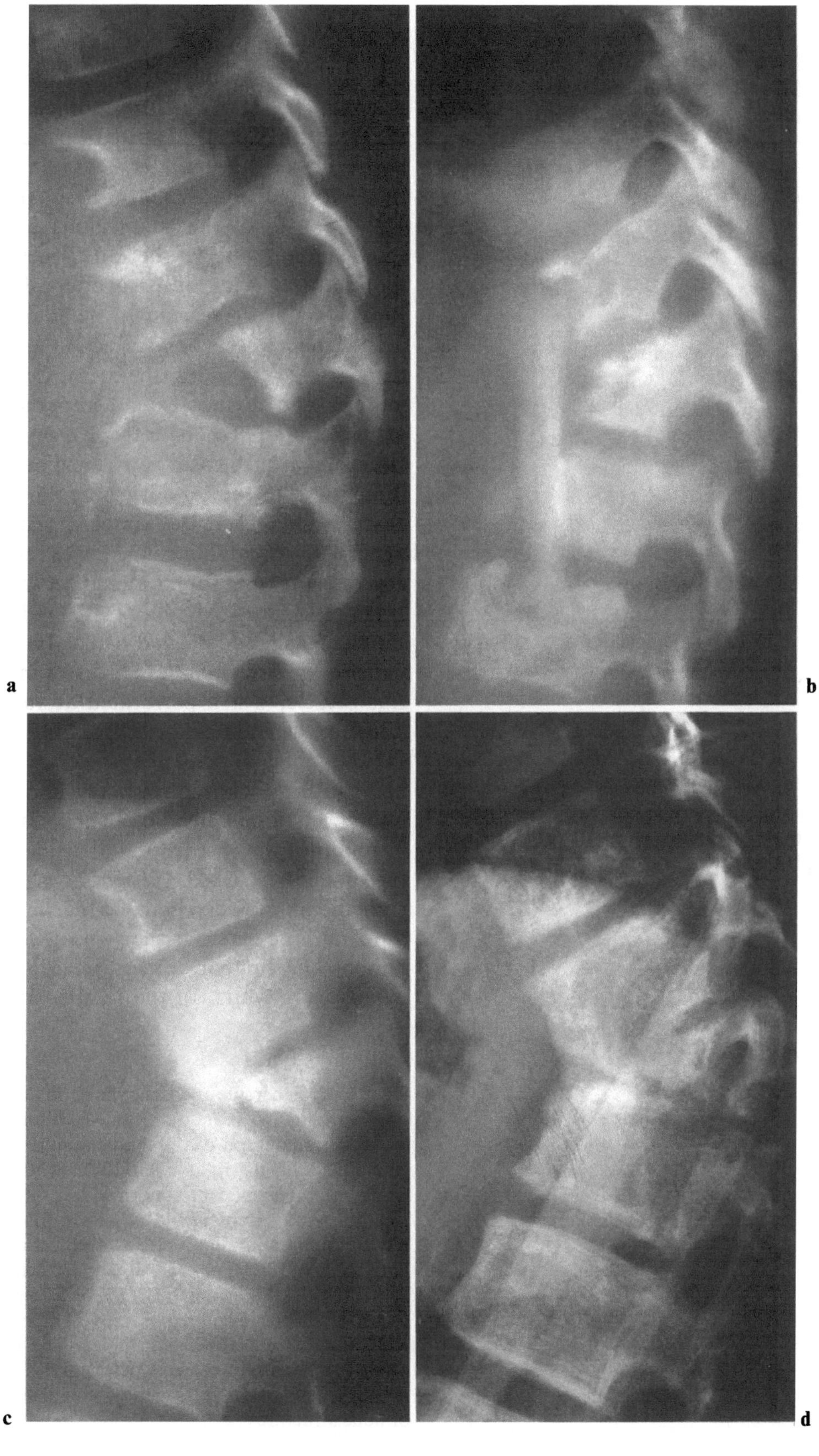
a
b
c
d

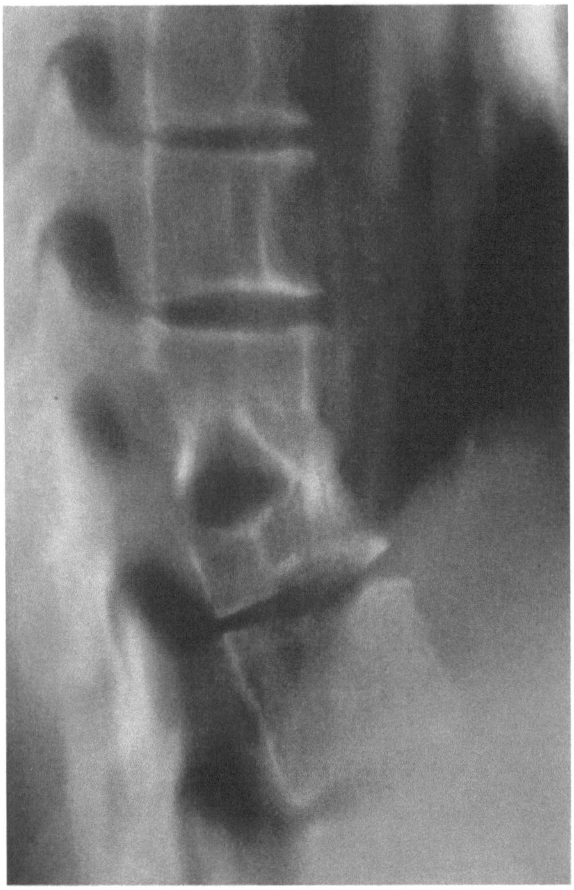

Fig. 8. Woman, 45 years old. Tuberculous process during healing. Spontaneous osseous fusion between vertebral bodies T-10 and T-11. Anterior gouge defect in T-8 and T-9. Slight kyphotic angle

5.3.1 Anterolateral Extension

Paravertebral abscesses caused by tuberculous spondylitis are frequently present, and they may become very large. In the thoracic spine they are fusiform, clearly identifiable, and visable on both sides of the spine. Sometimes the configuration looks like a "swallow nest" [8] (Figs. 9–11). The site of the tuberculous focus in the spine and anatomy of the soft tissues determine the characteristics of paravertebral abscesses. Burrowing abscesses caused by atlantooccipital foci of tuberculous bone affection are found retropharyngeally along the sternocleidomastoid muscles and do not extend into the posterior mediastinum [99]. The retropharyngeal soft tissue space in such cases is widened on the lateral radiograph of the cervical spine. Posteriorly an abscess may reach the vertebral canal. In patients with spondylitis in the lower cervical spine abscesses may be found along the scalenus and sternocleidomastoid muscles extending to the supraclavicular fossa and axilla. In one of our patients we saw bilateral abscesses in the trapezius muscle, which perforated at various locations on the shoulder and back. In the thoracic spine craniad to T-10 the abscesses usually remain rather localized and stay above the diaphragm. Lateral spread of an abscess may cause infection of the costovertebral articulations and the roots of the ribs [1] (Fig. 12).

If the abscess descends further in the caudal direction, the extent is the same as for thoracolumbar and lumbar abscesses caused by tuberculous spondylitis. In the lumbar area the ab-

Fig. 9a–e. Tuberculous spondylitis. Male immigrant from Surinam, 43 years old. Positive culture for *M. bovis*. **a** AP radiograph of the thoracolumbar spine: marginal defect on the right side of T-11 with rib erosion. Otherwise no significant abnormalities. Asymmetrically localized paravertebral cold abscess (*white arrows*). **b**, **c** With tomography: multiple involved vertebral bodies; both sides of T-11 are eroded. Central defects in T-12 and L-1 with sequestrum in L-1 (*black arrow*). The intervertebral discs are spared. **d** After 4 months: healing with ringlike central reossification in the bone cavern of T-12. The lateral concave defect of T-11 diminishes gradually. **e** After 6 years almost complete restoration of bone structures ▶

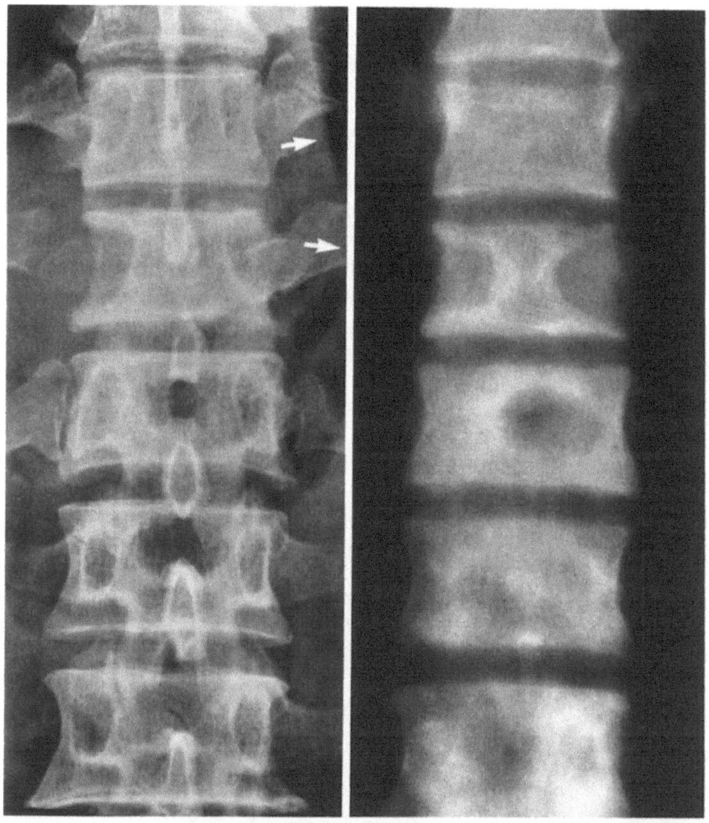

a, b

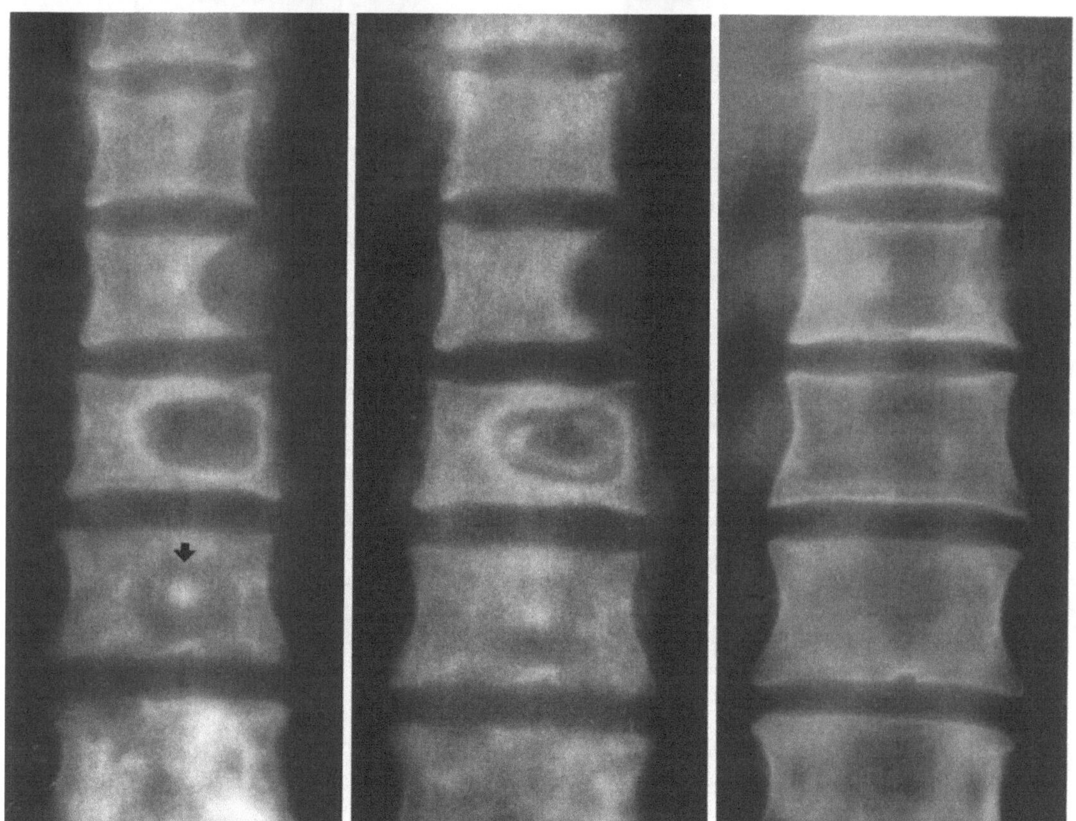

c–e

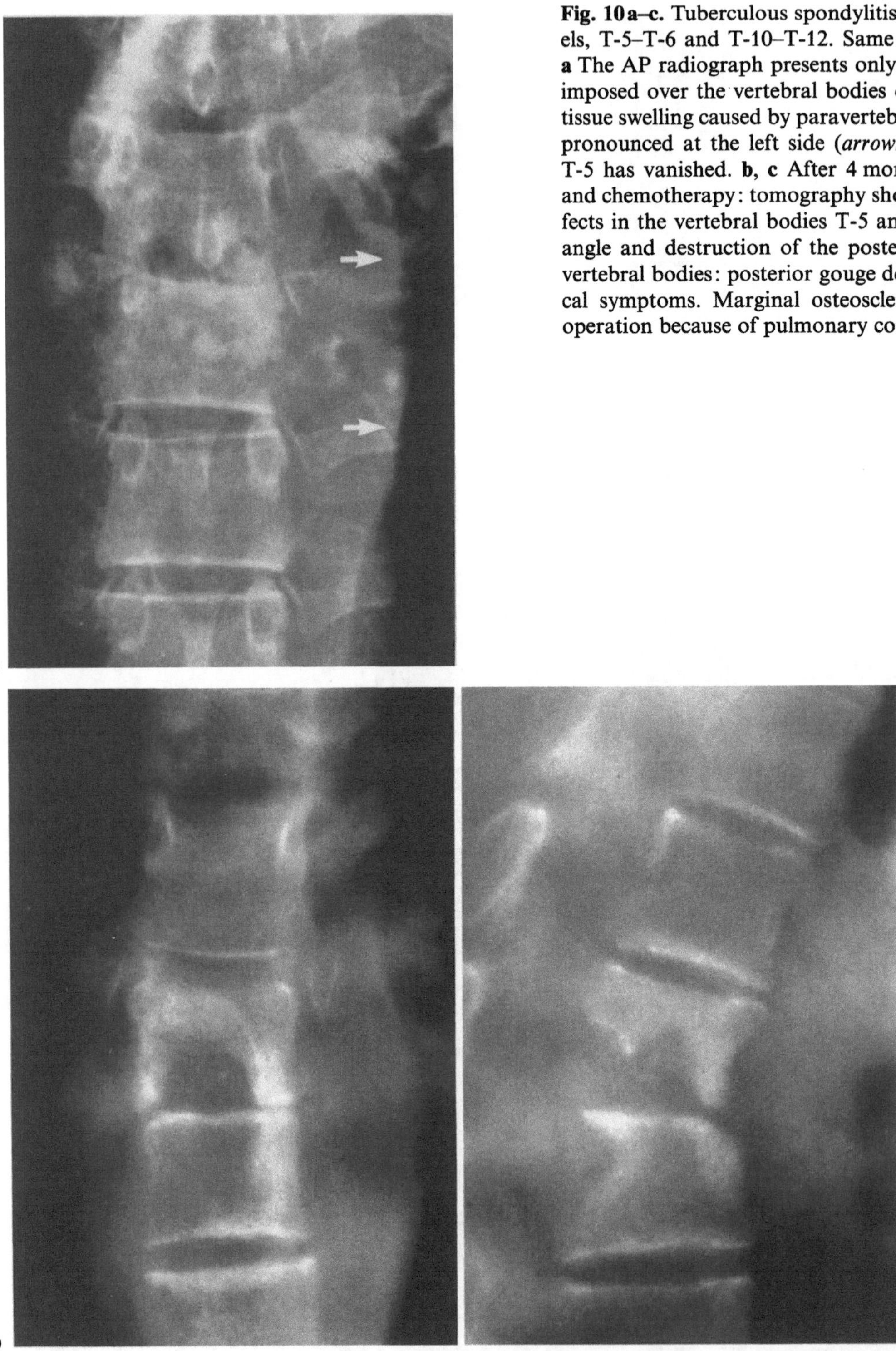

a b c

Fig. 10a–c. Tuberculous spondylitis at two different levels, T-5–T-6 and T-10–T-12. Same patient as in Fig. 1. **a** The AP radiograph presents only calcifications superimposed over the vertebral bodies of T-5 and T-6. Soft tissue swelling caused by paravertebral abscess and more pronounced at the left side (*arrows*). Left pediculus of T-5 has vanished. **b, c** After 4 months, immobilization and chemotherapy: tomography shows large osseous defects in the vertebral bodies T-5 and T-6 with kyphotic angle and destruction of the posterior contours of the vertebral bodies: posterior gouge defects. No neurological symptoms. Marginal osteosclerosis. No stabilizing operation because of pulmonary complications

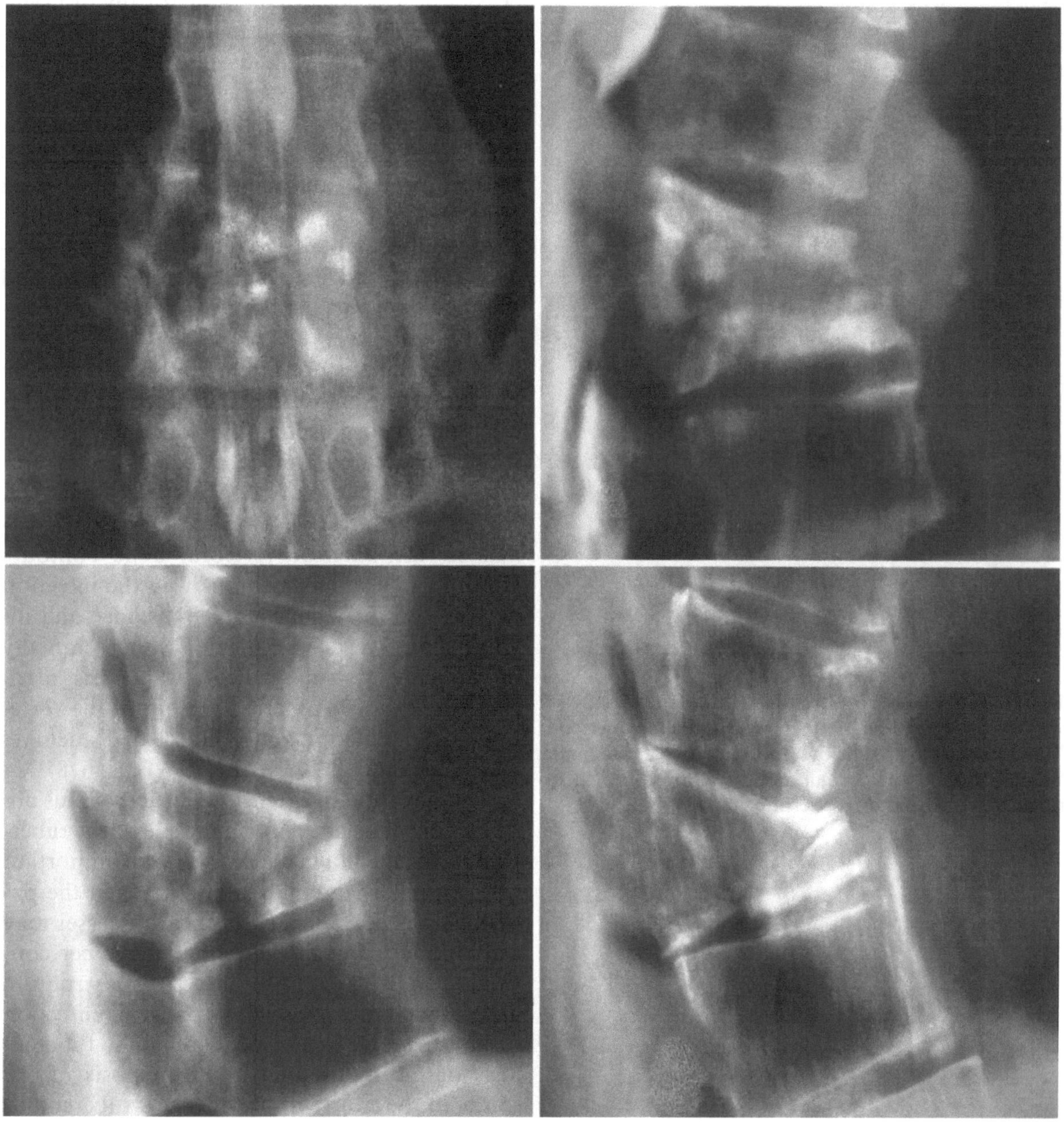

a b c d

Fig. 11a–d. Tuberculous spondylitis. Man, 63 years old. Previous history of pulmonary tuberculosis and cervical lymphadenitis. Tuberculous spondylitis was finally diagnosed after 5 years of back pain! On admission, incomplete spinal cord lesion. **a, b** Tomography of the lower thoracic spine presents affection of the vertebral bodies T-8–T-10. Severe destruction and paravertebral abscess laterally as well as ventrally. The remnants of the vertebral bodies T-9 and T-10 together have about the same height as a single normal vertebral body. Myelography demonstrates an obstruction in the vertebral canal at the lower border of T-8. **c** After 2 years: gradual healing with formation of a block vertebra, composed by the remnants of the vertebral bodies T-9 and T-10. **d** Five years after **a**: healed tuberculous process with block vertebra and small gibbus

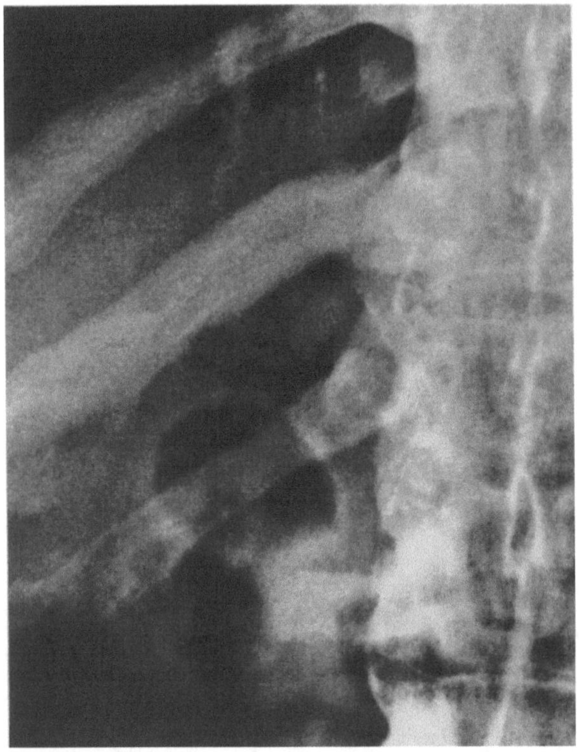

Fig. 12. Tuberculous rib affection secondary to spondylitis T-5–L-1, originating in the prechemotherapy period. Man, 56 years old. Previous tuberculous pleuritis and fistulas on the thoracic wall and sacral area. The 11th rib is thickened and osteosclerotic

scesses may be localized symmetrically or asymmetrically in the paravertebral region. Burrowing abscesses following the sheaths of the psoas muscles and the large vessels may appear in the pelvis, ischiofemoral region (along the anterior iliac artery), iliofemoral region (beneath Poupart's ligament), and even in the popliteal fossa (Figs. 13, 14). Presentation of an abscess through the lumbar trigonum (between the latissimus dorsi and external oblique muscles and the iliac crest) on the back of the patient is another possibility.

A tuberculous prevertebral abscess is usually not very large and dissects the anterior longitudinal ligament, infecting the adjacent vertebrae by subligamentous spread of bacilli per continuitatem. Infection of the vertebral bodies is caused by infiltration through the vascular canals in the anterior vertebral bone contours [159]. In this subligamentous way the infection may extend for a considerable distance and involve many vertebrae, located either cranially or caudally. A subligamentous abscess often causes a scalloped anterior contour of the vertebral body: anterior gouge defect or "aneurysmal syndrome" [1, 73, 142, 169] (Figs. 6–8).

The direction of extension of tuberculous abscesses depends not only on the site of the tuberculous focus; gravity also plays an important role, especially in children [147]. When the patient is in bed, especially thoracic abscesses may ascend and infect the vertebrae above per continuitatem [98, 147, 174]. Abscesses may rupture and form sinuses. Secondary pyogenic infection of sinuses seems to be more common in tuberculosis of the limbs than in tuberculosis of the spine. In the course of the disease a tuberculous abscess shrinks, with a fibrotic wall, and calcifications may occur during healing (Figs. 14–16, 26, 32). The centers of these abscesses may still contain active bacilli if the patient is not treated adequately with bactericidal antituberculous drugs.

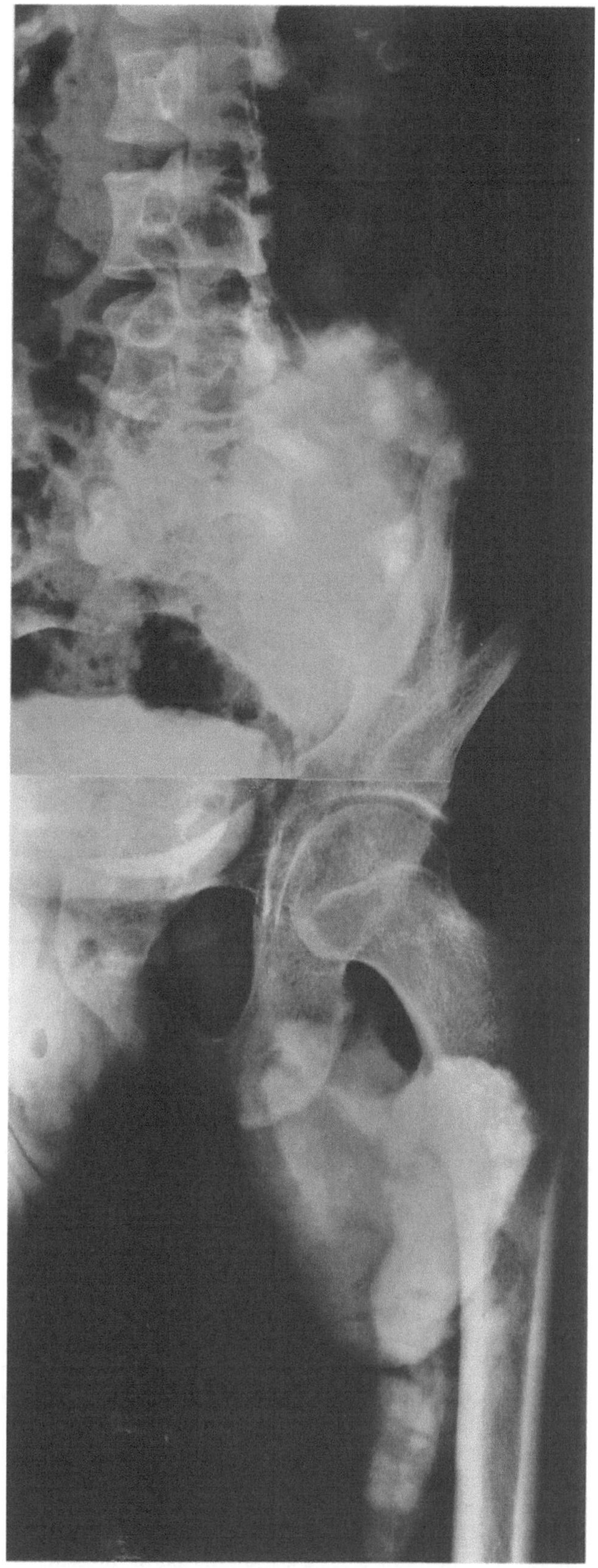

Fig. 13. Tuberculous burrowing abscess. Man, 22 years old. Two years previously, low back pain and radiologic changes considered to be an old spondylitis. On admission, cavernous pulmonary tuberculosis and a 3-month history of low back pain. Radiography after abscess punction and injection of contrast medium. Huge abscess in the left iliac fossa caused by *M. tuberculosis* with extension in the thigh

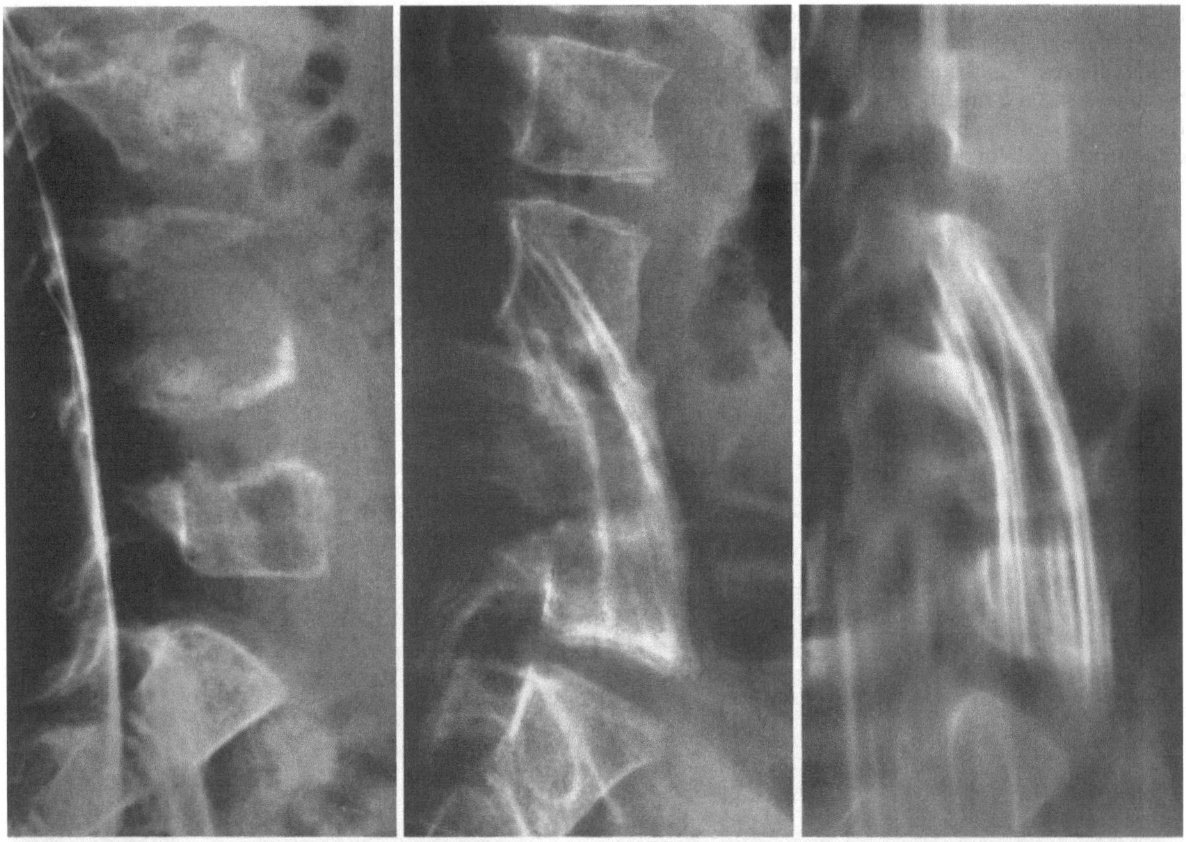

a–c

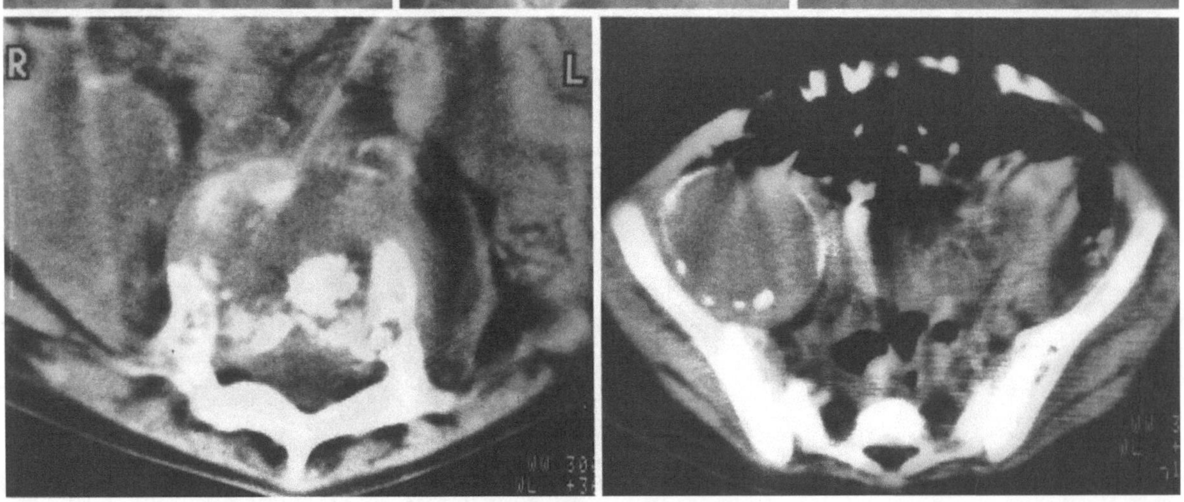

d, e

Fig. 14a–e. Tuberculous spondylitis. Adopted Haitian girl, 5 years old. Previous medical history unknown. **a** Involvement of the vertebrae L-2–L-5 and especially extensive destruction of the vertebral bodies L-3 and L-4. **b, c** After 6 months, chemotherapy and spondylodesis anterior: restoration of the vertebral body L-2 and beginning bony fusion of the flattened vertebrae L-3 and L-4. **d** CT at the same time as **a** demonstrates the destruction of the vertebral body L-4 and the paravertebral abscess on the right side. **e** CT of the pelvis presents a large abscess with calcifications in the right iliac fossa

Fig. 15a, b. Calcified psoas abscess. Woman, 37 years old. During the Second World War cavernous pulmonary tuberculosis. Eight years later, spondylodesis posterior because of tuberculous spondylitis. On admission, right-sided renal tuberculosis and calcifications in an old burrowing abscess on the left side ▶

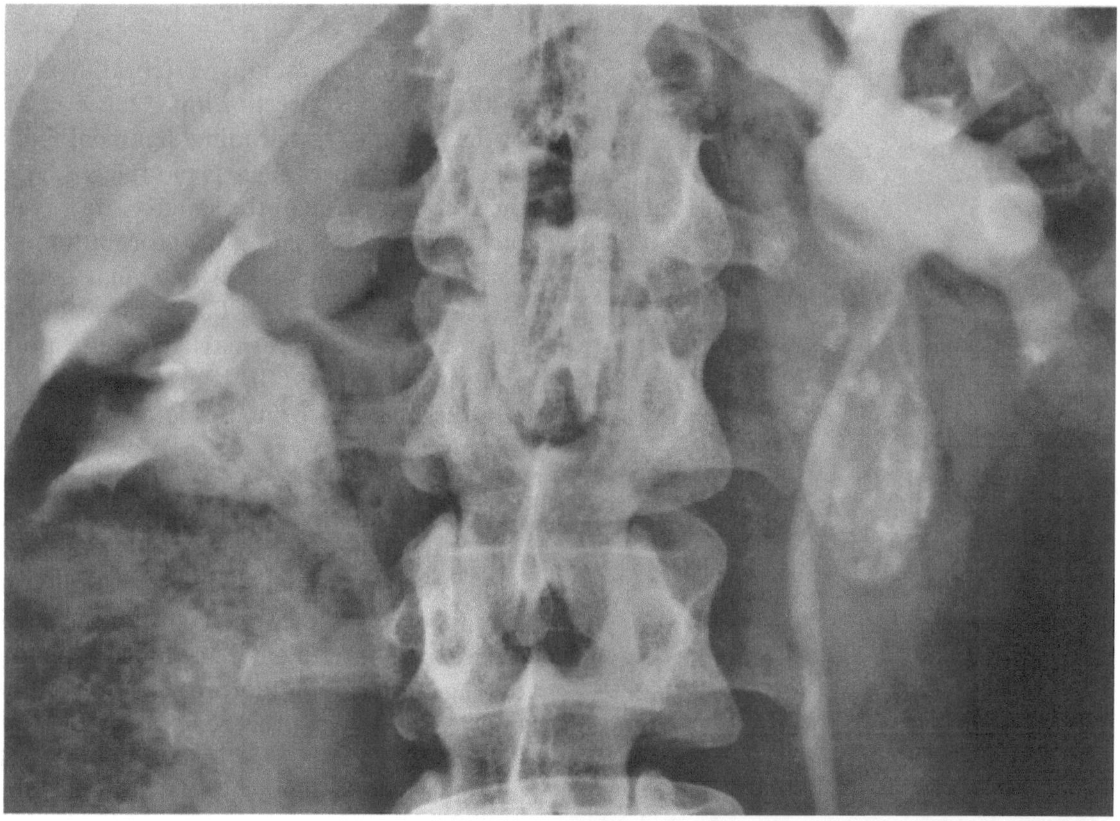

a

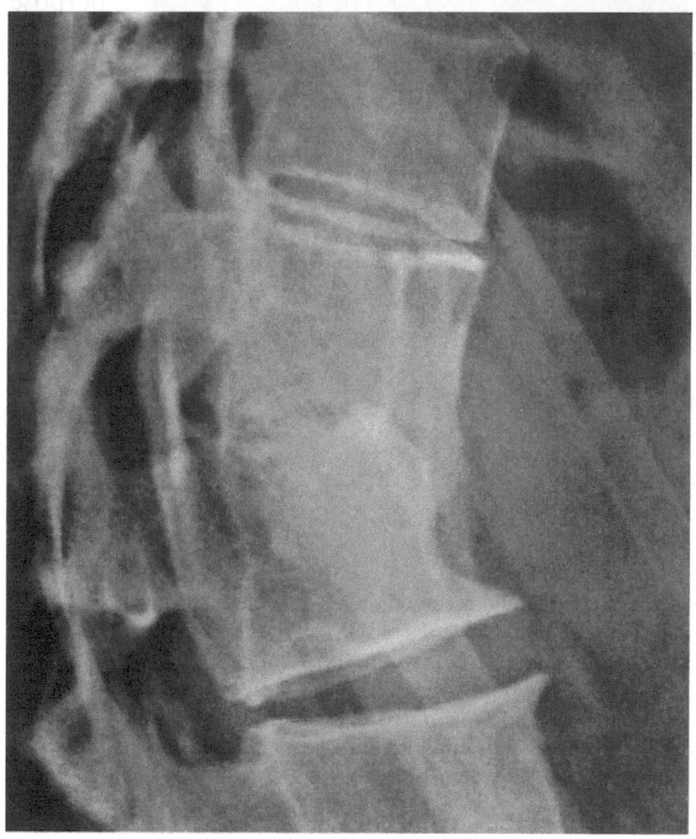

b

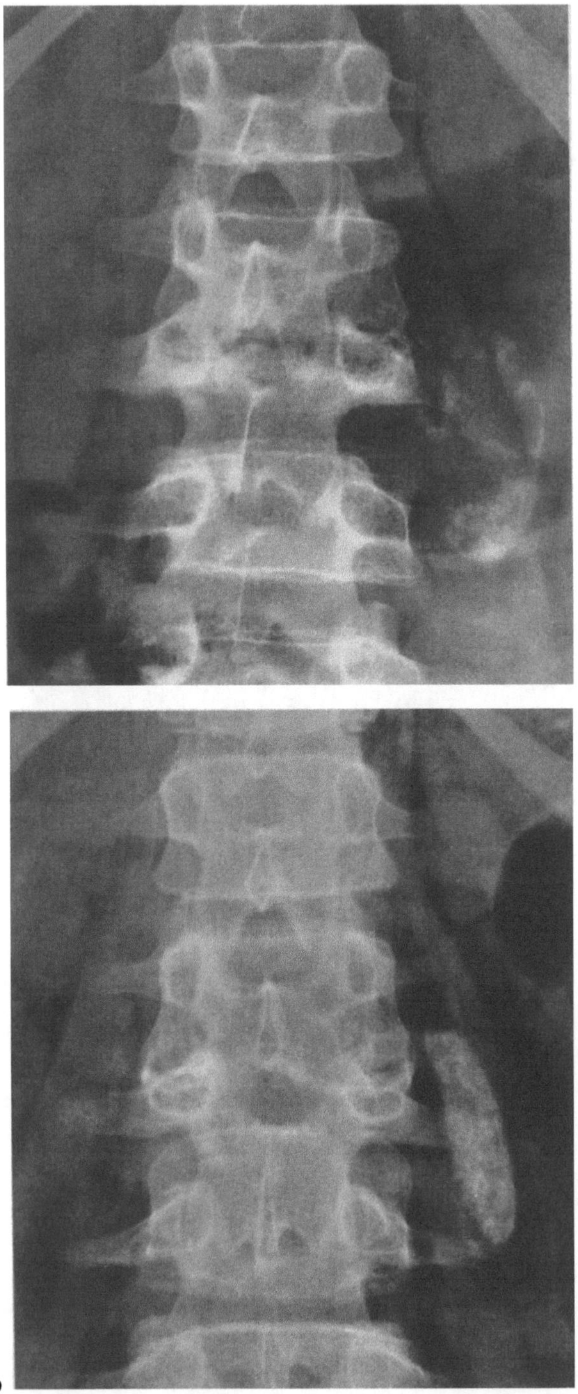

a

b

Fig. 16a, b. Tuberculous spondylitis and calcifications in psoas abscess. Boy, 10 years old. Primary tuberculosis at the age of 5 years. On admission, tuberculous spondylitis at L-2–L-3. **a** Spondylitis at L-2–L-3 with psoas abscess on the left side. Scattered calcifications. **b** After 2 years: the abscess has diminished in size, and the calcifications are close together. Bony fusion L-2–L-3

5.3.2 Posterior Extension

Extension of tuberculous vertebral involvement in the posterior direction may cause dissection of the posterior longitudinal ligament and medullary disturbances such as paraplegia, by extradural compression of the spinal cord. Myelography, CT, or MRI can give information in such patients about the site(s) of spinal cord compression (Figs. 11, 21). Posterior scalloping of the vertebral bodies may be seen: posterior gouge defects (Figs. 10, 17) [169].

Other reasons for neurological features in tuberculous spondylitis are perifocal circulatory disturbances or a prolapse of discal material. A polyneuropathy may be the result of isoniazid. Especially diabetics and alcoholics are prone to this complication. Vertebral collapse and infections of the spinal cord or the meninges seem to be infrequent reasons for spinal cord damage. CT is an important tool for evaluating the degree of canal encroachment [65, 69, 81, 92, 95, 107, 138, 175, 177]. Of course, MRI is also able to give important information for this purpose (Fig. 21).

a b

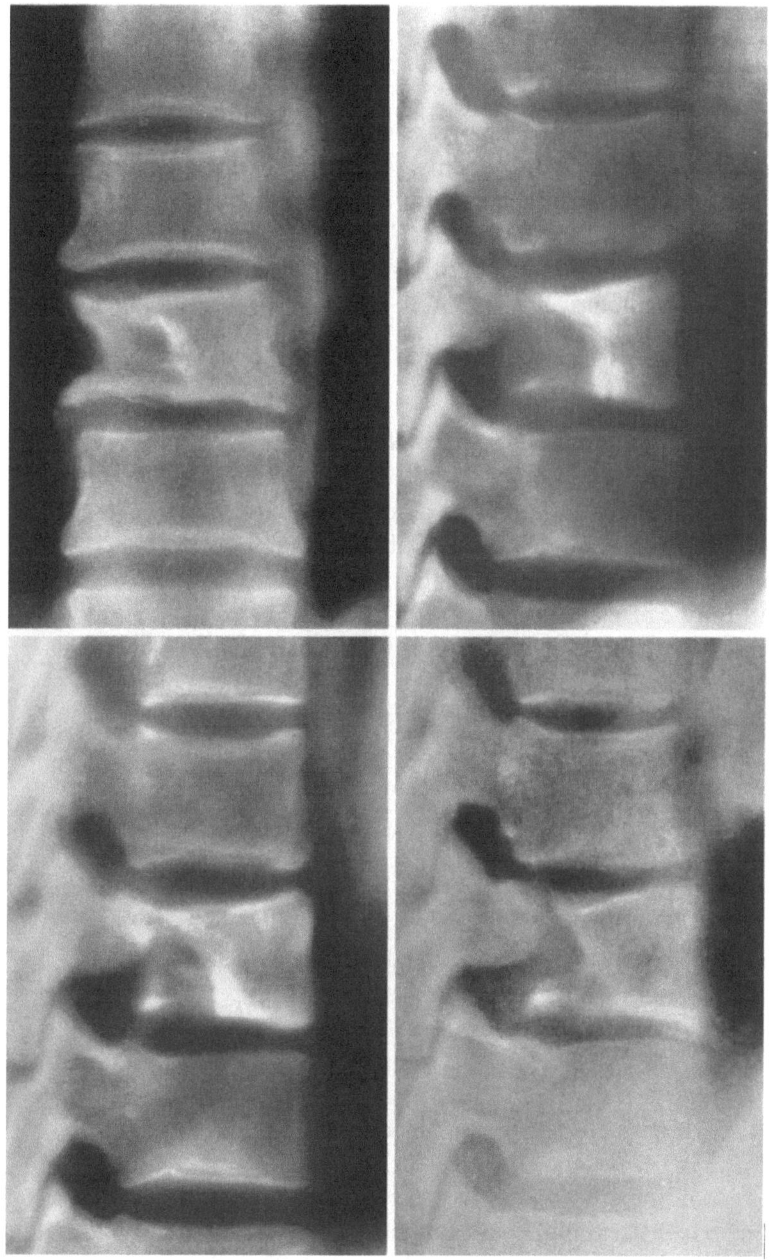

c d

Fig. 17a–d. Tuberculous spondylitis T-7–T-9. Male refugee from Surinam, 27 years old. Other foci of tuberculous spondylitis were localized at C-7–T-2, L-3–L-4, and sternum. Traumatic lesions after torture may have played a role in an endogenous reactivation of tuberculosis in the affected regions. **a, b** Tomography: affection of the vertebral body T-9 especially on the right and posterior side. The adjacent intervertebral discs seem not to be affected. The lesions in T-7 and T-8 are not visible on these radiographs. **c** Four months after **a**, during immobilization and chemotherapy: better delineation of the osseous focus. **d** Ten months after **a**. Separation between the pedicle and vertebral body. Posterior gouge defect still present

5.4 Radiologic Findings

5.4.1 Osseous Cavity in a Vertebral Body

The formation of an osseous cavity in a vertebral body usually occurs centrally, close to the anterior contour of the vertebral body, and near the subchondral bone plate (Figs. 1–4). This bone cavity is sometimes hardly visible on conventional radiographs, while tomography shows the lesion clearly (Figs. 1, 3, 10).

5.4.2 Intervertebral Disc Space Narrowing

Extension of the tuberculous lesion in the direction of the disc and destruction of the bone plate cause discal herniation into the vertebral body and may cause contamination of the discal material. Disc space narrowing may be the only initial finding [129] (Fig. 1).

5.4.3 Osseous Defects in Adjacent Vertebral Bodies and Intermediate Disc Destruction

A classic finding in tuberculous spondylitis is that of osseous defects in adjacent vertebral bodies, with intermediate disc destruction (Figs. 1, 2, 4, 23).

5.4.4 Absence of Disc Space Narrowing

It is not uncommon to find no narrowing of disc space; particularly in nonwhite patients, although adjacent vertebral bodies are affected [164, 169, 175] (Figs. 5, 9). The disc space may even be widened as a result of bone plate compression and granulation tissue within the disc [169]. We have also noticed these features in several of our white patients.

5.4.5 Collapse of Vertebral Bodies

Anterior collapse is the most frequent type of vertebral body collapse in the thoracic region,

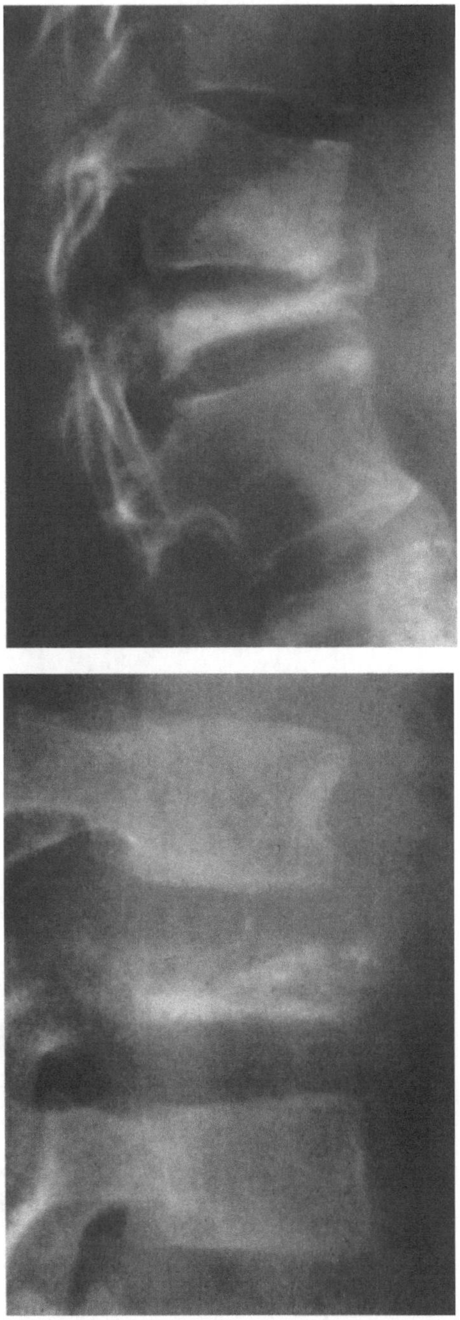

a

b

Fig. 18a, b. Two different patients with vertebra plana caused by tuberculous spondylitis. By courtesy of Dr. W.P. Cockshott, Hamilton, Ont., Canada. **a** Significant flattening of the vertebral body T-12 and a kyphotic angle; the latter is possibly related to the more oblique position of the intervertebral joint spaces in the thoracic vertebral column. The adjacent intervertebral discs are affected. **b** Typical vertebra plana in L-3. The cranial intervertebral disc is involved, and L-2 shows a superficial anterior spondylitis followed by lateral and posterior collapse (Figs. 6, 7, 10, 11, 14, 16, 23, 24). Especially in the tropics, vertebra plana types of collapse have been found [140]. Usually vertebra plana are present in the lumbar spine (Fig. 18). This phenomenon can be explained by the position of the intervertebral joints. In the thoracic spine the direction of these joint spaces is arranged oblique to the longitudinal axis of the spine. In the lumbar spine the joint spaces are arranged in a more parallel direction with the longitudinal axis of the spine. Gravity and the specific anatomy of the intervertebral joints together may be responsible for the higher rate of vertebra plana in the lumbar spine [174]. When the patient is in bed, reconstruction of the vertebral body may be possible [147].

5.4.6 Kyphosis, Pott's Gibbus

Wedge-shaped collapse of the vertebral body is most pronounced in the thoracic spine (Figs. 19, 20).

5.4.7 Scoliosis

Scoliosis may be caused by asymmetric destruction of the vertebral bodies and discs (Fig. 20).

5.4.8 Paravertebral Abscess

Detection of paravertebral abscesses is fairly easy in the thoracic spine but more difficult in patients with neck or retroperitoneal abscesses (Figs. 10, 25, 32). In the lumbar region the abscesses may be large, and the paravertebral soft tissues must be depicted sufficiently on conventional radiographs. In patients with abscesses ultrasonography, CT, and MRI may be helpful. On CT scans abscesses present as low-density paravertebral masses. After the application of contrast medium the hypervascular and partially fibrous wall can usually be clearly seen. The abscesses may be multiloculated and may present calcifications (Figs. 13–16, 26, 32). Visualization of the spread to the superficial dorsal soft tissues is also improved by the use of CT and MRI.

5.4.9 Anterior Scalloping of Vertebral Bodies (Anterior Gouge Defect, "Aneurysmal Syndrome")

Extension of a tuberculous abscess beneath the anterior longitudinal ligament, possibly together with the transmission of aortic pulsations, may be the cause of the so-called anterior gouge defect [73, 94, 169] (Figs. 6–8). Other causes of anterior scalloping include lymphadenopathy from metastasis, lymphoma, and aneurysm of the aorta.

5.4.10 Posterior Scalloping of Vertebral Bodies (Posterior Gouge Defect)

Extension of a tuberculous abscess beneath the posterior longitudinal ligament, frequently in combination with medullary compression, may cause scalloping [5] (Figs. 10, 17). Other causes of posterior scalloping are congenital disorders, neurological diseases, and acromegaly.

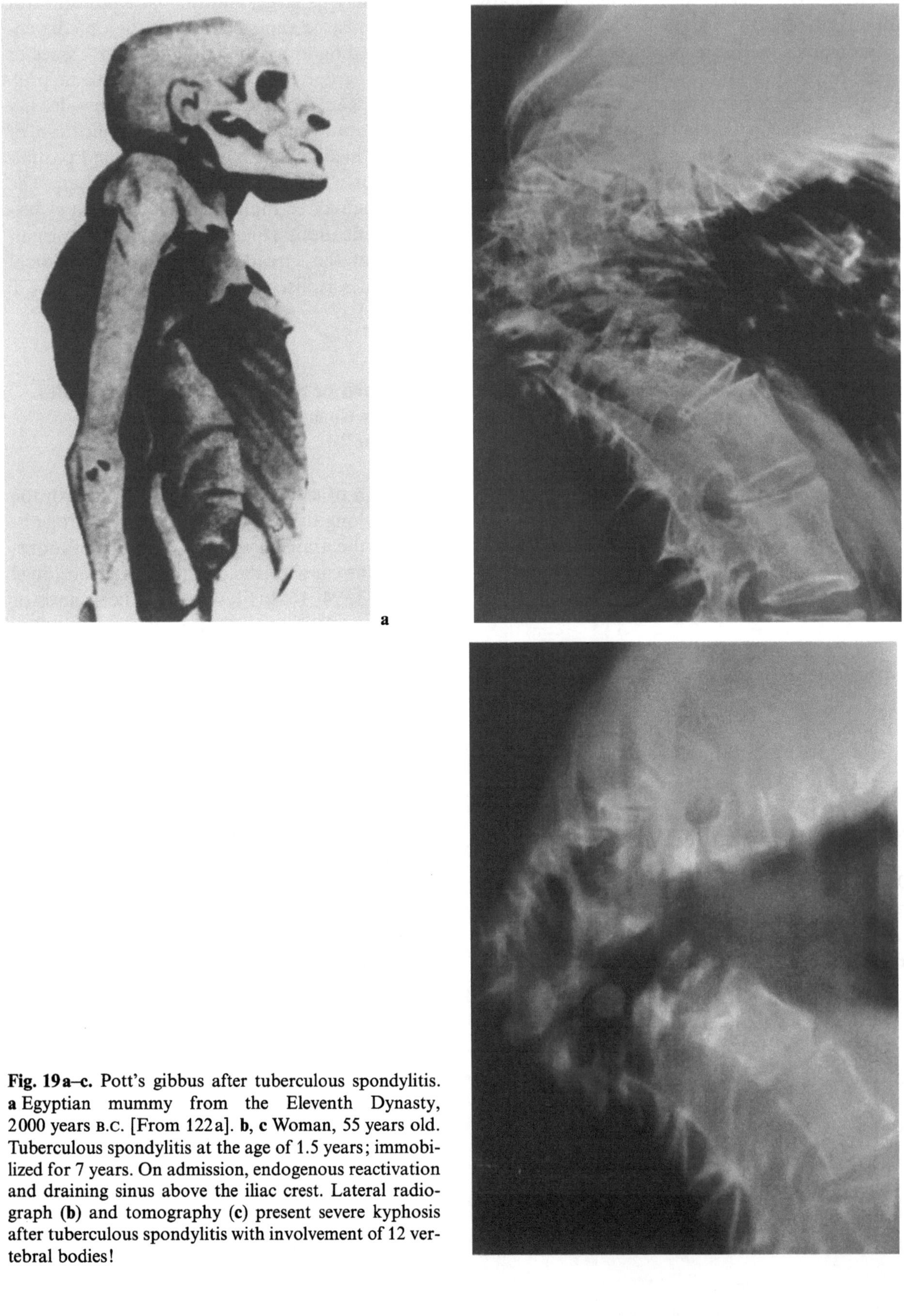

Fig. 19a–c. Pott's gibbus after tuberculous spondylitis. **a** Egyptian mummy from the Eleventh Dynasty, 2000 years B.C. [From 122a]. **b, c** Woman, 55 years old. Tuberculous spondylitis at the age of 1.5 years; immobilized for 7 years. On admission, endogenous reactivation and draining sinus above the iliac crest. Lateral radiograph (**b**) and tomography (**c**) present severe kyphosis after tuberculous spondylitis with involvement of 12 vertebral bodies!

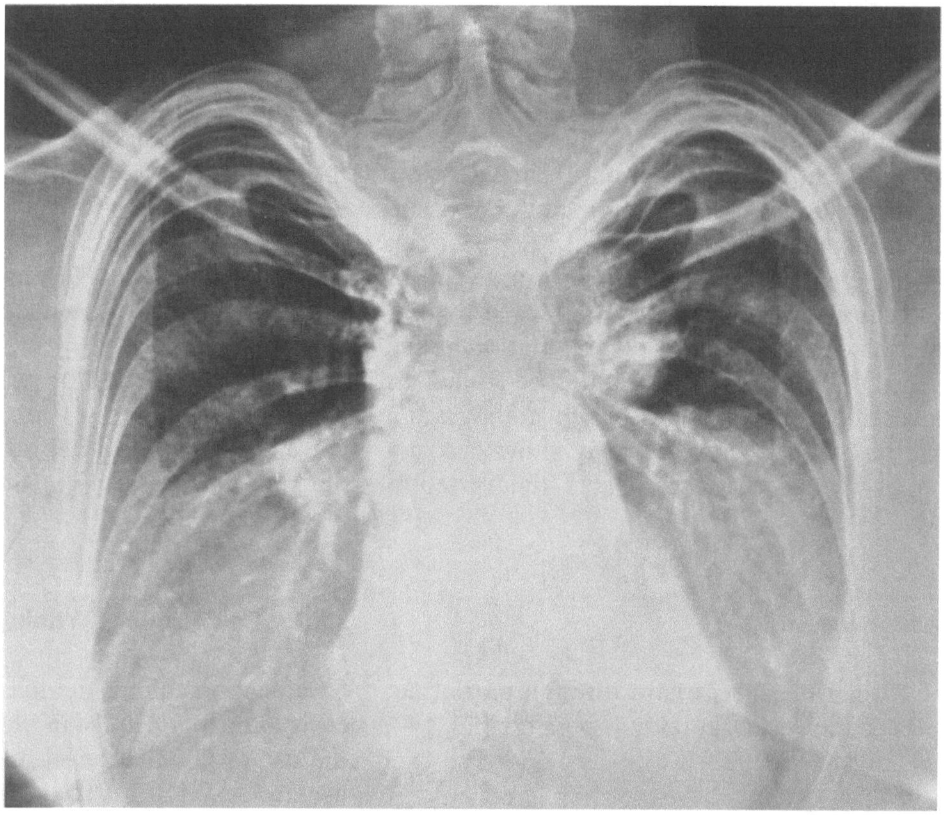

a

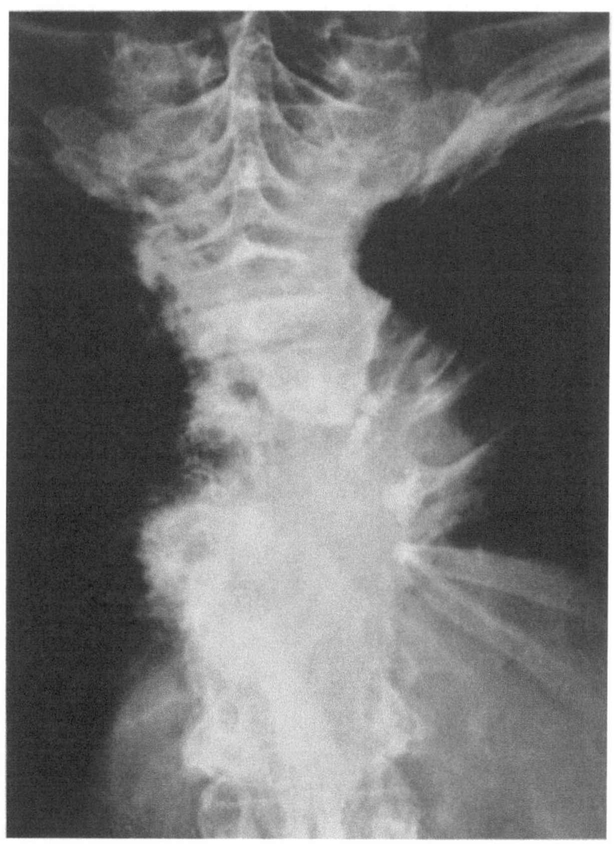

b

Fig. 20 a, b. Same patient as in Fig. 19 b. Fanlike configuration of the ribs as a result of multiple collapsed vertebrae. Note the peculiar position of the posterior spinal processes of the cervicothoracic vertebrae

5.4.11 Protrusion into the Vertebral Canal

Fragmentation and dislocation of a vertebral body may sometimes cause canal encroachment and medullary compression [175], but neurological complications usually result from extension of a tuberculous abscess or of granulation tissue into the spinal canal [140, 175] (Figs. 11, 22, 23]. CT and MRI provide more information in these cases if the compression is caused by disc material or the presence of granulation tissue (Fig. 21). These materials cannot be found on conventional radiographs or on tomograms; these techniques, however, may show destruction of the posterior border of the vertebral body.

5.4.12 Sequestra

The formation of sequestra through partial necrosis of the vertebral body is possible [99, 147, 175] (Figs. 3, 6, 9, 23).

5.4.13 Osteosclerosis

Osteosclerosis is a sign of healing. It is more frequent in yet untreated patients living in temperate climates and is usually located perifocally [140] (Figs. 1, 3, 5, 6, 9).

5.4.14 Destruction of Costovertebral Joints and/or Roots of the Ribs

Either initial infection or secondary infection by paravertebral abscesses are the reason for involvement of costovertebral joints and roots of the ribs [95, 129, 147]. Rib notching may be present (Fig. 12).

5.4.15 Calcifications Within Abscesses

Calcifications along the margins of the abscess cavity are found only in chronic disease. With the use of CT the detection of calcifications is usually easy [107, 138, 175, 177] (Figs. 14–16, 26, 32).

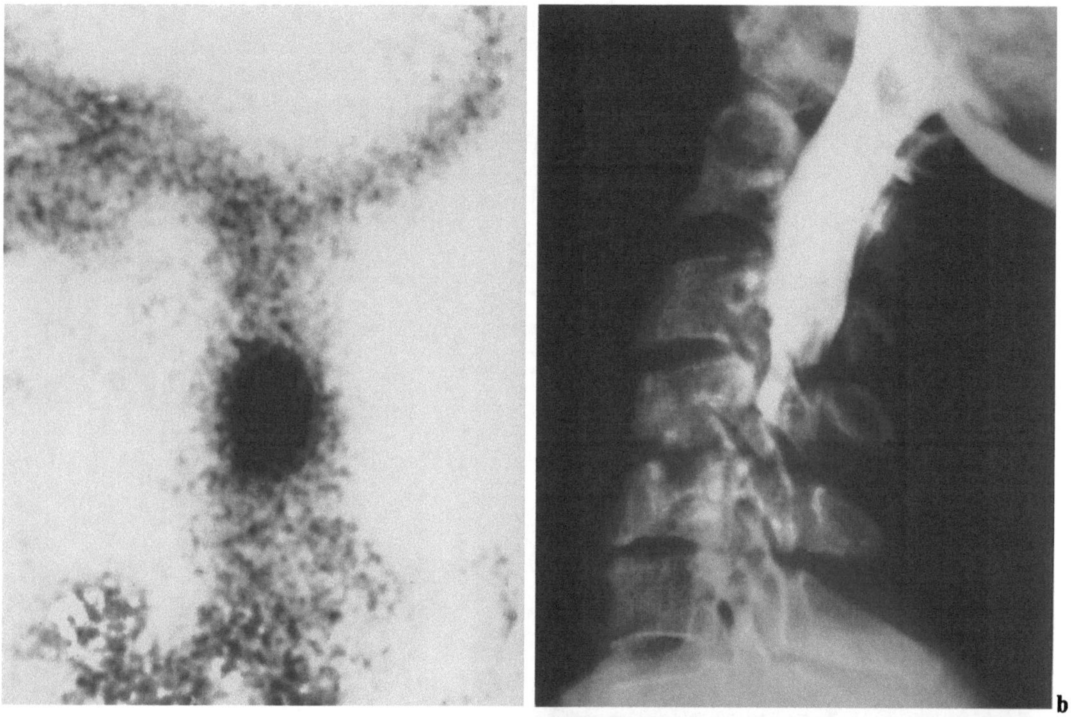

a b

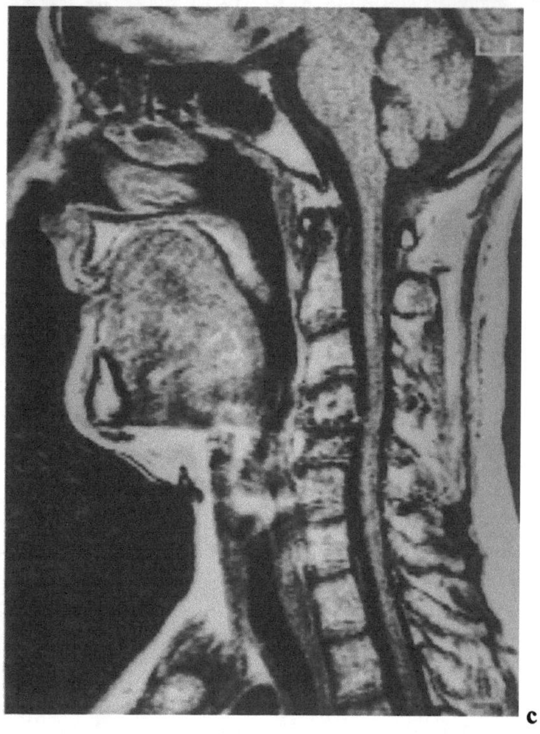

c

Fig. 21 a–c. Tuberculous spondylitis of the cervical spine and right sacroiliac joint. Woman, 67 years old. Previous tuberculous pleuritis. **a** Scintigraphy: high uptake in the region of the active tuberculous focus. **b** Myelography demonstrates an obstruction in the cervical vertebral canal at the level of C-4. The vertebral bodies C-4 and C-5 are involved. The intermediate disc is narrowed. **c** After 2 months, immobilization and chemotherapy: T1-weighted MRI clearly demonstrates decreased signal intensity of C-4 and C-5, as well as narrowing of the vertebral canal anteriorly. No prevertebral abscess

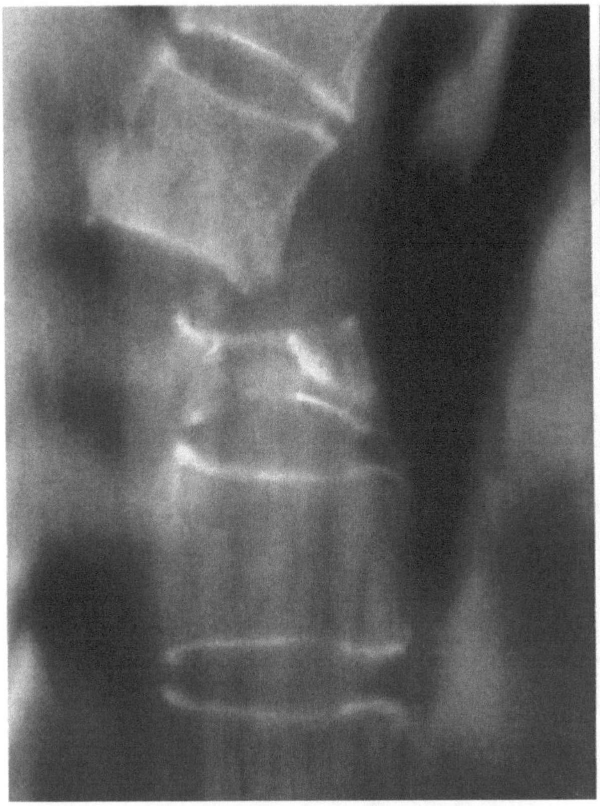
a

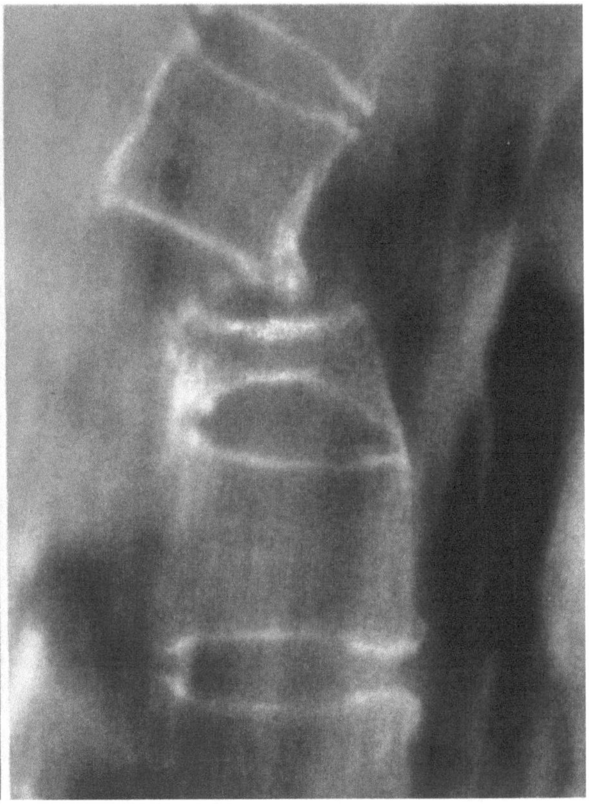
b

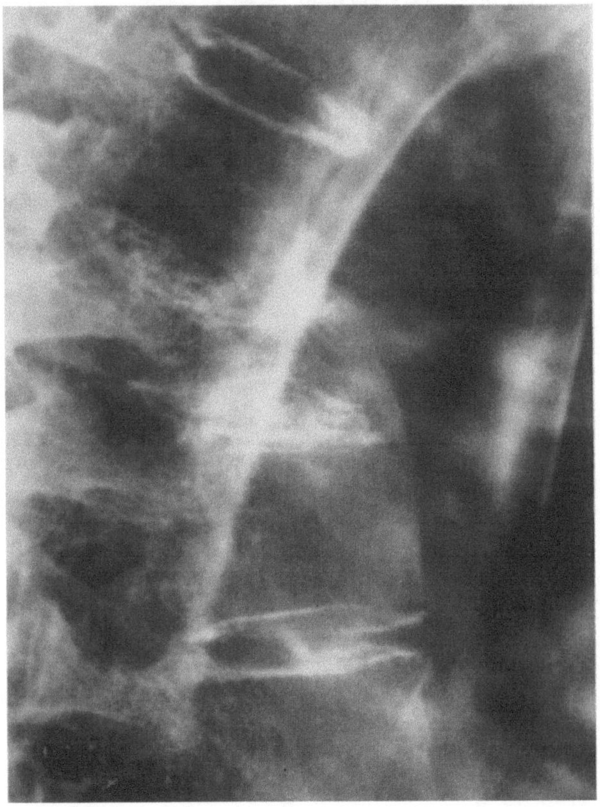
c

Fig. 22a–c. Tuberculous spondylitis in T-4–T-6. Indonesian woman, 49 years old. No previous history of tuberculosis. On admission, paraparesis. After laminectomy the neurological features disappeared. **a** Displacement of the upper part of the thoracic spine above the level of T-6 in dorsal direction. The vertebral body of T-6 is flattened, presenting an osseous lesion, and the lower bone plate is eroded, as is the anterior inferior corner of T-4. The vertebral body of T-5 proved to be completely vanished! **b** After 1 year, chemotherapy, spondylodesis posterior, and immobilization: remineralization and repair of T-6. Well-defined lower bone plate. Syndesmophytelike ossification between T-6 and T-7. Blunt osteophyte at the inferior edge of T-4. **c** Four months after **b**: healed tuberculous process with gibbus and without neurological sequelae

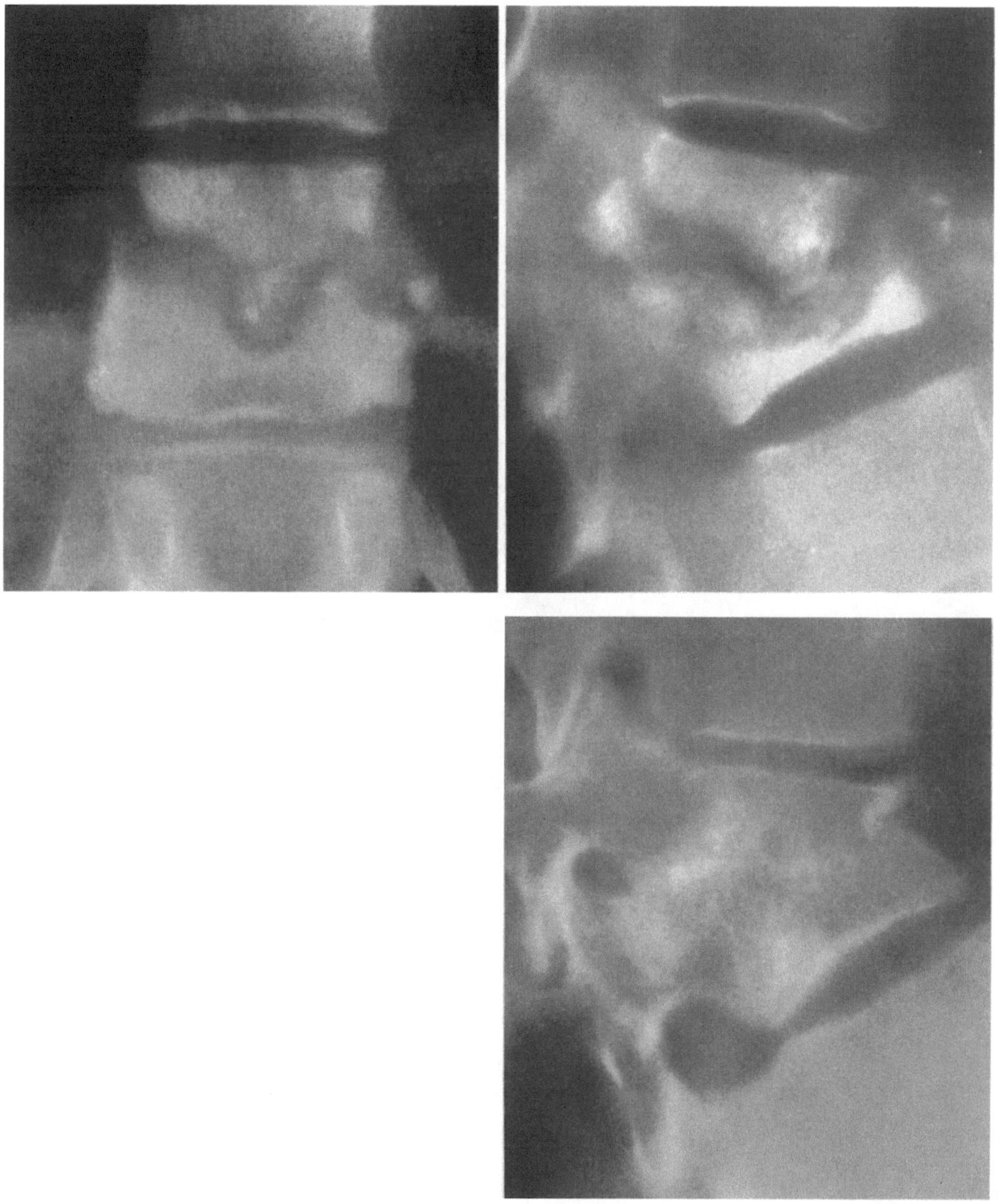

a b c

Fig. 23a–c. Tuberculous spondylitis. Woman, 47 years old. Thirty years before admission, cervical lymphadenitis and tuberculous pleuritis. **a, b** Tomography presents destruction of the vertebral bodies T-11 and T-12, with loose bone fragments and displacement of bone fragments in the direction of the vertebral canal. Kyphotic angle. No neurological complications. **c** One year after radical excision of necrotic tissue with implantation of bone graft: bony fusion with formation of a block vertebra

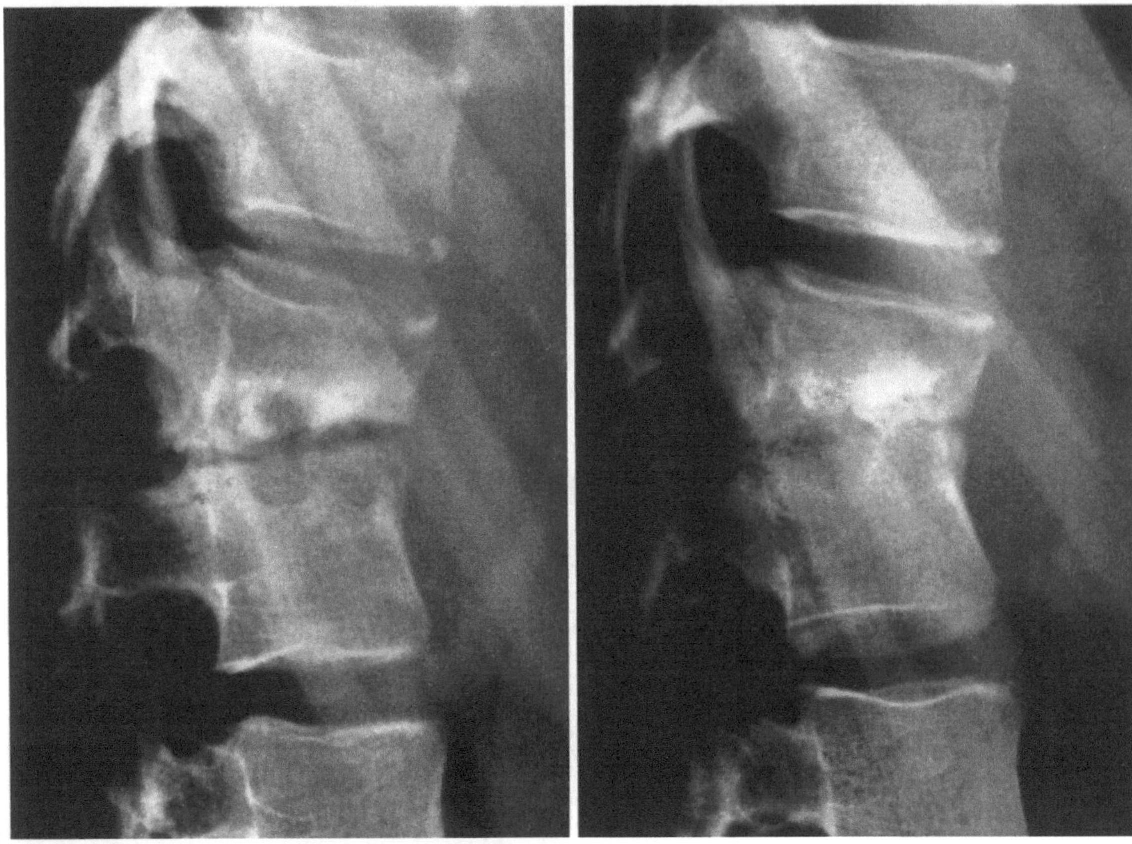

a b

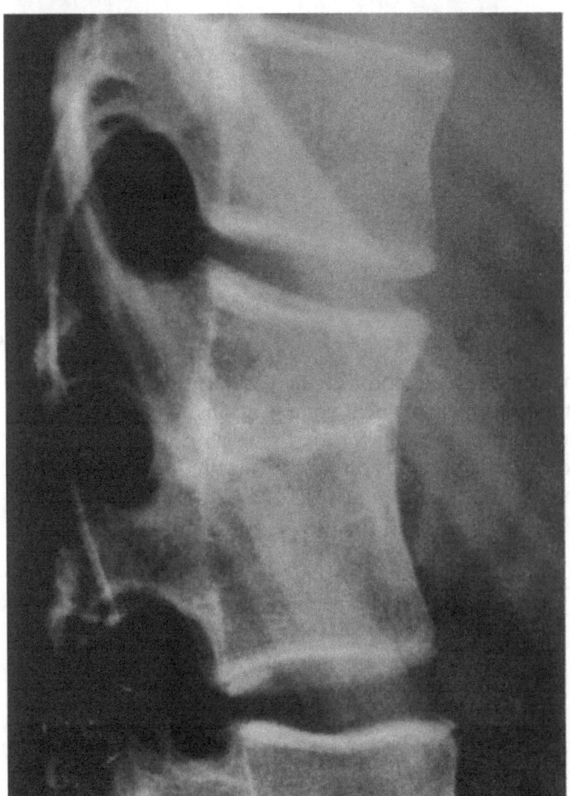

c

Fig. 24a–c. Tuberculous spondylitis. Man, 26 years old. Active pulmonary tuberculosis. **a** Tuberculous involvement of the vertebral body L-1 and similar lesions on the opposite side of L-2. Wedge-shaped vertebral body L-1. Narrowing of the intermediate intervertebral disc. Slight kyphotic angle. **b** After 3 months, chemotherapy and immobilization: improvement of the infectious process and tendency to bony fusion. **c** One year after **a**: spontaneous bony fusion and only slight kyphosis

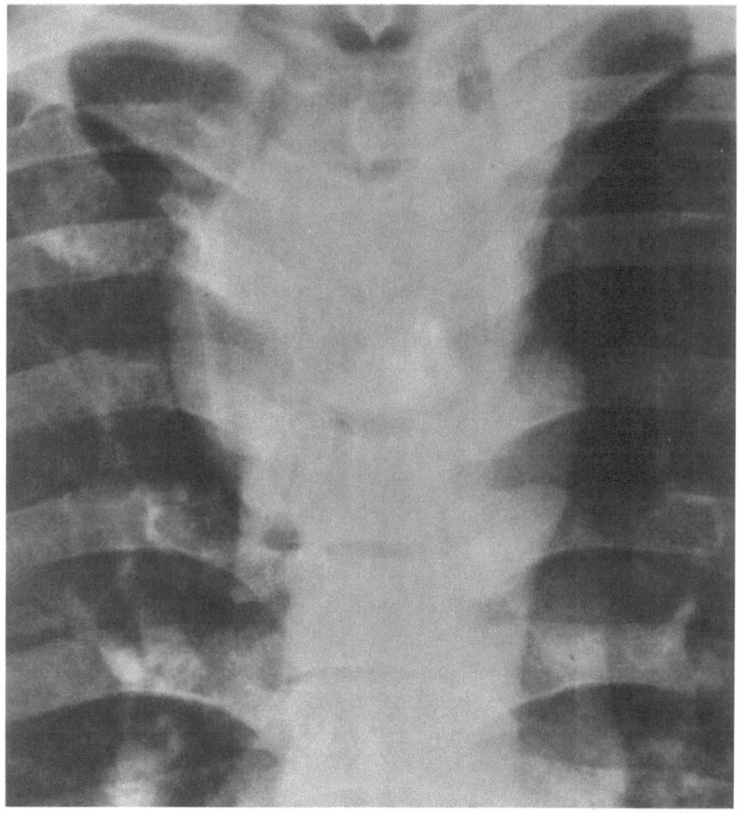

a

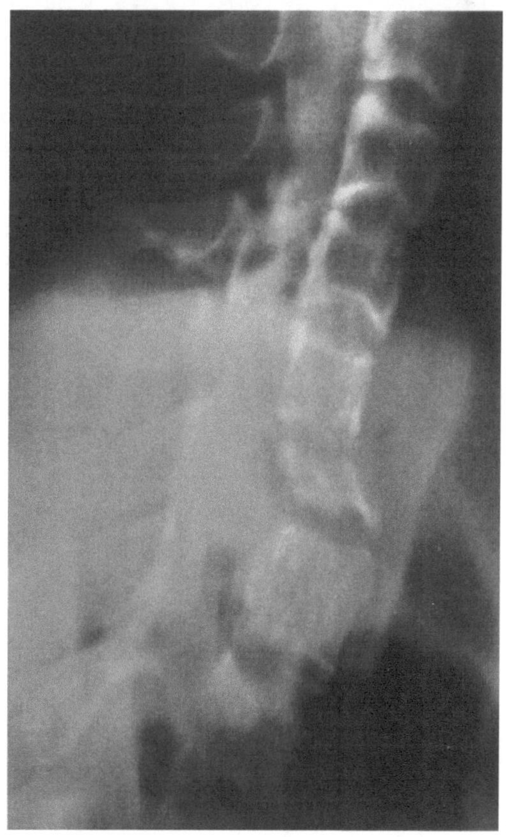

b

Fig. 25a, b. Tuberculous spondylitis at two levels, C-6–C-7 and T-1–T-4. Sailor from the Philippines, 27 years old. No previous history of tuberculosis. Pathological reflexes but no paresis. **a** Paravertebral abscess, most pronounced on the right side. **b** Involvement of the vertebral bodies C-6 and C-7, with prevertebral abscess. Kyphotic angle at that level with compensatory lordotic angle at C-7–T-1 a–c

d–f

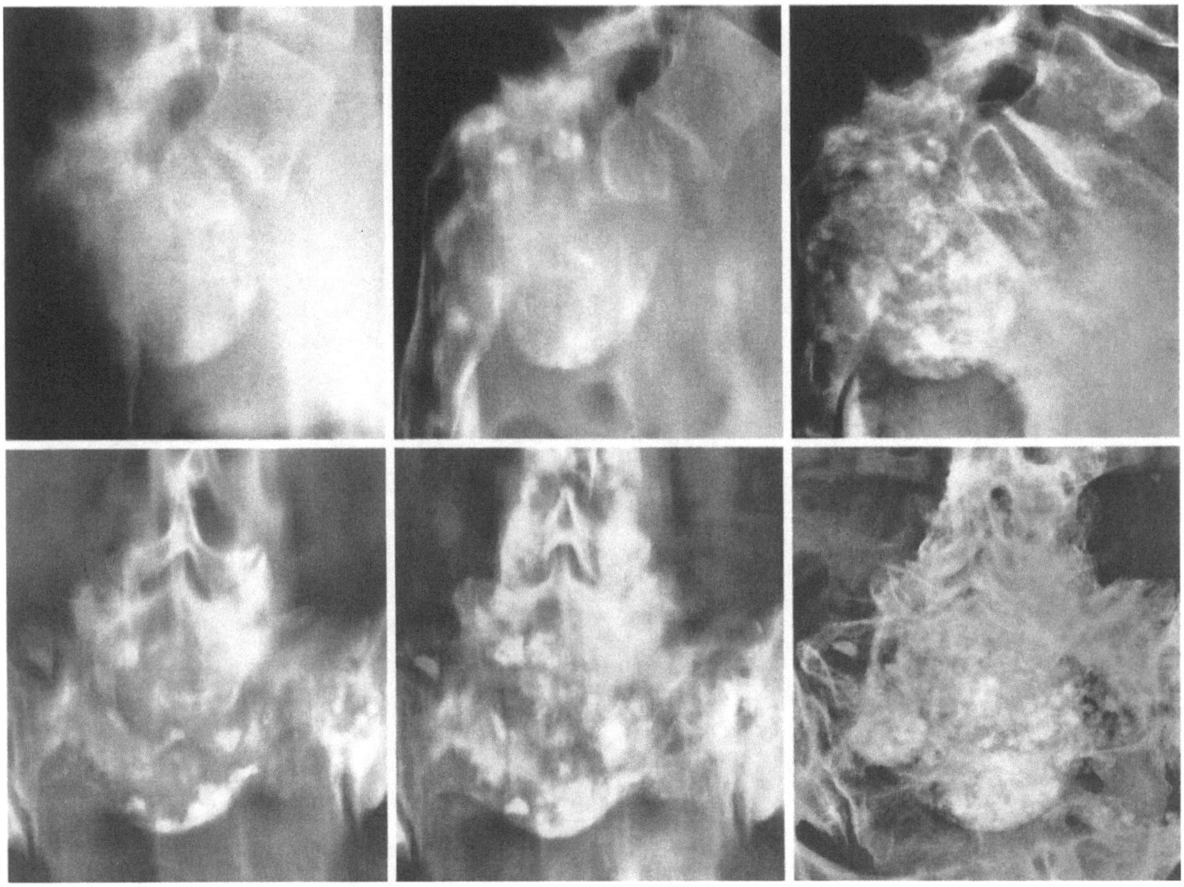

Fig. 26a–f. Tuberculous spondylitis of the sacrum. Woman, 44 years old. At the age of 10 years, tuberculous spondylitis at L-5–S-2. Treatment with cytostatics and ^{131}I for follicular carcinoma of the thyroid. Shortly thereafter, reactivation of tuberculous lymphadenitis. Possibly because of inadequate treatment of this lymphadenitis, reactivation of the spondylitis was induced. **a**, **d** Destruction of the upper part of the sacrum with large presacral abscess and calcifications. **b**, **c** After 1 year: tomography and lateral radiograph present sacrum destruction and abscess formation. The number of calcifications has increased. **e** Two years after **a**, **d** and posterior spondylodesis with implantation of bone chips. **f** Seven years after **a**, **d**: healed tuberculous process. The abscess is extensively calcified

5.4.16 Affection of Vertebral Arch and Appendages

Initial affection of the vertebral arch and appendages is rare; predominantly this is encountered in adult and in nonwhite patients – it was found in two of our nonwhite patients [8, 11, 91, 168] (Figs. 27, 30). In general, the compact bone structures of the vertebral arches are probably not ideal sites for the tuberculous bacilli. In 10% of patients with tuberculous spondylitis, secondary vertebral arch infections are found [8, 19, 97] (Fig. 28). Also in these cases, tuberculous granulomatous tissue may compress the spinal cord or the cauda equina from the dorsal or lateral aspect. The intervertebral discs are usually relatively spared, but extensions to other parts of the arches, ribs, or vertebral bodies may occur [11]. Extraosseous chronic tuberculous granulation tissue in the vertebral canal may initially present with neurological symptoms and without radiographic abnormalities of the vertebrae [8, 84].

5.4.17 Cervical Spine Affection

Affection of the cervical spine is not uncommon in nonwhite patients [99, 124, 164] (Figs. 21, 25, 30–32). We have noticed it in only one of our white patients. There is a high risk of serious neurological features, especially in atlanto-occipital localization of tuberculosis. The dens and the articulations in this region may undergo destruction. Sudden death may occur by dislocation and/or extension of the abscess into the spinal canal.

5.4.18 Ossification of the Anterior Longitudinal Ligament

Marked anterior and lateral bony bridging is described in patients from the tropics and may simulate ankylosing spondylitis [1, 81] (Fig. 29).

5.4.19 Solitary Vertebral Involvement

Involvement of single vertebrae is not uncommon in nonwhite patients but is also seen in whites [29]. The adjacent intervertebral discs may be entirely normal. Paravertebral abscesses may be scanty or absent [169] (Fig. 5).

5.4.20 Healing Stages of Vertebral Spondylitis

In reviewing the series of radiographs from an individual patient with spondylitis, the lack of progression in radiologic abnormalities may indicate that healing has started [140]. Better demarcation of the osseous defects by bone formation around the tuberculous focus is found. Later, intrafocal bone structures become visible. Bony fusion is not an early radiologic feature. Spontaneous bony fusion usually did not occur in adults before the use of chemotherapy; fibrous ankylosis was the rule. After the use of antituberculous chemotherapy spontaneous bony fusion presents frequently and has even been reported in 60% of cases [110]. Spondylodesis may be necessary (Figs. 4, 7, 14, 15, 22, 23, 33, 34). In the healing phase of tuberculous spondylitis, extensive osteosclerosis sometimes results in the formation of an ivory vertebra.

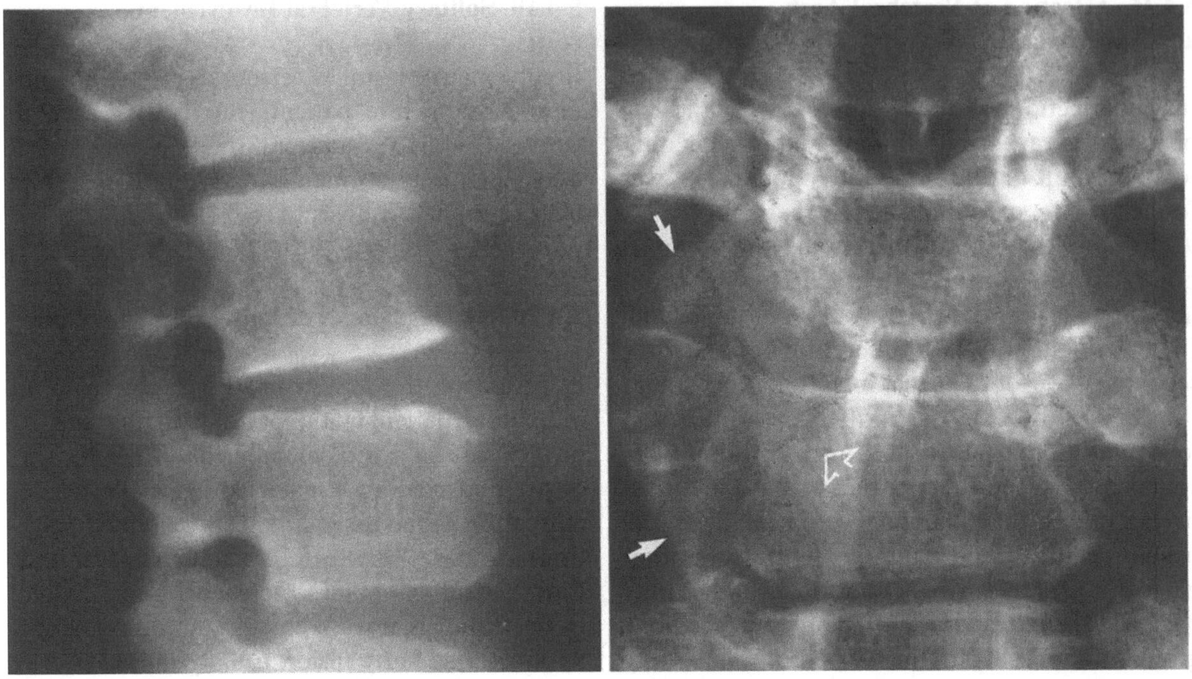

a b

Fig. 27 a, b. Pedicle involvement in tuberculosis. **a** Same patient as in Fig. 9. Tomography demonstrates well-defined osteolytic lesion in the vertebral arch of L-2. At the left side of the same vertebra another bone cavern and superficial spondylitis on the anterior contours of L-2 and L-3 were present. (See also Fig. 9). **b** Vanished right predicle (*open arrow*) caused by tuberculous involvement of T-5 posteriorly and paravertebral abscess (*solid arrows*). Inferior bone plate of T-4 possibly also eroded, intervertebral disc T-4–T-5 not significantly narrowed. (By courtesy of Dr. W.P. Cockshott, Hamilton, Ont., Canada.)

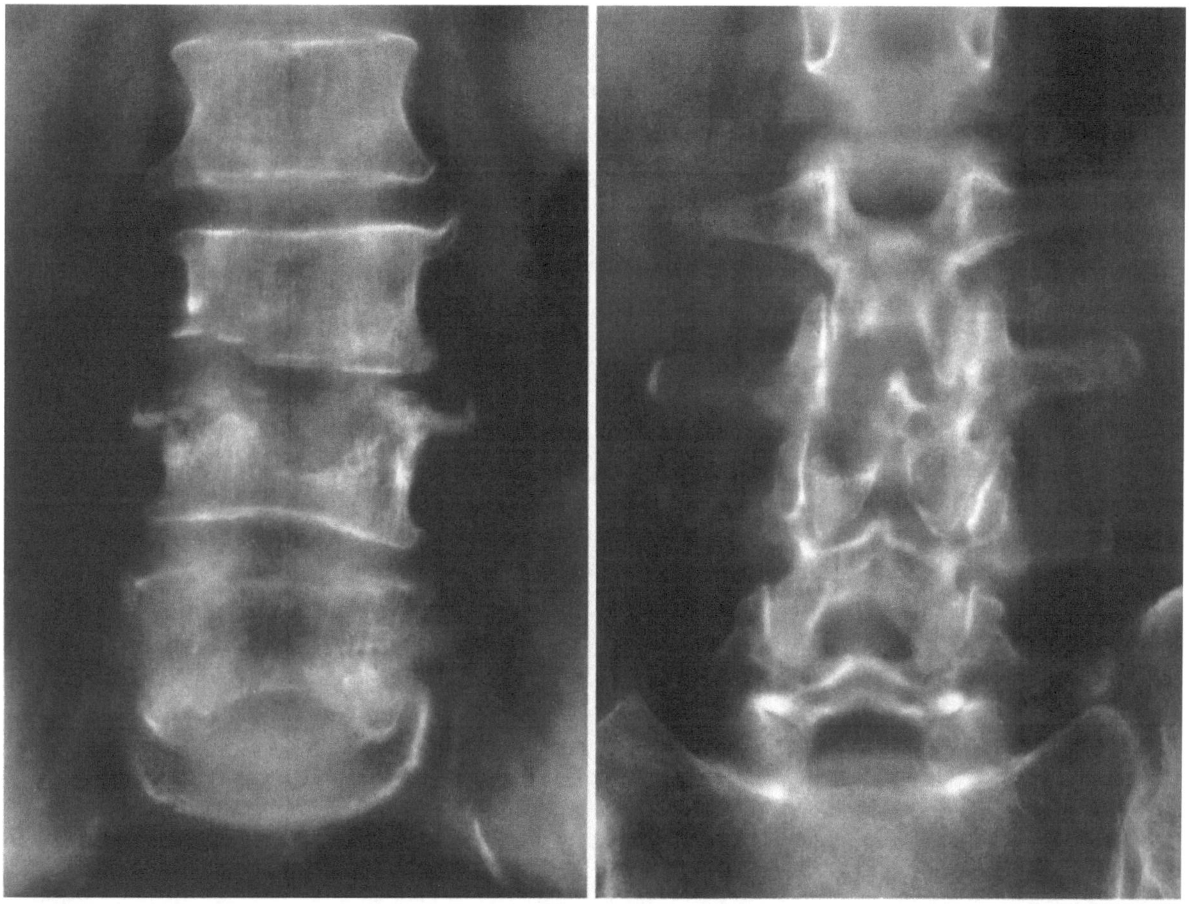

a b

Fig. 28a, b. Tuberculous spondylitis. Woman, 68 years old. Family history of tuberculosis. Previous history of vulva carcinoma. Bone biopsy presented positive histologic findings for tuberculosis. Tomography presents destruction especially of the vertebral arch L-3 and the vertebral body of L-4. The intermediate disc is involved. These radiologic findings are more suspicious for spondylitis than for metastasis because of the affection of the intervertebral disc and the destroyed adjacent bone plates

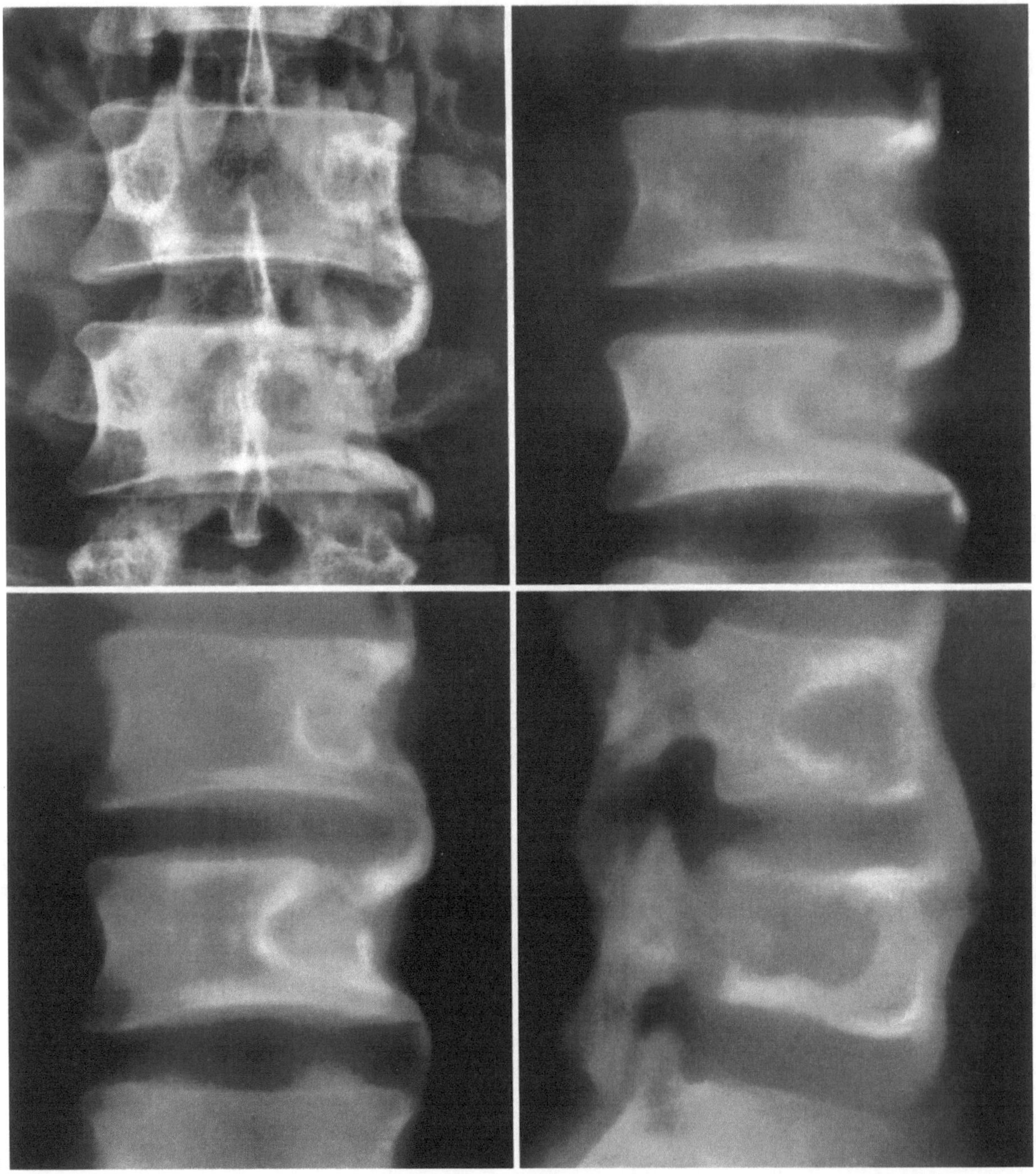

a b c d

Fig. 29a–d. Tuberculous spondylitis. Same patient as in Fig. 17. Other sites of tuberculous spondylitis at C-7–T-2 and T-7–T-9. **a, b** AP radiograph and tomography present osseous lesions on the left side of the vertebral bodies L-3 and L-4. Tomography improves the visualization of the bone lesions. Osteosclerosis in L-4. Ossification of the anterior longitudinal ligament. The intervertebral disc is only slightly diminished in height. **c** After 1 year: the osseous lesions are surrounded by marginal osteosclerosis. Healing process. **d** Three months after **a, b**: tomography in sagittal direction presents extensive ossification of the anterior longitudinal ligament. The osseous defects are bordered by marginal osteosclerosis. Posterior contour of L-4 is destroyed

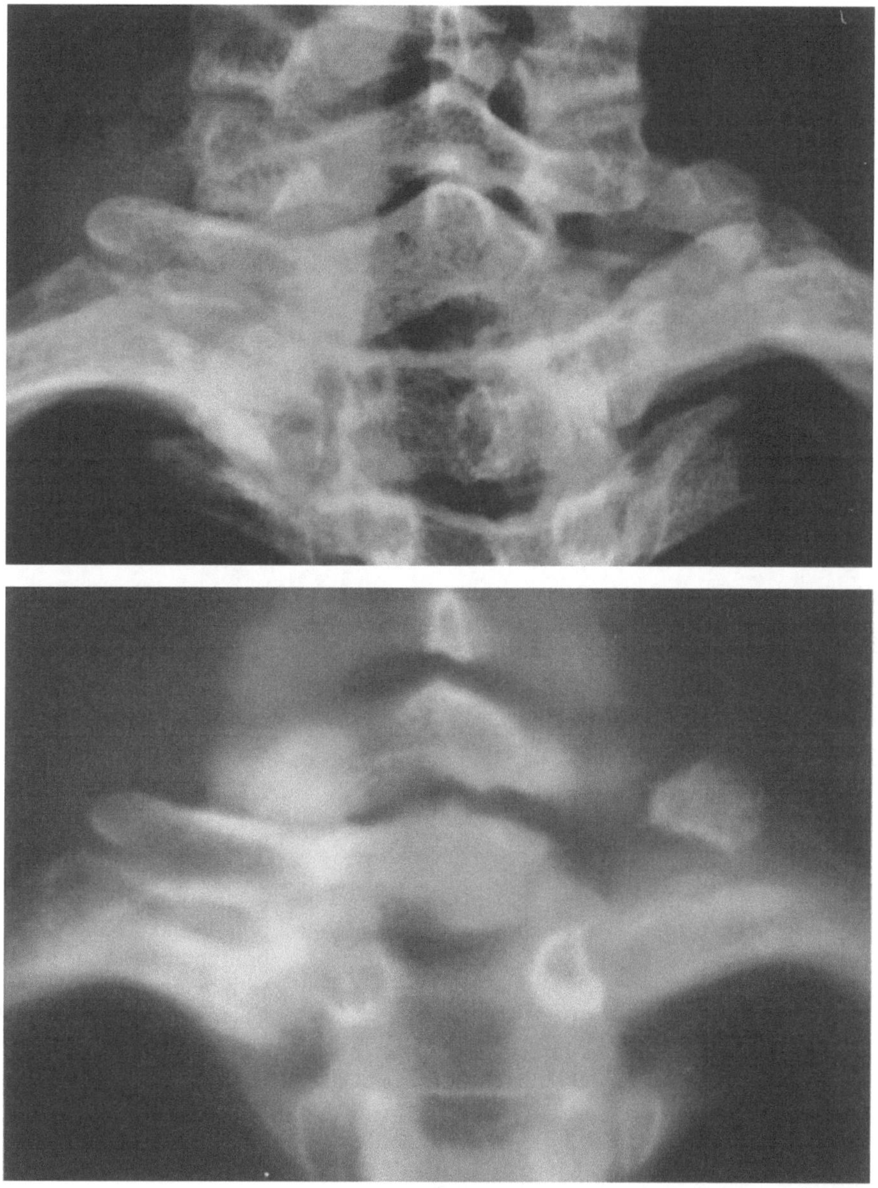

a

b

Fig. 30 a, b. Tuberculous spondylitis. Same patient as in Figs. 17 and Fig. 29. AP radiograph and AP tomography present destruction of the vertebral arch of T-1 and the left transverse processus, with dislocation

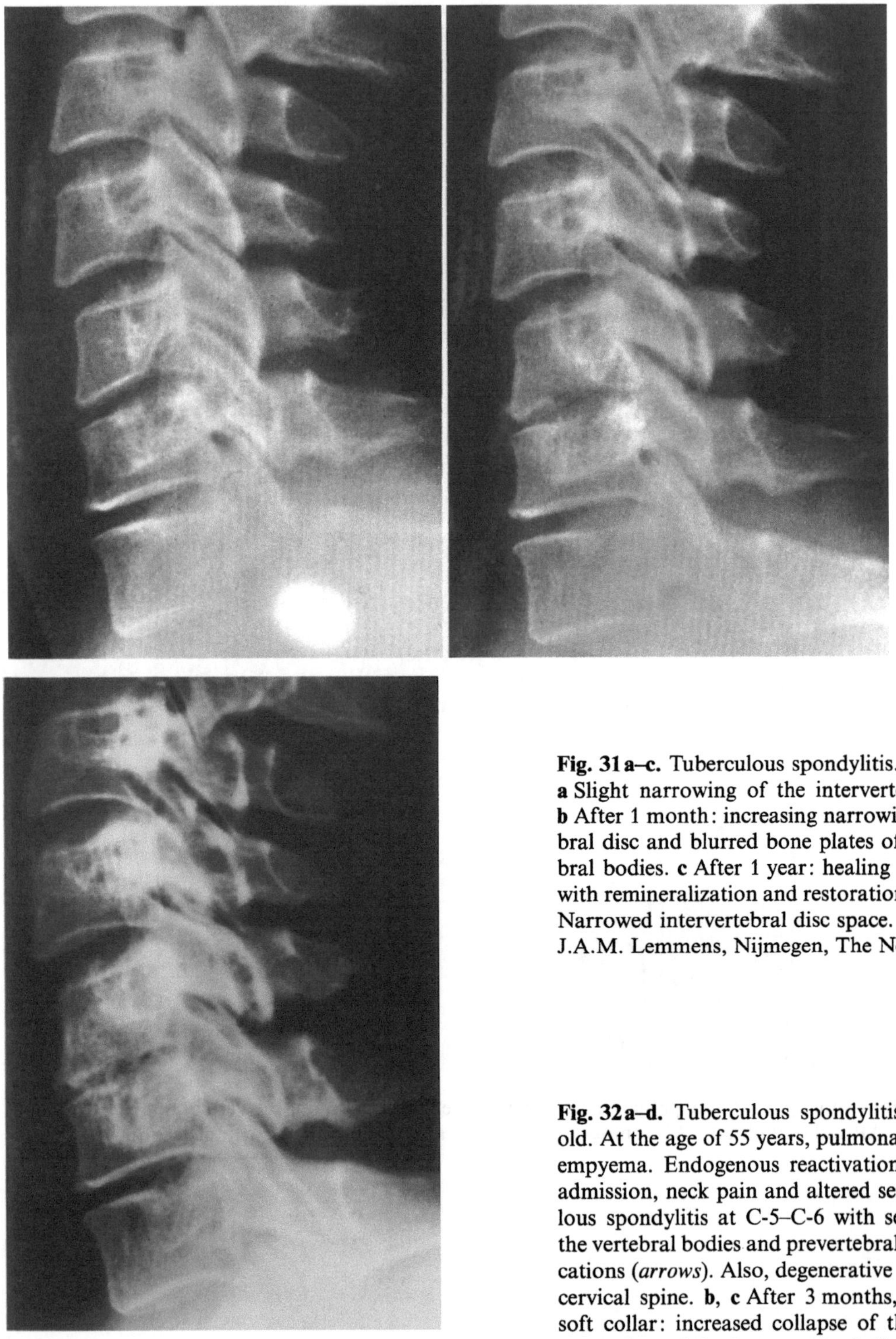

a b c

Fig. 31a–c. Tuberculous spondylitis. Man, 45 years old. a Slight narrowing of the intervertebral disc C-5–C-6. b After 1 month: increasing narrowing of the intervertebral disc and blurred bone plates of the adjacent vertebral bodies. c After 1 year: healing tuberculous process with remineralization and restoration of bone structures. Narrowed intervertebral disc space. (By courtesy of Dr. J.A.M. Lemmens, Nijmegen, The Netherlands.)

Fig. 32a–d. Tuberculous spondylitis. Woman, 88 years ▶ old. At the age of 55 years, pulmonary tuberculosis with empyema. Endogenous reactivation after 11 years. On admission, neck pain and altered sensibility. a Tuberculous spondylitis at C-5–C-6 with severe destruction of the vertebral bodies and prevertebral abscess with calcifications (*arrows*). Also, degenerative abnormalities in the cervical spine. b, c After 3 months, chemotherapy and soft collar: increased collapse of the vertebral bodies, narrowing of the intervertebral disc and improved demarcation of the tuberculous focus with increasing osteosclerosis. Kyphotic angle at C-5–C-6. d One and a half years, after a: spontaneous bony fusion of the vertebral bodies with kyphotic angle at the C-5–C-6 level. Ossification of the anterior longitudinal ligament. Healed tuberculous process

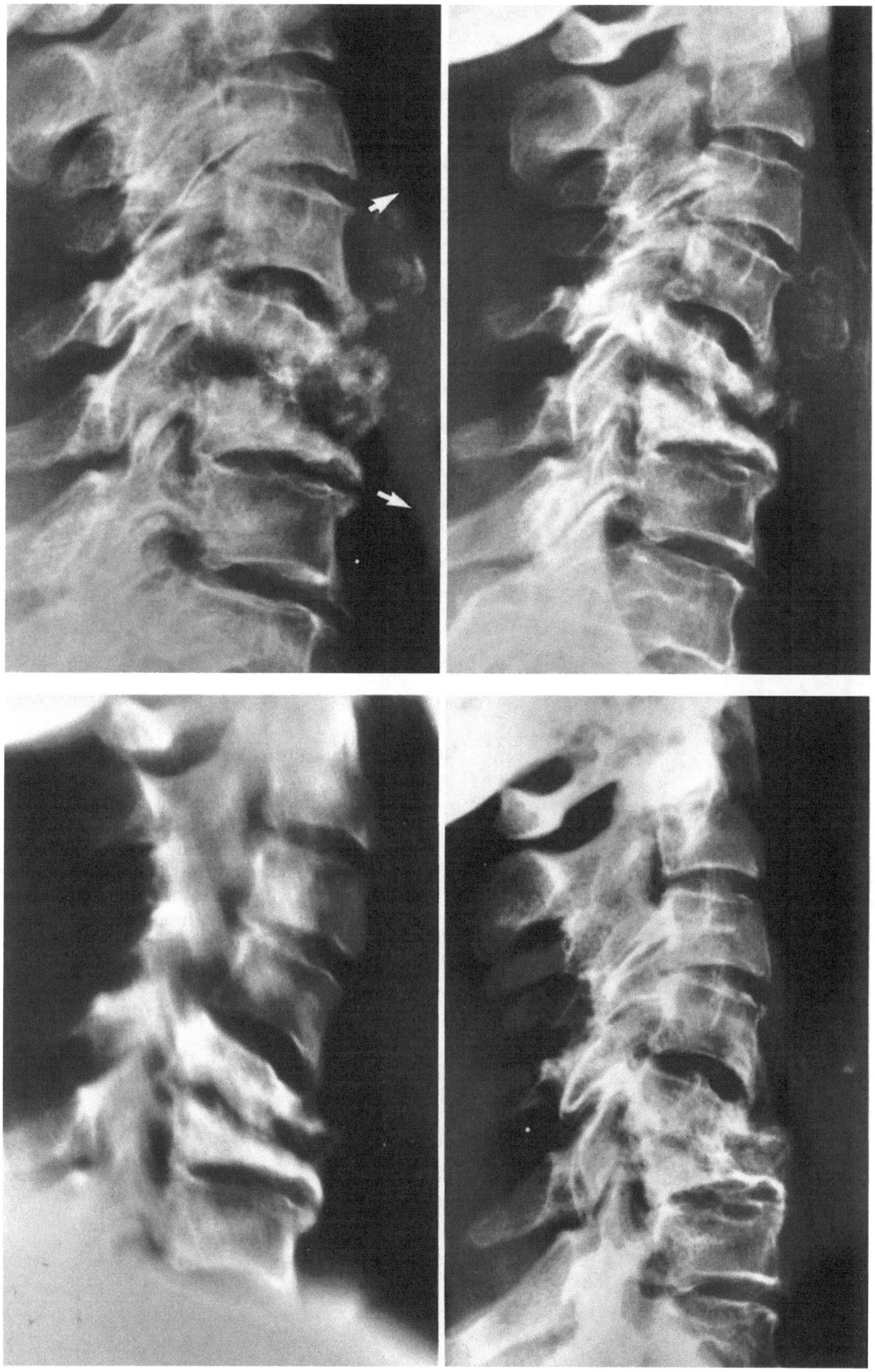

a b c d

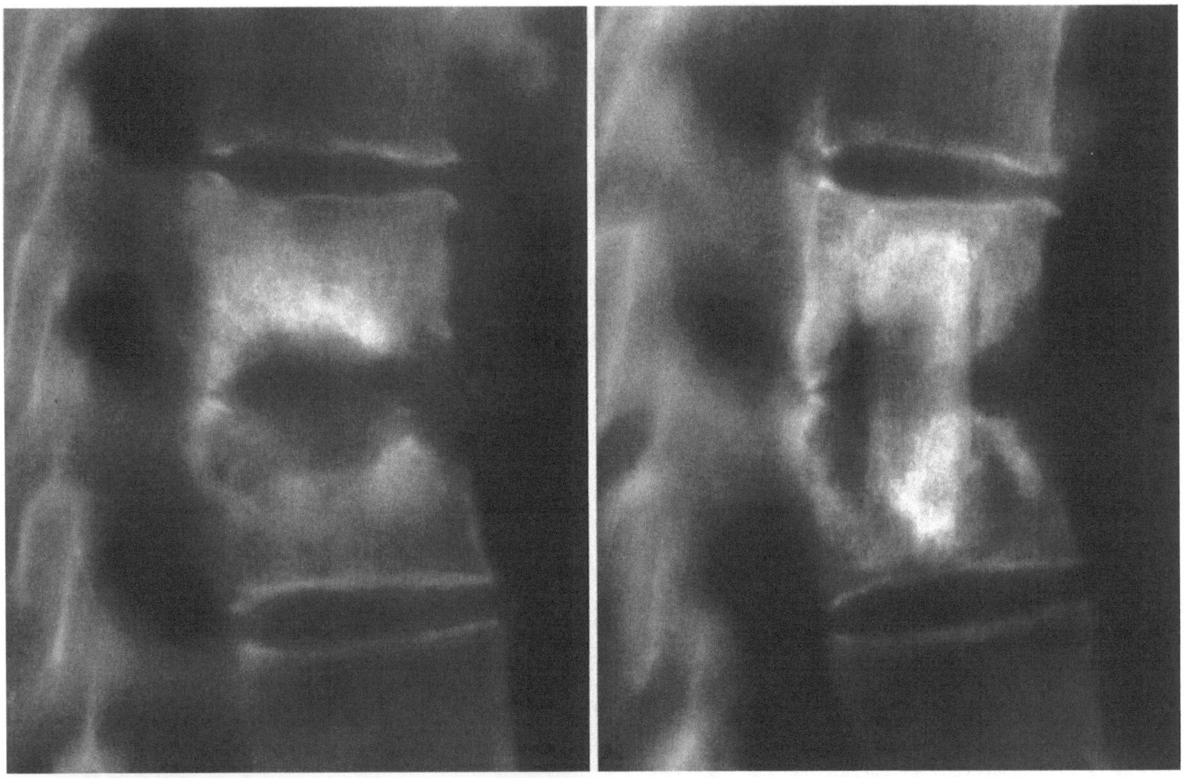

a b

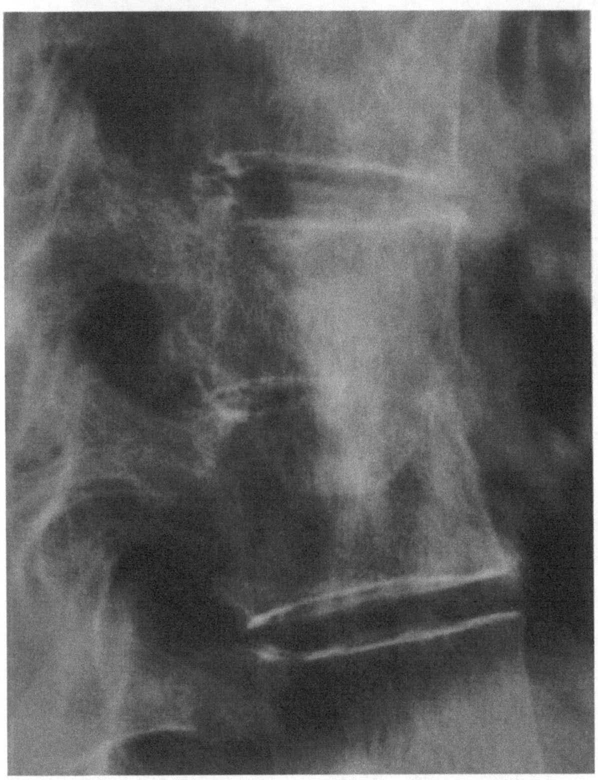

c

Fig. 33a–c. Tuberculous spondylitis. Woman, 70 years old. Family history of tuberculosis (*M. bovis*). **a** Characteristic findings of tuberculous spondylitis at T-8–T-9. Affection of two adjacent thoracic vertebrae and destruction of the intermediate intervertebral disc. **b** Six months after **a**: chemotherapy, immobilization, and radical operation with bone graft spondylodesis anterior. **c** Two years after **a**: bony fusion without collapse. Normalization of the bone structures and only slight kyphotic angle

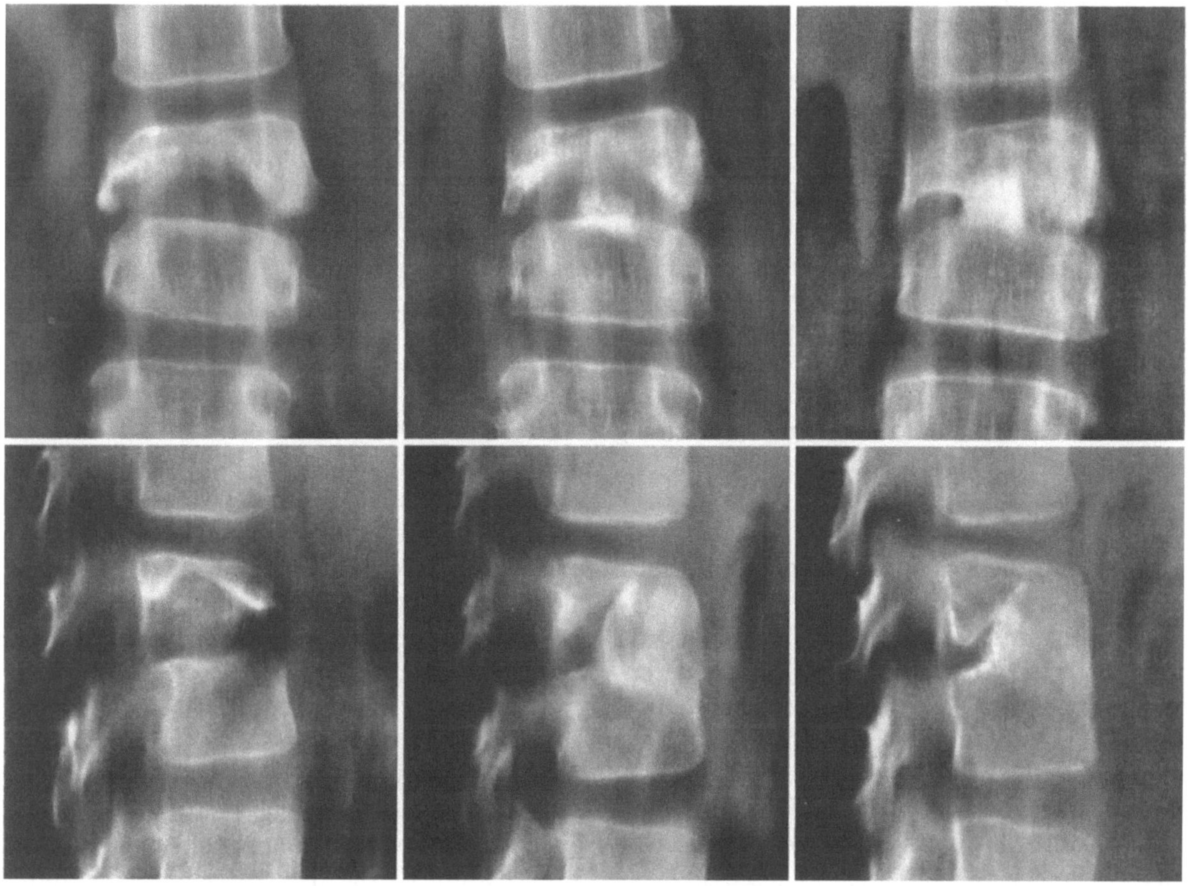

Fig. 34a–f. Tuberculous spondylitis. Boy, 5 years old. Conversion of tuberculin skin test. Recurrent infections (gastrointestinal and pulmonary). Positive culture for tuberculosis of the bone biopsy. **a, d** Active tuberculous spondylitis of the vertebral body L-2 and the right side of the superior bone plate of L-3. Extensive destruction. **b, e** After 4 months, chemotherapy, excision of necrotic bone tissue, anterior spondylodesis, and immobilization: beginning bony fusion. **c, f** One year after **a**: bony fusion and only small residual cleft posteriorly

5.5 Differential Diagnosis

5.5.1 Pyogenic Spondylitis

Pyogenic forms of spondylitis (e.g., staphylococci, salmonella, Escherichia coli, β-hemolytic streptococcus, Bang's brucella) [69] may result in considerable, rapid and progressive discovertebral destruction; usually, however, such lesions are rarely destructive and heal early, with repair of bony structures, osteosclerosis, and osteophytes [104, 109]. Abscesses are often absent or smaller than in tuberculosis, and the forming of block vertebrae is less common (Figs. 35–37).

5.5.2 Primary or Secondary Tumors of the Spine

Destruction due to primary or secondary tumors of the spine (eosinophilic granuloma, aneurysmal bone cyst, myeloma, metastasis, chordoma, etc.) is confined to the medullary bone and spares the "white line" and the intervertebral disc. The cortical white line and the intervertebral disc may be destroyed only in the later stages. There is no paravertebral abscess.

5.5.3 Fractures of the Vertebrae

Fractures of the vertebrae may have their origin in a primary trauma, or they may occur secondarily to a preliminary disease. Paravertebral hematomas may be present and mimic tuberculous abscesses.

5.5.4 Scheuermann's Disease

Schmorl's nodules may simulate a tuberculous affection of the vertebral bodies [20]. They are usually located in the middle or the lower part of the thoracic spine. The intervertebral discs may be slightly narrowed, but otherwise the discs are intact.

5.5.5 Intervertebral Disc Degeneration

5.5.6 Sarcoidosis

In sarcoidosis lesions of the vertebrae and intervertebral discs are sometimes found, although rarely. The radiologic features may mimic those of tuberculous spondylitis (Fig. 38). In sarcoidosis, however, there is never an abscess.

5.5.7 Hydatid Disease of the Spine

Ill-defined hydatid lesions of the spine, appearing as a "bunch of grapes," may be difficult to differentiate from tuberculous vertebral involvement [126]. Osteosclerosis and advanced bone lesions with destruction of the cortex and a spread to the soft tissues may be present. The intervertebral discs are not affected.

5.5.8 Actinomycosis

In actinomycosis subligamentous spread with preservation of the disc spaces may be found [29].

Fig. 35 a–d. Differential diagnosis: spondylitis of unknown origin. Man, 51 years old. Positive tuberculin skin test. Acute onset with severe back pain and fever. No biopsy was done to confirm the diagnosis. **a, c** Two months after first clinical symptoms, characteristic findings of spondylitis at L-2–L-3 with disc involvement and irregular bone plates. **b, d** Four months after **a, c**, antituberculous chemotherapy and immobilization resulted in spontaneous bony fusion. The clinical course is inconsistent with tuberculous infection because of the rapid healing with osteosclerosis and the formation of osteophytes ▶

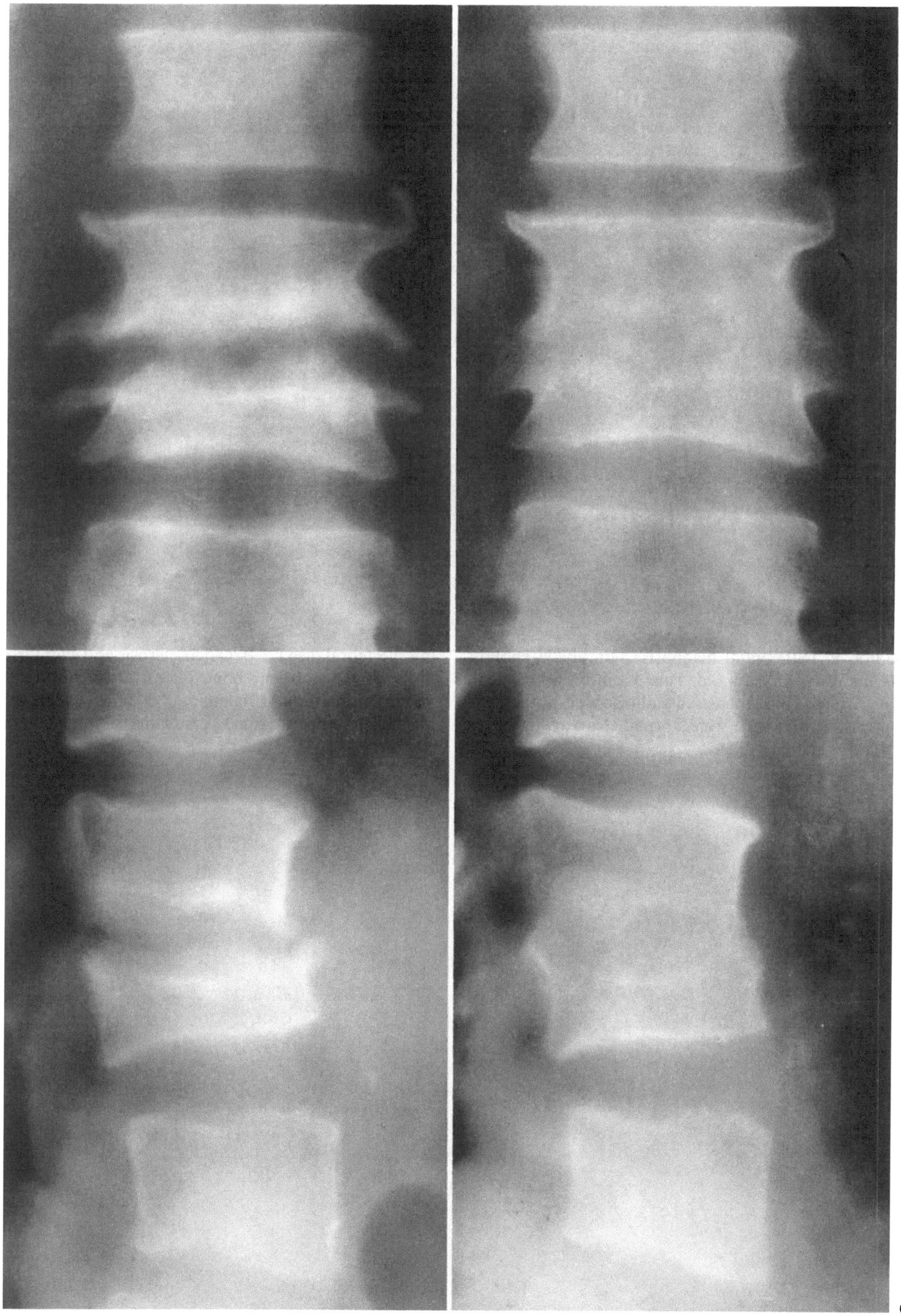

a b c d

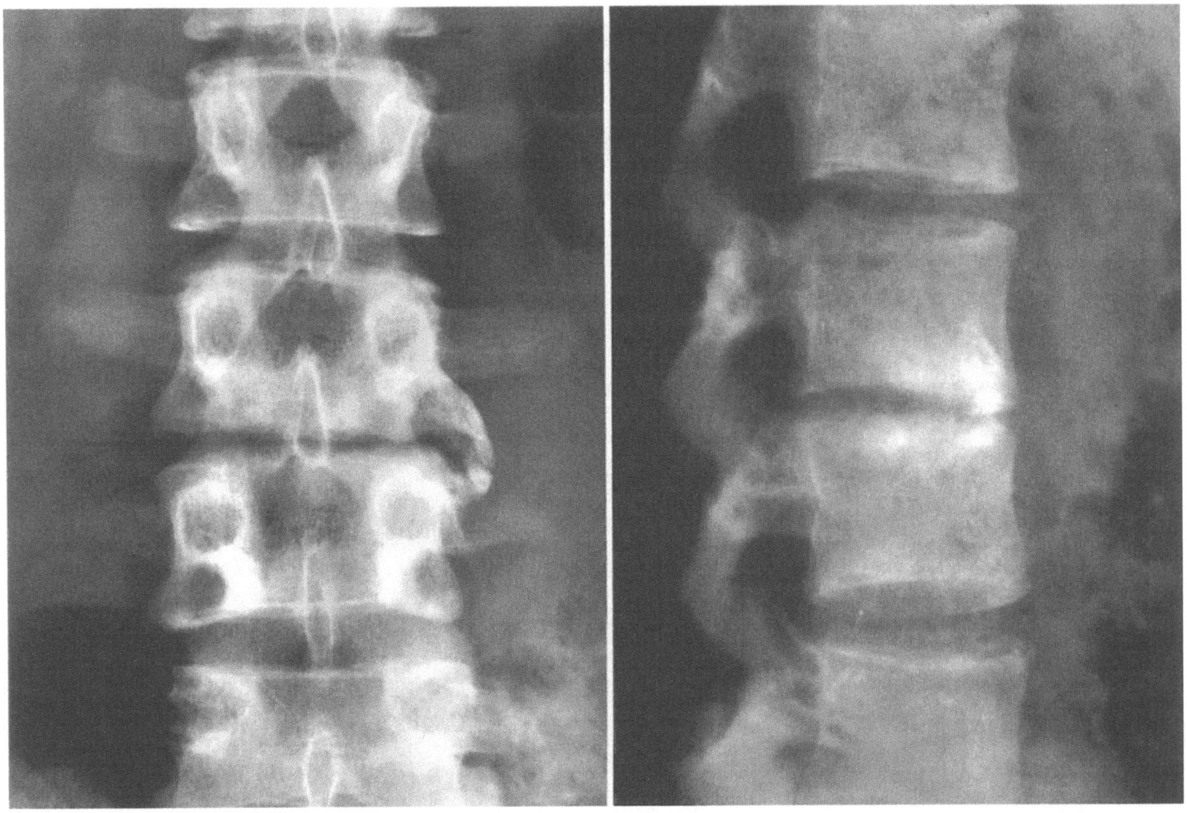

a b

Fig. 36a, b. Differential diagnosis: salmonella spondylodiscitis. Boy, 17 years old. Four months earlier, acute onset of back pain. Increased radioisotope uptake; radiographs at that time were normal. Narrowing of the intervertebral disc L3–4. Osteosclerosis and slight irregularity of the adjacent bone plates. Ossification of the anterior longitudinal ligament. No bony fusion of the affected vertebrae. After 1 year, same radiologic findings

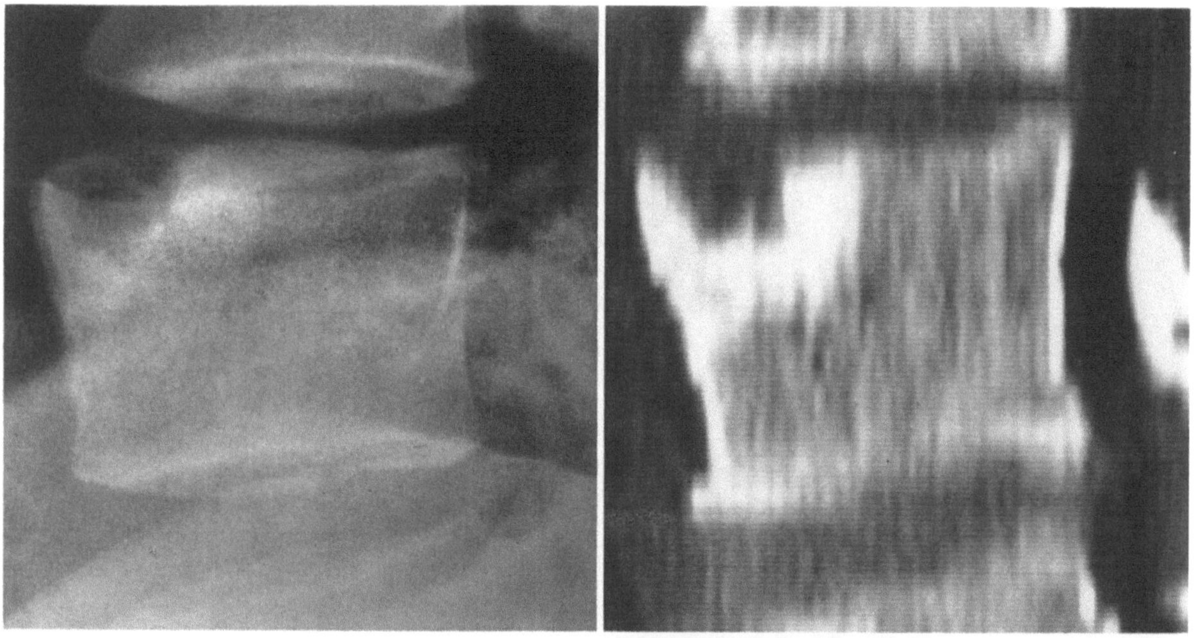

a b

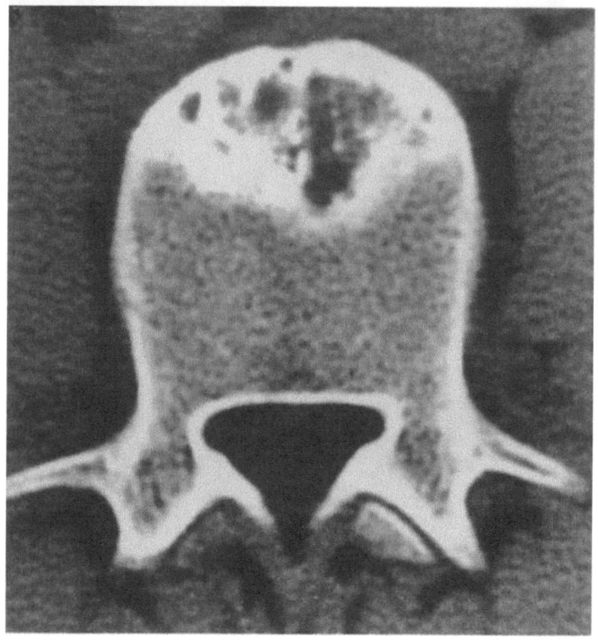

c

Fig. 37 a–c. Differential diagnosis: brucella spondylitis. **a** Adult man with significant osseous defect at the anterior superior border of L-4, with marginal osteosclerosis, disc space narrowing, and periosteal bone formation at L-4 anteriorly. **b** CT reformation in sagittal projection presents same findings as **a**. **c** CT in transverse projection clearly demonstrates a multilocular osseous lesion with extensive osteosclerosis. (By courtesy of Riyadh Armed Forces Hospital, Saudi Arabia.)

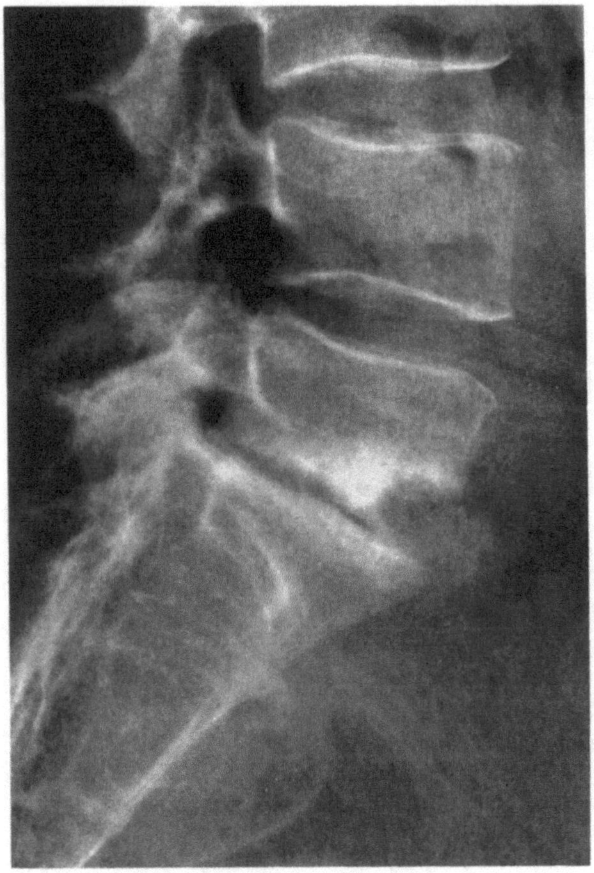

Fig. 38. Differential diagnosis: sarcoidosis. Woman, 50 years old. Spondylodiscitis at L-5–S-1 with erosions of the adjacent bone plates and osseous defect with osteosclerosis in the lower part of L-5

6 Tuberculous Arthritis

6.1 General Remarks

The course of tuberculosis of the skeleton is often different in the white and nonwhite races (Chap. 4).

Spondylitis is the most common form of tuberculous bone involvement [12, 48, 64, 93, 129, 147, 175], followed in frequency by arthritis of the weight-bearing joints of the lower extremities (Table 1, see p. 11). In cases of vertebral involvement the disease often starts in two adjacent vertebrae. Usually only a single joint is affected at any time, in contrast to generalized arthritides. In most reviews the hip and knee joints are reported to be those most frequently affected. In 30 patients with tuberculous gonitis 75% were under the age of 18 years [31]. In older publications the presence of preexistent or simultaneous pulmonary tuberculosis or pleuritis and tuberculous bone lesions are described in 46%–71% of patients and in 79% of autopsies [62]; in more recent publications these rates are lower – 25% [48] and 20%–50% [56], respectively.

Warns [174] identified pleuritis in 76% of his patients with skeletal tuberculosis. The manifestation of tuberculous foci in bones and joints is thought to depend on certain pathogenetic factors. After hematogenous and/or lymphogenous spread of bacilli to many different organs of the body, including the skeleton, these foci may remain dormant until recrudescence occurs [64, 103]. Subsequent local trauma or recurrent microtraumata may be the cause of a modification in the state of local resistance, followed by activation of the tuberculous infection [56, 80, 103, 147]. This could be an explanation for the preferential involvement of the spine and the joints of the lower extremities, because these are the parts of the skeleton with the most weight bearing. Although this theory is not totally proven, tuberculous infections in unusual sites of the skeleton may also be activated by a trauma [64]. Generalized debility is mentioned as being another pathogenetic factor in the activation of dormant tuberculous bacilli [56].

Tuberculous osteomyelitis after BCG inoculation is rare and is almost always found within 2 years after vaccination [148]. In cases of generalized infection caused by BCG, especially if severe immunologic deficiency is present, the prognosis was reported to be bad [145], however nowadays the infection can be cured. Hematogenous spread of *M. bovis* BCG to the skeleton mostly affects the epiphyseal and metaphyseal areas of the long bones. Arthritis is usually not found [145].

6.2 Radiologic Modalities

In most cases conventional radiologic modalities (anteroposterior and lateral radiographs and tomography) are sufficiently reliable for the detection and follow-up of tuberculous involvement of bones and joints. Radionuclide bone scan is useful in the initial stages when radiographs do not yet demonstrate characteristic abnormalities. CT may be indicated if conventional radiographic techniques do not have the ability to give sufficient information about bone destruction or soft tissue involvement. MRI is an expensive but reliable modality in demonstrating early inflammatory foci, and it also gives an excellent depiction of the para-articular soft tissue structures. Para-articular abscesses are easily detected, especially by ultrasonography,

CT and MRI. Sinography may indicate the trajectory of a sinus and the location of the inflammatory lesion, but it is often unreliable because of very narrow and multiple sinuses. Opacification of abscesses after puncture and the injection of contrast medium may be indicated (Figs. 13, 100).

6.3 Correlation Between Pathology and Radiology

The incubation period of tuberculosis may extend up to the length of a lifetime. A latent period varying in length from several months to many decades [12, 147] may be found before the diagnosis of skeletal tuberculosis is made. The time that elapses between initial complaints and positive radiologic findings may be from a few weeks up to several months. The initial infection of a joint by tuberculous bacilli may occur in the synovial membrane, in the epi/metaphyseal bone area, or in both simultaneously. In most cases the affected joint is swollen and painful, but sometimes the findings are subtle, some erosions are present, and no effusion is evident: caries sicca.

On the basis of radiologic findings of tuberculous arthritis, four stages can be indicated [109]:

Stage I. Demineralization with or without some widening of the joint space caused by affection of the synovial membrane, either specific or nonspecific (Fig. 39).

Stage II. One or more osseous foci or erosions usually in combination with a slight narrowing of the joint space by initial cartilage destruction. In this stage the thickened synovial membrane fills the joint space, and bone erosions develop at sites of attachment of the joint capsule (Fig. 40).

Stage III. The whole joint is involved, several osseous lesions are present, the joint space is strongly narrowed, but there is no gross anatomical destruction of the joint (Fig. 41). In this stage the joint space is filled with the thickened synovial membrane and pus. The joint cartilage, capsule, and ligaments are destroyed. Abscesses and sinuses may be present and readily detected, especially in the more superficial joints. Immediate treatment may still preserve the joint.

Stage IV. Further destruction of the joint takes place, with gross deformation (Fig. 42). Complete restoration is no longer possible.

Fig. 39a–c. Tuberculous gonitis, stage I. Woman, 20 years old. **a** Periarticular demineralization. **b** After 7 months: osteoporosis. Joint space intact. **c** One year after **a**: slight osteoporosis; otherwise no abnormalities ▶

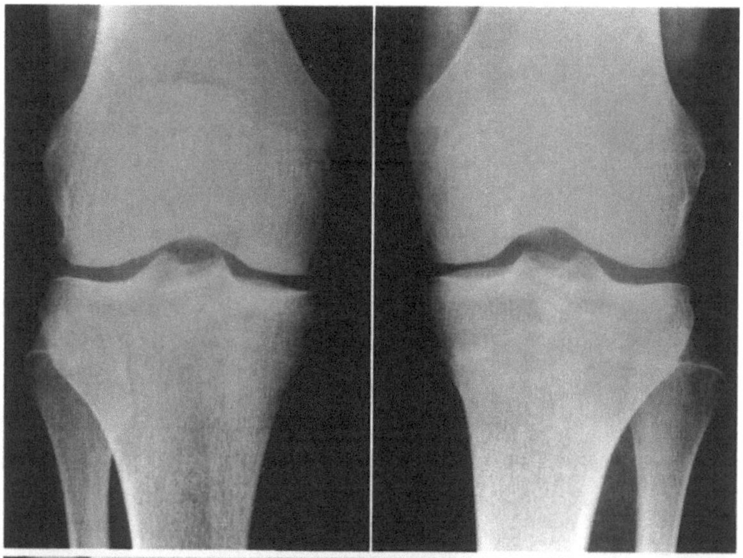

a

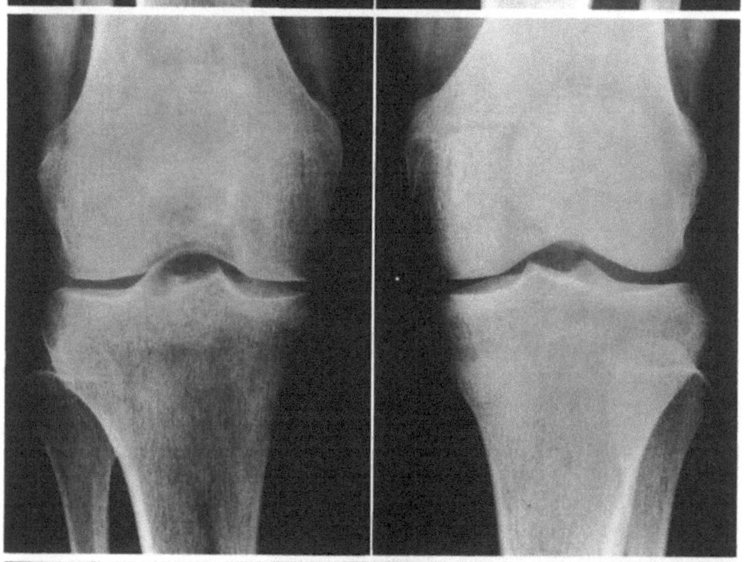

b

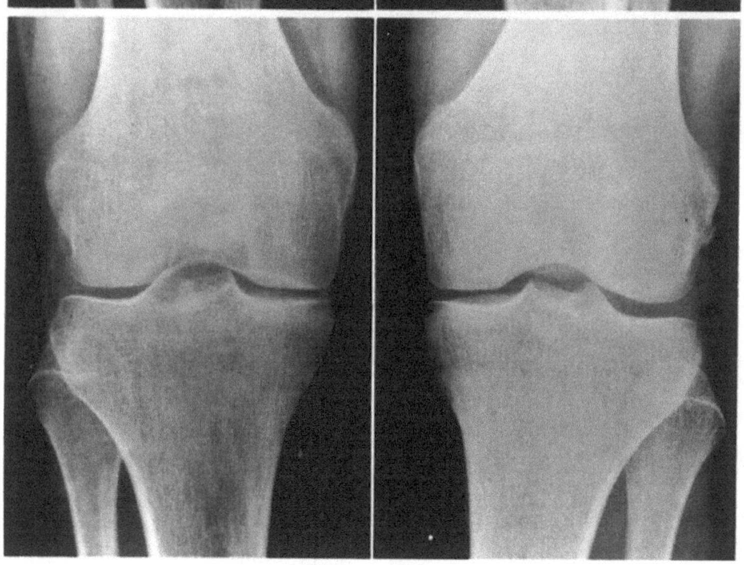

c

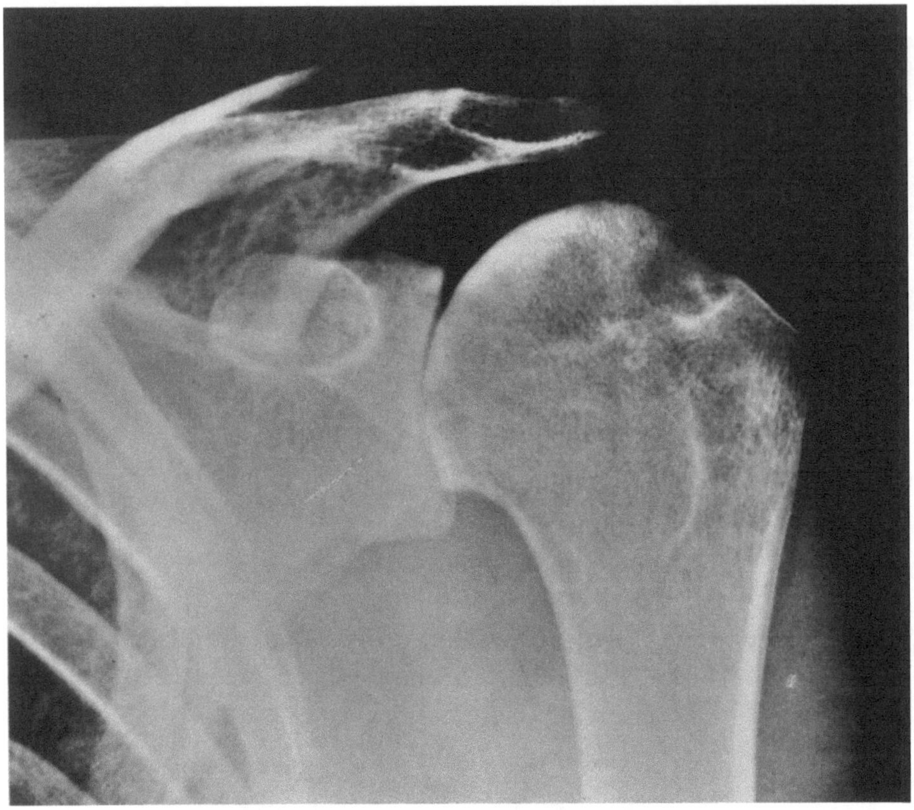

▲
Fig. 40. Tuberculosis of the shoulder, stage II. Man, 21 years old. Positive histologic findings of tuberculosis. Initial synovitis with joint space narrowing and small erosions. Large marginal erosion in the anatomic neck

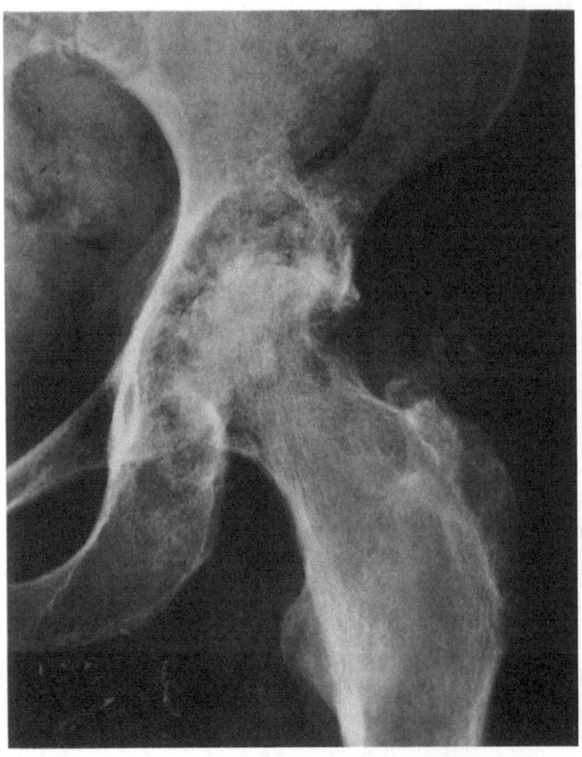

Fig. 41. Tuberculosis of the hip, stage III. Man, 59 years old. Periarticular demineralization, joint space narrowing, marginal erosions in femur, and destruction of the acetabulum

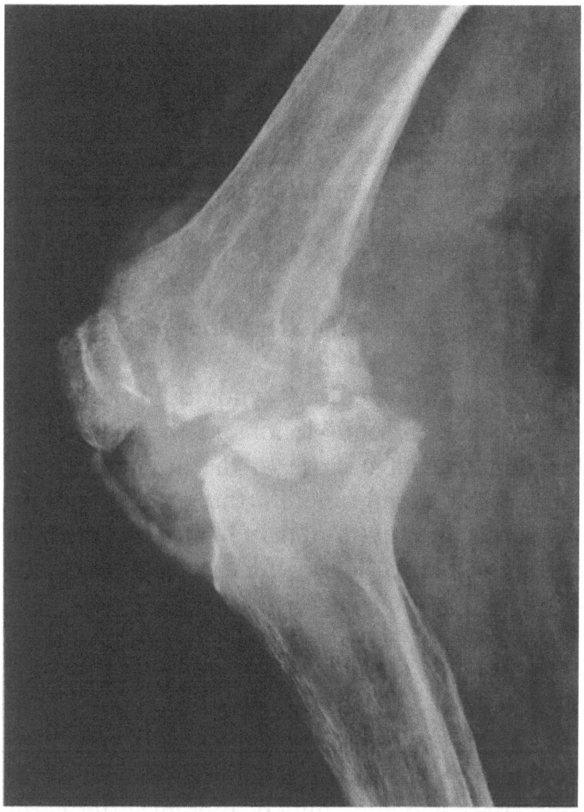

Fig. 42. Tuberculous gonitis, stage IV. Woman, 58 years old. Severe destruction of the knee joint, swelling, and blurred contours

6.3.1 Infection of Synovial Membrane

If the synovial membrane is initially infected, it becomes hypertrophic, and joint effusion occurs by perifocal hyperemia. Tuberculous granulation tissue develops at the margins of the joint cartilage close to the sites of synovial membrane attachment, and progressive subchondral destruction of osseous structures occurs. In the beginning the joint cartilage is not completely covered with tuberculous granulation tissue, thus the function of the joint and, especially, the area of contact and pressure between the articulating bones are preserved. In later stages the subchondral granulations attack the central part of the joint cartilage, and the nutrition of the cartilage by the synovial fluid becomes deficient. In the meantime, the tuberculous granulation tissue invades the subchondral bone, followed by detachment and destruction of the joint cartilage. The affection of the synovial membrane and joint capsule results in focal capsular destruction and the creation of pathways for the extension of tuberculous abscesses to more superficial areas. Destruction of the joint may be the result of these mechanisms [110]. Weight bearing has a negative influence.

6.3.2 Infection of Bone

If infection starts in the bony structures of the joint, this is located in the majority of cases in the epi/metaphyseal area. The tuberculous focus may be confined to the bone or invade the cortex, affecting the synovial membrane secondarily. In this way the same sequence of events occurs as described in Sect. 6.3.1. Evolution of tuberculous arthritis depends on the severity of the disease in the affected patient and on the moment of medical intervention. The degree of osteoporosis, joint effusion, joint space narrowing, focal joint lesions, joint destruction, para-articular abscesses, and periostitis may differ widely in individual patients because of such factors as patient's and doctor's delay, race, age, prevalence for tuberculous infection, and effects of treatment. For this reason the radiologic manifestations of tuberculous arthritis may differ widely, ranging from only slightly abnormal to completely destroyed joints.

6.4 General Radiologic Findings

In the early stages of tuberculous arthritis plain radiographs may be normal, although tomography may already show lesions. Abnormalities become manifest only after a number of weeks.

6.4.1 Synovitis

6.4.1.1 Demineralization/Osteoporosis

Perifocal hyperemia provokes local acidosis, which frees calcium salts and causes juxta-articular demineralization (Fig. 39). In addition, a diminution in the number of bone trabeculae occurs, giving rise to enlargement of the spaces between them and a decrease in their resistance. The normally sharp cortical outline becomes blurred, and in cases of extensive osteoporosis it is even invisible. Osteoporosis is especially marked in the hyperergic forms of tuberculous arthritis with rapid and severe joint destruction. In patients with tuberculous synovitis, osteoporosis usually starts in the epi/metaphyseal area. Recalcification of the bony structures of the joint is an important sign and indicates healing. In a tuberculous infection this proceeds rather slowly compared to infections of other origin.

6.4.1.2 Hydrops

Perifocal hyperemia causes both osteoporosis and overproduction of synovial fluid. In joints of the extremities hydrops can usually be suggested on conventional radiographs because displacement of the para-articular soft tissues is present. Small amounts of synovial fluid are easily detectable by MRI.

6.4.1.3 Soft Tissue Swelling

Hypertrophy of the synovial membrane and overproduction of synovial fluid are responsible for this feature early in the infection. Later, an abscess may be responsible for soft tissue swelling.

6.4.1.4 Erosions of the Joint Margin

In cases of tuberculous synovitis, granulation tissue causes osseous lesions at the margins of the joint cartilage close to the attachments of the synovial membrane. Further extension of tuberculous granulation tissue into the medulla is responsible for larger bone defects (Figs. 40–42).

6.4.1.5 Joint Space Narrowing

In the early stages of joint involvement some joint space widening may be present; afterwards deficient nutrition of the joint cartilage and subchondral lesions are responsible for the destruction of articular cartilage and for joint space narrowing (Figs. 40–42). In comparison to pyogenic arthritis, joint space narrowing is usually a relatively late feature and may be slight or even absent [64]. The radiologic features are slowly developing thinning of joint cartilage, periarticular osteoporosis, and peripheral erosions at the synovial attachment, known as Phemister's triad [42, 60]. In healing stages, destroyed articular cartilage may be replaced by fibrocartilage [31].

6.4.2 Osseous Focus

6.4.2.1 Bone Cavities

Cavities in focal bone lesions caused by the hematogenous spread of tuberculous bacilli vary widely. In cases with severe periarticular osteoporosis the initial infectious focus may hardly be visible, even with the aid of tomography. In another group of patients the foci are easily detected within an area of perifocal osteoporosis. Caseous transformation of the focus may take place with a calcified ring [147]. In patients with rapid caseous necrosis the infectious focus becomes ischemic or anemic from circulatory deficiency and maintains the same density or even increases in density compared to the surrounding bone tissue (sequestrum). If this caseous lesion is infiltrated by granulomatous tissue, a bone cavern is formed, and abscess formation and draining sinuses may occur. Sometimes tuberculous foci are more cystic, with a distinct demarcation, with or without scant osteosclerosis [1, 47, 172].

6.4.2.2 Demineralization/Osteoporosis

Focal or severe periarticular osteoporosis may be found. In the latter, detection of the initial bone lesion may be very difficult.

6.4.2.3 Sequestra

In cases of caseous foci and bone caverns sequestra may be present.

6.4.2.4 Marginal Osteosclerosis

In the beginning stages of osseous tuberculosis, marginal osteosclerosis is seen only in the more caseous lesions.

6.4.2.5 Periosteal Bone Formation

Periosteal bone formation is rarely an early feature. It is caused by periosteal granulations which invade cortical bone by infiltrating the lymph spaces. In this way a subperiosteal abscess is formed, and periosteal new bone may form secondarily. The degree of periostitis varies widely and depends on the localization of the tuberculous focus and the severity of the infection.

6.4.3 Abscesses and Sinuses

Epi/metaphyseal foci may extend to the neighboring soft tissues and cause para-articular abscesses. Increase in size is a sign of abscess activity. Reduction in size and calcifications within the abscess are favorable features. The trajectory of a sinus can sometimes be determined by sinography. Secondary infection of the joint cavity via a discharging sinus is usually a cause of increasing pain and further cartilage destruction [31].

6.4.4 Disturbances in Growth and Ossification

Affection and destruction of the epiphyseal plate by a tuberculous process is the cause of impaired longitudinal growth in children. On the other hand, a metaphyseal focus crossing the epiphyseal plate may infect the epiphysis and enlarge or damage the epiphyseal bone center [172]. Spread of a pyogenic infection across an epiphyseal plate is uncommon, but in tuberculosis this type of spread is commonly encountered (Figs. 78, 86). Foci near the epiphyseal plate may stimulate increased bone length by perifocal hyperemia, and hypertrophy of bone trabeculae is possible.

6.4.5 Osteosclerosis

Later in the course of disease osteosclerosis is caused by bone reparation and recalcification. Increasing bone density by remineralization is usually a feature of healing.

6.4.6 Joint Destruction

The destruction of joints is seen in the more advanced cases.

6.4.7 Calcifications of Soft Tissues

Calcifications are encountered in healing para-articular tissues.

6.4.8 Bone Fusion

Bone fusion is a late feature in tuberculous arthritis. Fusion may be fibrous or osseous.

6.5 Differential Diagnosis

Depending on the localization and the radiologic features of tuberculous arthritis, a number of other diseases must also be excluded.

- Pyogenic arthritis and osteomyelitis.
- Rheumatoid arthritis.
- Seronegative arthritis (juvenile rheumatoid arthritis, psoriatic arthritis, reactive arthritis).
- Osteoarthrosis.
- Hematoma.
- Metastasis.
- (Pseudo)gout.
- Myeloma.
- Hyperparathyroidism.
- Neuropathic joint disease.
- Primary neoplasms.
- Villonodular synovitis.
- Chronic recurrent multifocal osteomyelitis [14, 36, 137].
- Lymphoma.
- Osteonecrosis.
- Hydatid cysts.

More specific differential diagnoses are presented in the chapters concerned with tuberculous arthritis in the various joints.

7 Tuberculous Affection of the Upper Limb Joints

7.1 Shoulder

Among patients with tuberculosis of bones and joints, tuberculous involvement of the shoulder is rather rare and is encountered in 1.0%–3.0% of cases [48, 64, 93, 96, 109, 120] (Table 1, see p. 11). In our material 17 patients (3.7%) with tuberculous arthritis of the shoulder were present. Multifocal bone lesions are described in the majority of patients with tuberculosis of the shoulder [147]. In our material 5 of the 17 patients presented multifocal tuberculous osseous foci, situated in the elbow (two cases), in the sacroiliac joint (two cases) and in the contralateral shoulder (one case). Adult patients are more frequently affected than children [90, 109, 120, 147, 161, 171], and previous or active pulmonary tuberculosis or pleuritis as a sign of hematogenous spread of bacilli is found in the majority of cases [147, 174].

7.1.1 Pathology

As with tuberculous involvement of other joints, either initial synovitis or a tuberculous osseous focus is the abnormality originally found (Chapt. 6).

7.1.1.1 Initial Synovitis

The joint capsule is infiltrated by tuberculous granulomatous tissue, and a varying amount of synovial fluid is present. Infectious flocculi, released by the synovial membrane and deposited intra-articularly, collect mostly at the edges of the joint cavity in close connection to the joint capsule. The consequence of this tuberculous synovitis may be an invasion of the lymph vessels of the cortical bone at the sites of attachment of the joint capsule and osseous involvement. In the humerus these osseous defects are found in the anatomic neck. In an analogous way osseous defects in the scapula caused by primary synovitis are localized around the glenoid cavity (Figs. 43–46). Rapid healing of primary synovitis without osseous infiltration during chemotherapy does not cause distinct radiologic abnormalities. Arthritis sometimes develops, with rapid necrosis of joint cartilage, bare bone osteitis, and severe destruction of the joint (Fig. 45). In other patients clinical findings are subtle, no effusion is evident, and only some marginal erosions are found (caries sicca).

7.1.1.2 Osseous Focus

An initial osseous focus is usually localized in the epiphysis or metaphysis. Enlarging osseous lesions lead to deformation of the humeral head and/or the glenoid. In epiphyseal foci the possibility of perforation to the joint and of arthritis is present. In metaphyseal foci the chance of this is smaller because of the usually extracapsular localization, but infection of the joint cavity is still possible via the tendon sheath of the long biceps head, infection of the subacromial bursa or infection of the outer side of the capsule.

Abscesses and sinuses are less frequent than in other locations of joint tuberculosis. They usually occur late in the disease (Fig. 48). Migration of upper arm abscesses may follow the tendon sheath of the biceps muscle, or spread along the fasciae of the biceps and triceps muscles and must be looked for at these sites [120].

Abscesses and sinuses from osseous foci in the glenoid (Fig. 47) may present themselves in the axilla or along the fascia of the pectoralis major muscle at the lateral wall of the thorax [109, 147].

If fibrous adhesions in the joint cavity are formed, narrowing of the joint space results. Growth disturbances in infancy induced by tuberculous involvement may lead to deformation of the humeral head and/or the glenoid. Even hypoplasia of the arm may develop.

7.1.2 Radiologic Findings (Figs. 43–47)

7.1.2.1 Synovitis

- Demineralization/osteoporosis.
- Hydrops.
- Soft tissue swelling.
- Marginal erosions at the sites of capsule attachment.
- Joint space narrowing: usually a late feature.

7.1.2.2 Osseous Focus

- Bone cavities.
- Demineralization/osteoporosis.
- Marginal osteosclerosis.
- Sequestra: not a common finding.
- Periosteal bone formation: This is a sign of healing but may also be seen while the infection is still active at other sites in the affected joint.

7.1.2.3 Destruction of Humeral Head and/or Glenoid

In cases with arthritis of the shoulder joint severe destruction of the humeral head and/or glenoid may develop.

7.1.2.4 Abscesses and Sinuses

Presentation of abscesses is: axilla, lateral wall of the thorax, along the tendon sheath of the biceps and triceps muscles.

7.1.2.5 Healing and Healed Stages

- Osteosclerosis.
- Calcifications in the soft tissues.
- Bone fusion: Spontaneous bony fusion is very rare; fibrous ankylosis may occur.
- Disturbances in growth and ossification of the shoulder in childhood and adolescents.

7.1.3 Differential Diagnosis

- Adult rheumatoid arthritis (Fig. 49b).
- Juvenile rheumatoid arthritis.
- Rotator cuff degeneration.
- Pyogenic arthritis.
- Neuropathic joint disease.
- Amyloidosis (Fig. 49a).
- Primary bone tumors.
- Metastatic disease.
- Crystal-induced arthropathy (CPPD).
- Osteoarthrosis.
- Osteonecrosis.
- Villonodular synovitis.
- Progressive idiopathic chondrolysis [82].

a b c d

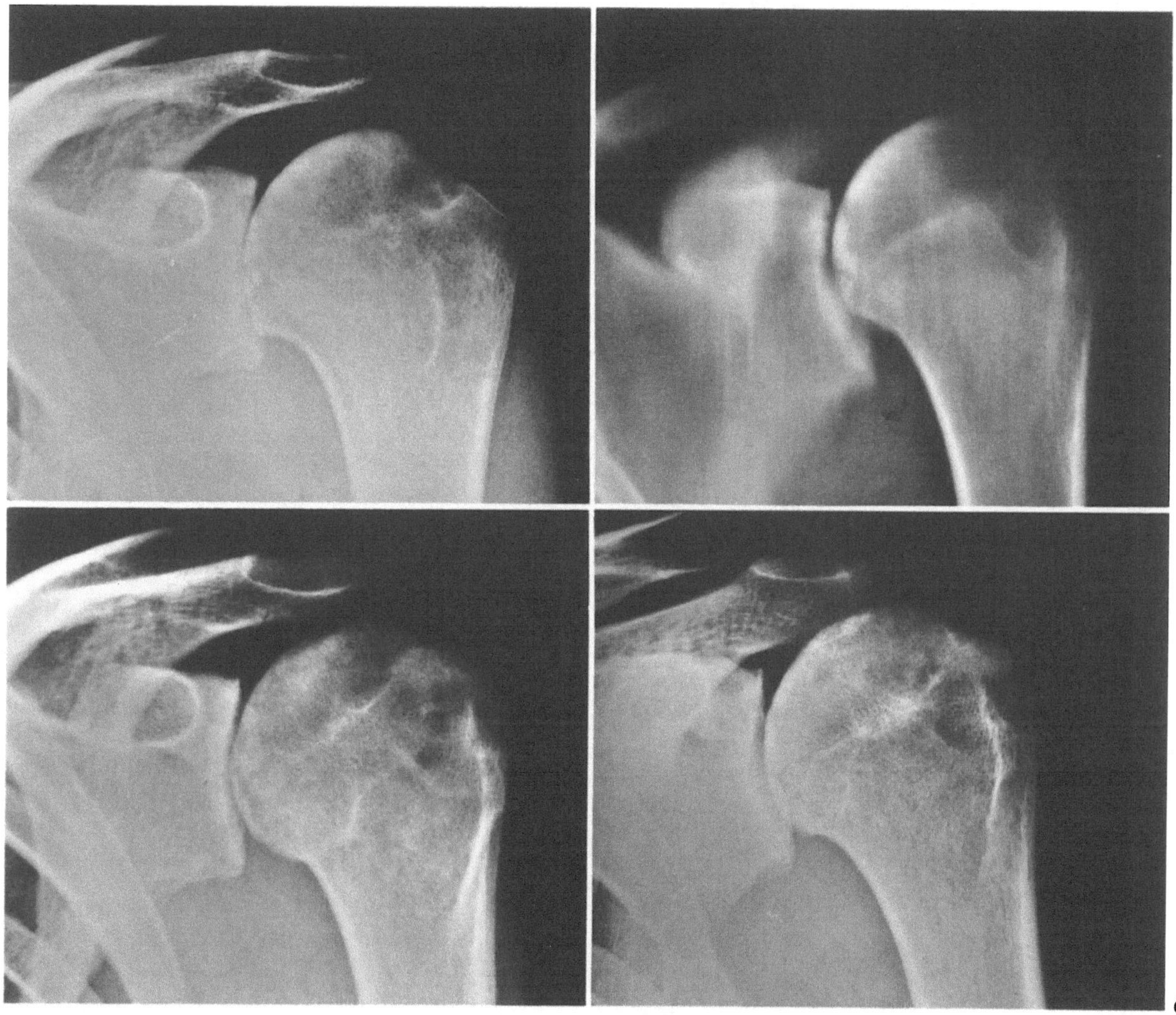

Fig. 43a–d. Tuberculosis of the shoulder. Man, 21 years old. Positive histologic findings of tuberculosis. **a, b** Initial synovitis with joint space narrowing and small erosions. Large marginal erosion in the anatomic neck. **c** One year after **a, b**: more demineralization and bone destruction with large erosions. **d** One and a half years after **a, b**: healing with remineralization and reossification. Some widening of the joint space

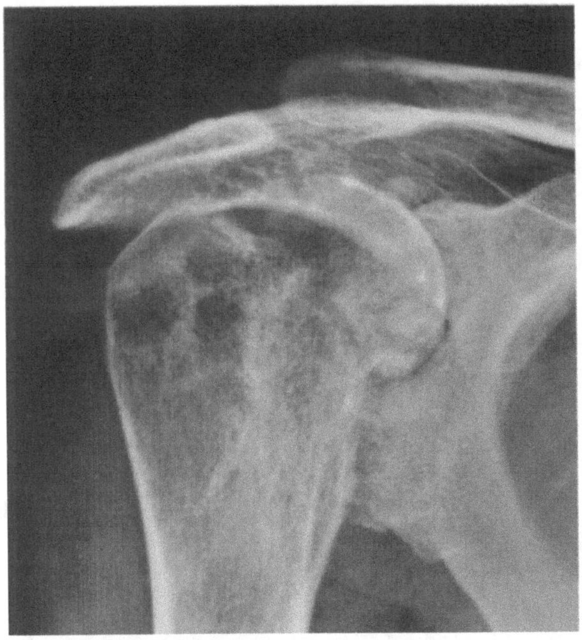

Fig. 44. Tuberculosis of the shoulder. Man, 57 years old. Marginal erosions in the humerus especially at the sites of attachment of the joint capsule. Destruction of the joint space and the glenoid. Demineralization

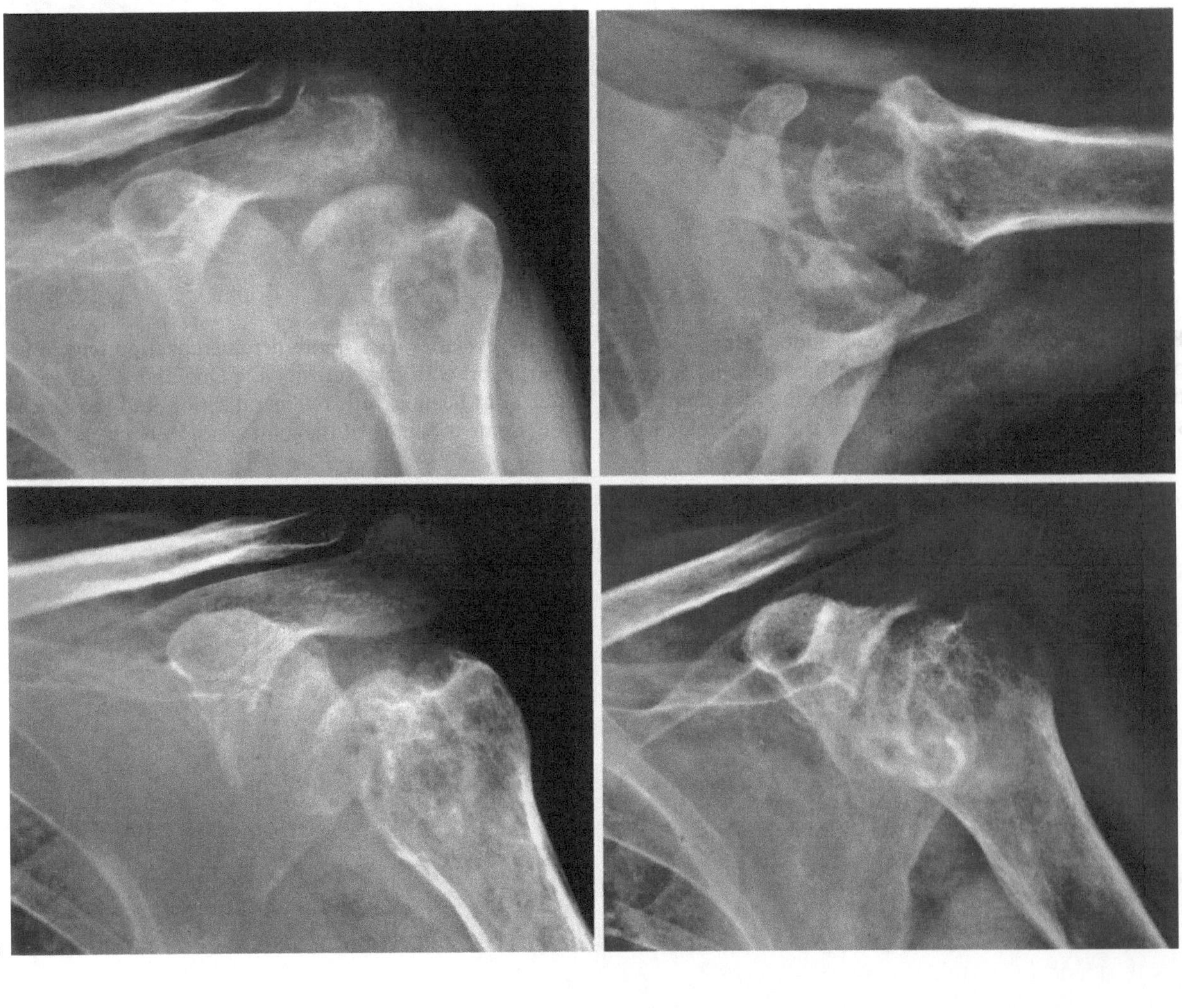

a b

c d

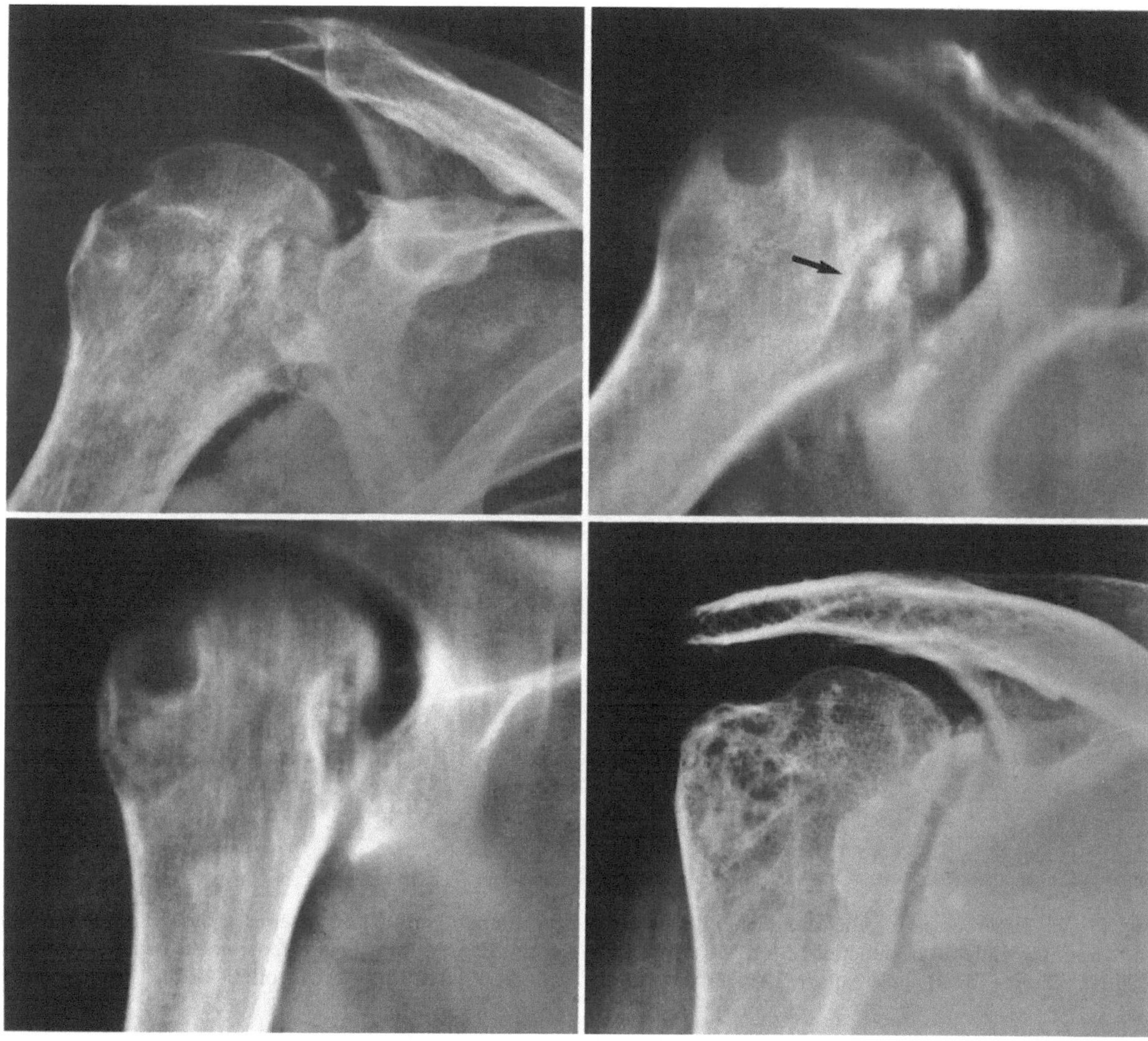

a b c d

◄ **Fig. 45a–d.** Tuberculosis of the shoulder and draining sinus anteriorly. Man, 70 years old. Tuberculous lymphadenitis 40 years earlier and tuberculous coxitis 30 years earlier. Positive histologic and bacteriological findings for tuberculosis. **a** Large marginal erosions, demineralization, and joint destruction. Glenoid ill-defined. Some periosteal bone formation along the humeral shaft. **b**, **c** After 6 months: progressive destruction of the shoulder joint but remineralization and increased bone density. **d** Seven years after **a**: healed tuberculous process. Impaired function of the joint

Fig. 46a–d. Tuberculosis of the shoulder and draining sinus anteriorly. Man, 71 years old. History of tuberculous pleuritis. **a**, **b** Severe destruction of the shoulder joint with erosions of humerus and glenoid. Sequestra in the humeral head (*arrow*). **c** One year after **a**, **b**: the sequestra seem to be fragmented and partly dissolved. **d** Six years after **a**, **b**: healed joint with slightly impaired function. Remineralization, reossification, and improved delineation of the bone contours

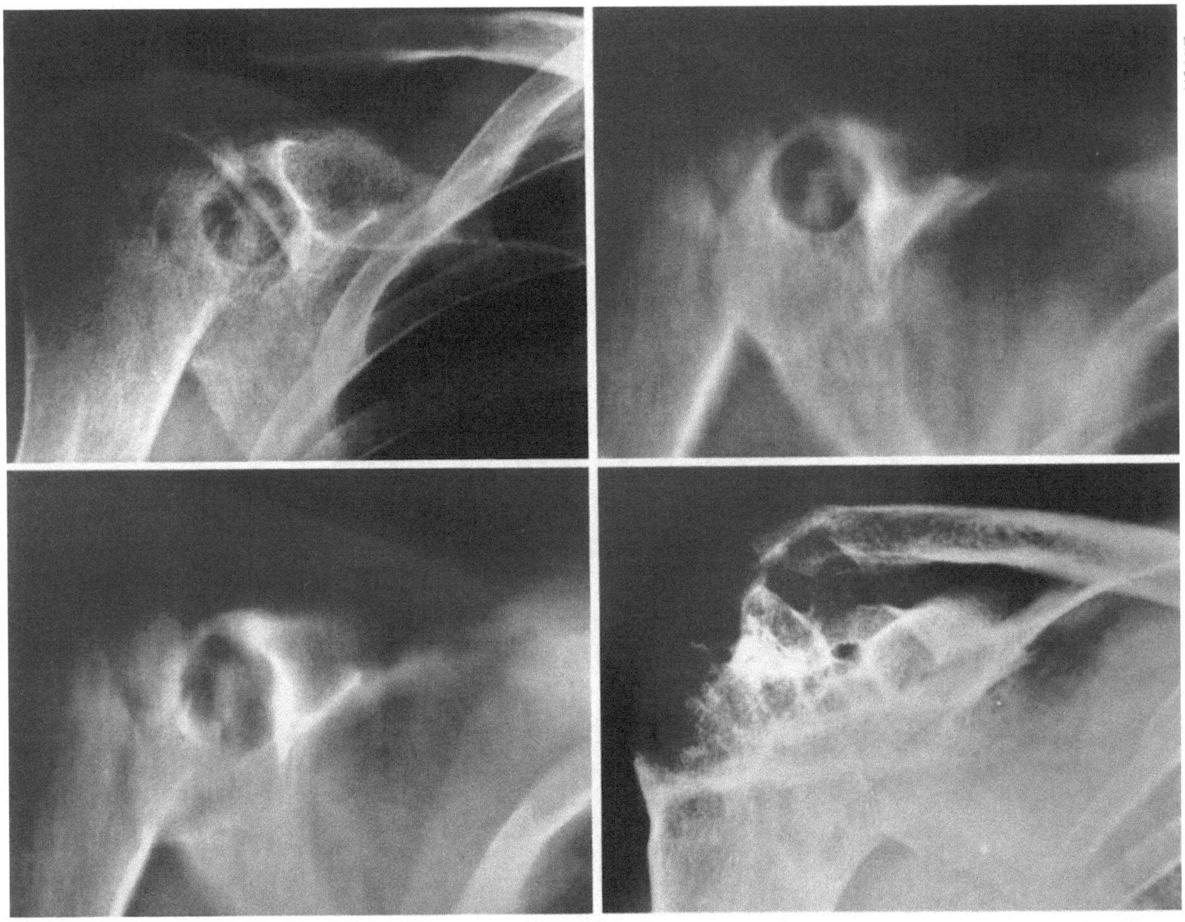

a b c d

Fig. 47 a–d. Tuberculosis of the shoulder with abscess and draining sinus after punction. Man, 36 years old. Positive cultures for *M. tuberculosis*. **a–c** Destruction of the humeral head and osseous focus with sequestrum in the glenoid. Marginal osteosclerosis around the bone cavity. **d** After 6 years: arthrodesis of the shoulder joint

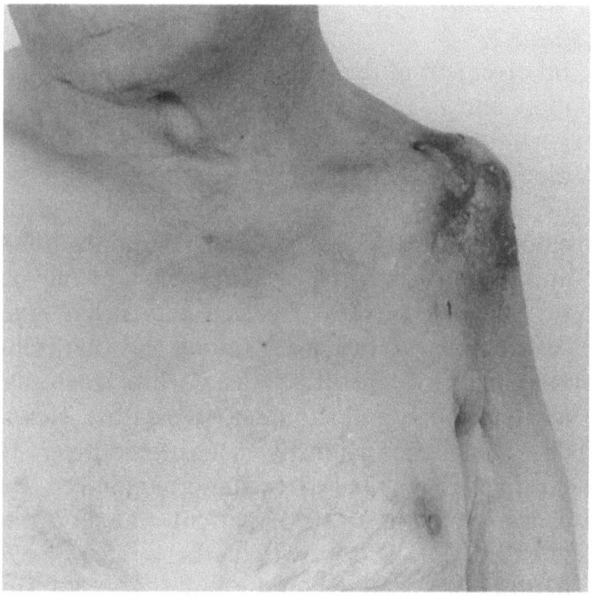
a

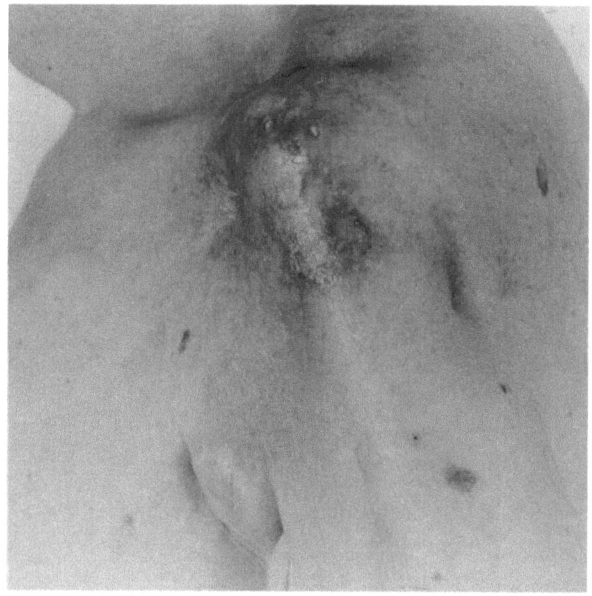
b

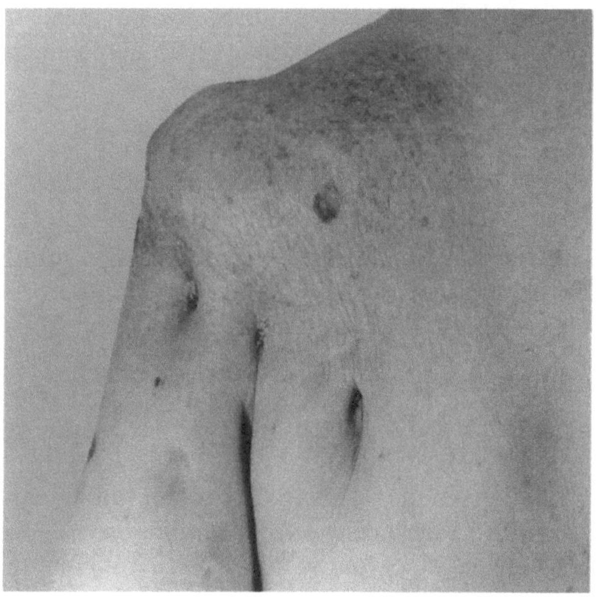
c

Fig. 48 a–c. Tuberculosis of the shoulder. Man, 56 years old. Previous pulmonary tuberculosis, tuberculous empyema, tuberculous gonitis, and tuberculous arthritis of the left shoulder with draining sinuses for 24 years. Atrophy of the musculature and impaired function. A number of sinuses are visible

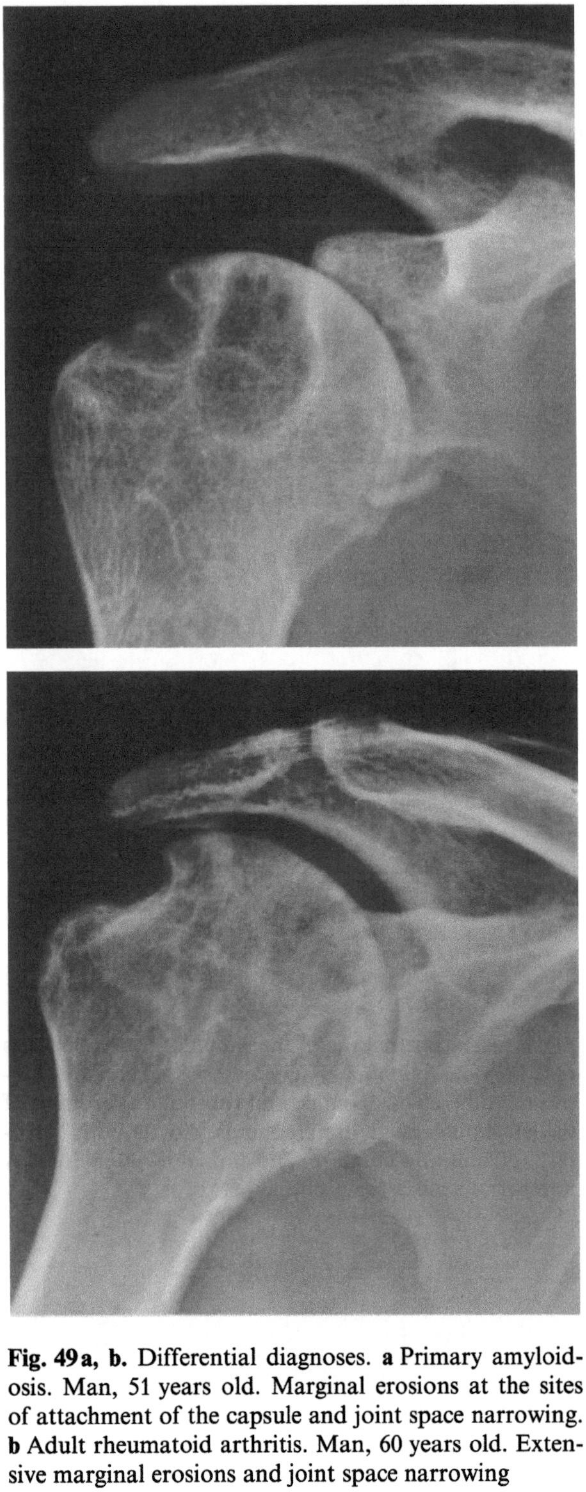

a

b

Fig. 49 a, b. Differential diagnoses. **a** Primary amyloidosis. Man, 51 years old. Marginal erosions at the sites of attachment of the capsule and joint space narrowing. **b** Adult rheumatoid arthritis. Man, 60 years old. Extensive marginal erosions and joint space narrowing

7.2 Elbow

Involvement of the elbow joint is rather uncommon and is reported in 0.5%–8% of cases of joint tuberculosis [48, 79, 93, 96, 109, 158] (Table 1, see p. 11). We reviewed eight adult patients (1.7%) with tuberculous affection of the elbow. Multifocal lesions are commonly found and are proven to be present in five of our patients [147]. In these five patients seven other tuberculous lesions were found together, situated in the spine (two cases), hip, sacroiliac joint, ischium, and shoulder (two cases). Nowadays the disease is mostly encountered in adults, but in the past most patients were children. Because of a long delay by patient and physician most patients present with rather severe abnormalities of the elbow joint on admission. Active or previous pulmonary tuberculosis or pleuritis is also found in many patients with involvement of the elbow.

7.2.1 Pathology

As with tuberculous involvement of other joints, either synovitis or a tuberculous osseous focus is the abnormality initially found (Chapt. 6).

7.2.1.1 Initial Synovitis

Initial synovitis seems to be uncommon in comparison to the presence of an initial osseous focus. In most of our patients with tuberculous affection of the elbow joint, it was impossible to track down the initial site of infection.

7.2.1.2 Osseous Focus

The predilection sites for tuberculous osseous foci are reported to be the epi/metaphyseal region of the radius, ulna, and humerus. In many cases the olecranon seems to be the initial site of the tuberculous focus [109]. The olecranon is also most exposed to (minor) traumata. A nonbacterial synovitis may develop small abnormalities in bone structure at the same time that the osseous focus heals. In many cases of nonspecific synovitis no bone sequelae are found. Depending on the specific localization of the foci, perforation to the joint space may occur. If so, a tuberculous arthritis develops, and rapid destruction of the joint is possible (Fig. 52).

Abscesses and sinuses caused by tuberculous affection of the elbow joint occur in the majority of patients [147].

7.2.2 Radiologic Findings (Figs. 50–53)

7.2.2.1 Synovitis

- Demineralization/osteoporosis.
- Hydrops.
- Soft tissue swelling.
- Marginal erosions.
- Joint space narrowing.
- Joint destruction: often very extensive, with or without subluxation.

7.2.2.2 Osseous Focus

- Bone cavities: usually of epi/metaphyseal localization in ulna, radius, and humerus.
- Demineralization/osteoporosis: localized or more extensive.
- Marginal osteosclerosis.
- Sequestra: uncommon.
- Periosteal bone formation.

7.2.2.3 Abscesses und Sinuses

7.2.2.4 Disturbances in Growth and Ossification

Disturbances in growth and ossification may occur in childhood, for example, accelerated skeletal maturation and enlarging epiphyseal centers. Cubitus valgus and varus deformities may be seen.

7.2.2.5 Healing and Healed Stages

- Osteosclerosis.
- Calcifications or ossifications in the soft tissues.
- Bone fusion: Spontaneous bony fusion occurs in about 20% of patients [65]; fibrous ankylosis is present in other patients.

7.2.3 Differential Diagnosis

- Adult rheumatoid arthritis (Fig. 54).
- Juvenile rheumatoid arthritis.
- Osteochondritis dissecans.
- Pyogenic arthritis.
- Primary bone tumor.
- Metastatic disease.
- Hemophilia.
- Neuropathic joint disease.
- Osteoarthrosis.
- Villonodular synovitis.

a–c

d–f

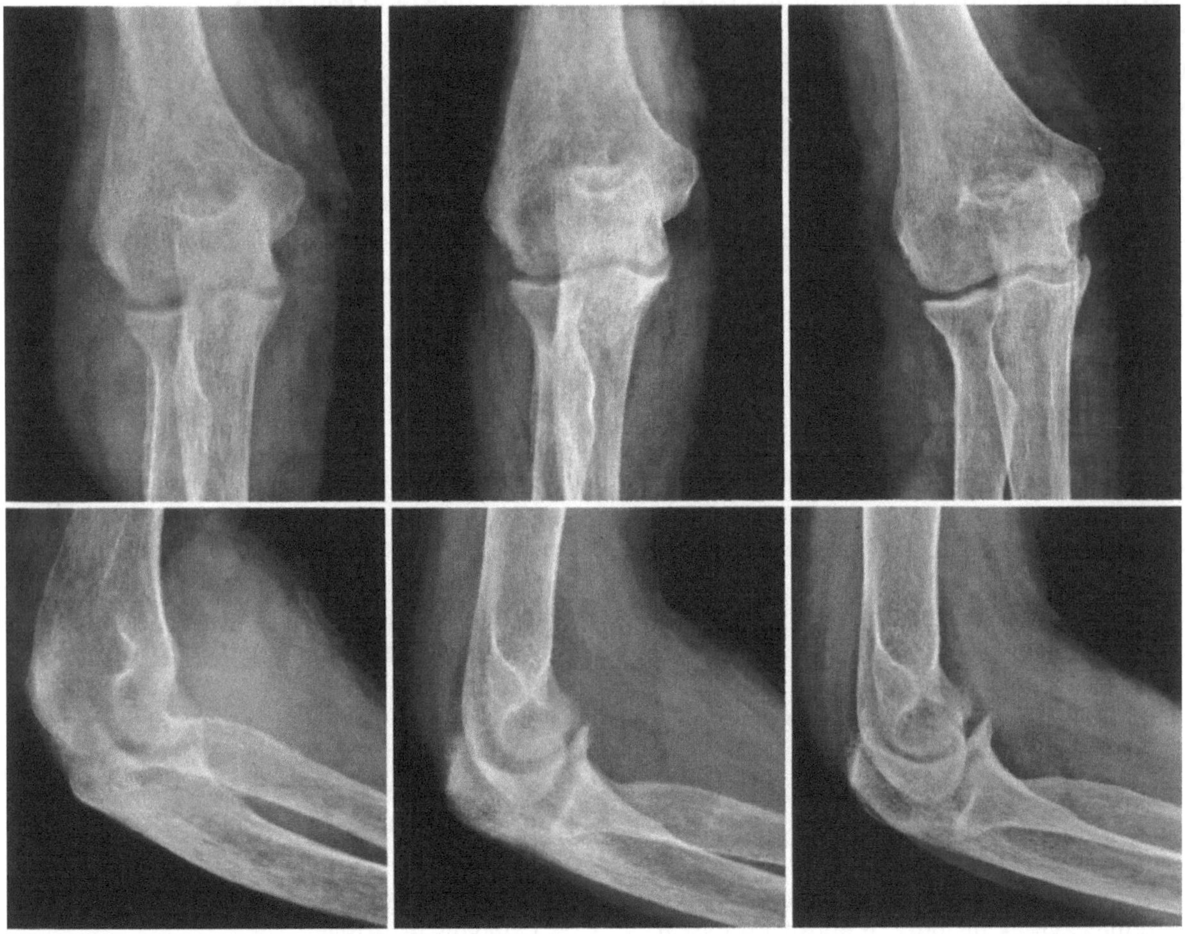

Fig. 50 a–f. Tuberculosis of the elbow. Turkish woman, 41 years old. Previous pulmonary tuberculosis. Involvement of the elbow with sinus laterally and positive culture of *M. tuberculosis*. **a, d** Synovitis with huge soft tissue swelling and blurred joint contours. Hydrops and periosteal bone formation along the proximal radius shaft. **b, e** One half year after **a**, immobilization and chemotherapy: healing stage. Decreased soft tissue swelling and some restoration of the joint margins. Hydrops. **c, f** One year after **a**: healed tuberculous process with residual marginal erosions of the radius and slight degenerative changes

Fig. 51 a–d. Tuberculosis of the elbow. Woman, 37 years old. Active renal tuberculosis and intermittent elbow complaints for 3 years. **a, c** Osseous focus in the proximal end of the ulna (*arrows*) and osteosclerosis in the lateral condyle of the humerus. **b, d** After 1.5 years: healing of the tuberculous process with remineralization and residual changes in the proximal part of the ulna ▶

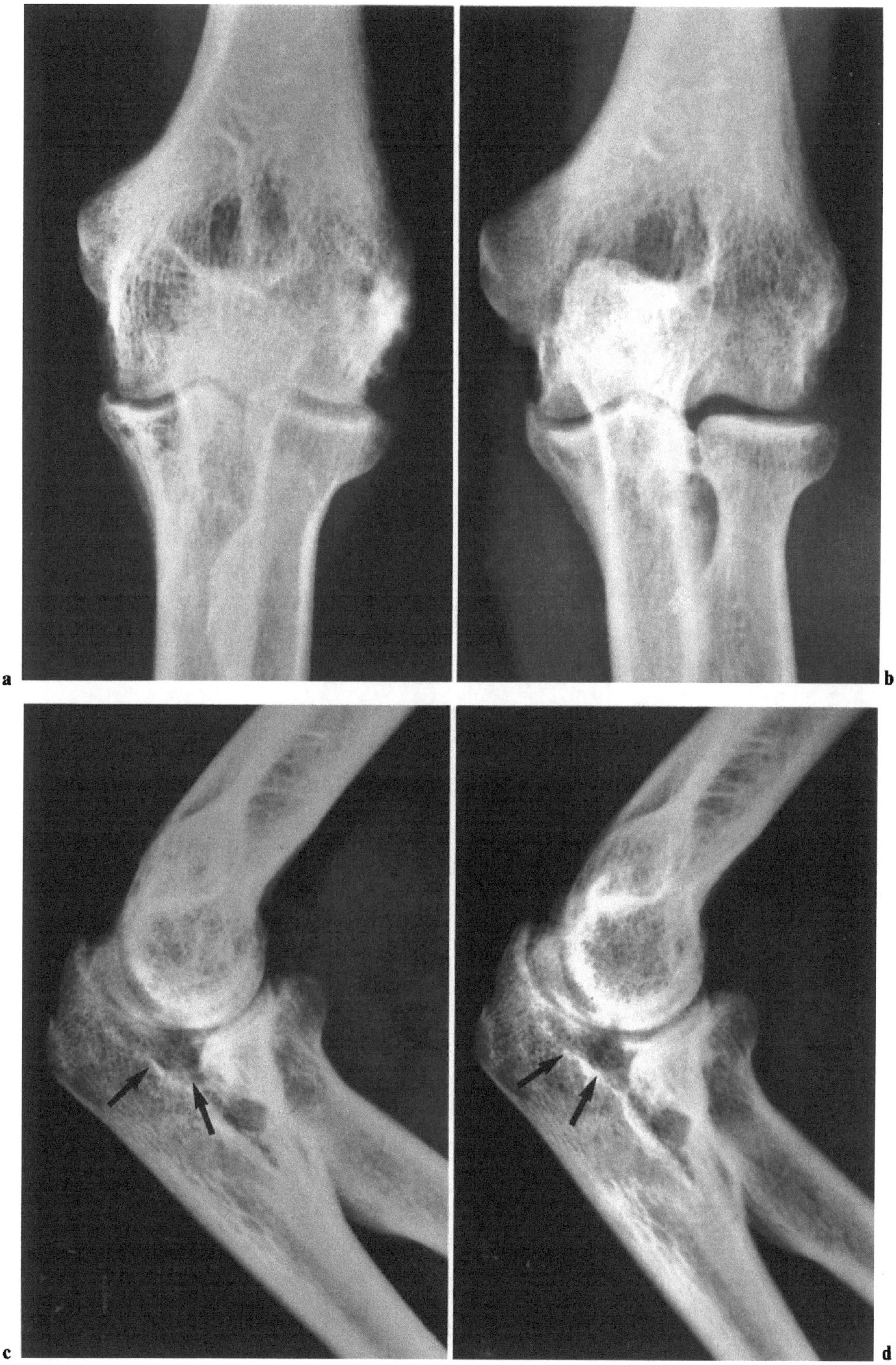
a
b
c
d

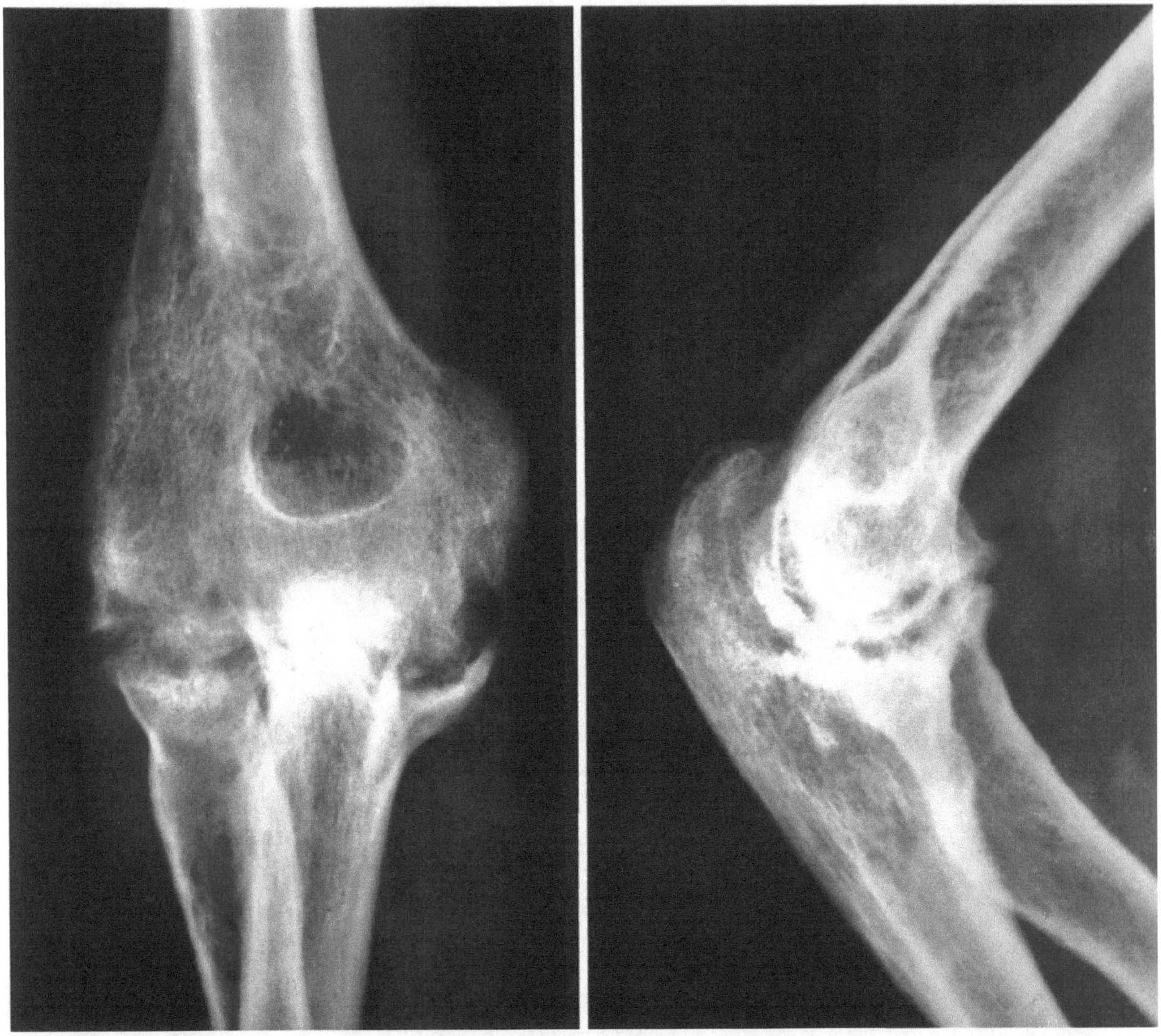

a b

Fig. 52a, b. Tuberculosis of the elbow. Man, 37 years old. Eight years previously, elbow complaints with positive culture for *M. tuberculosis*. On admission for cavernous tuberculosis and spondylitis of the lumbar spine. Inactive disease in the elbow. Severe destruction of the elbow joint after healing. Extensive osteosclerosis

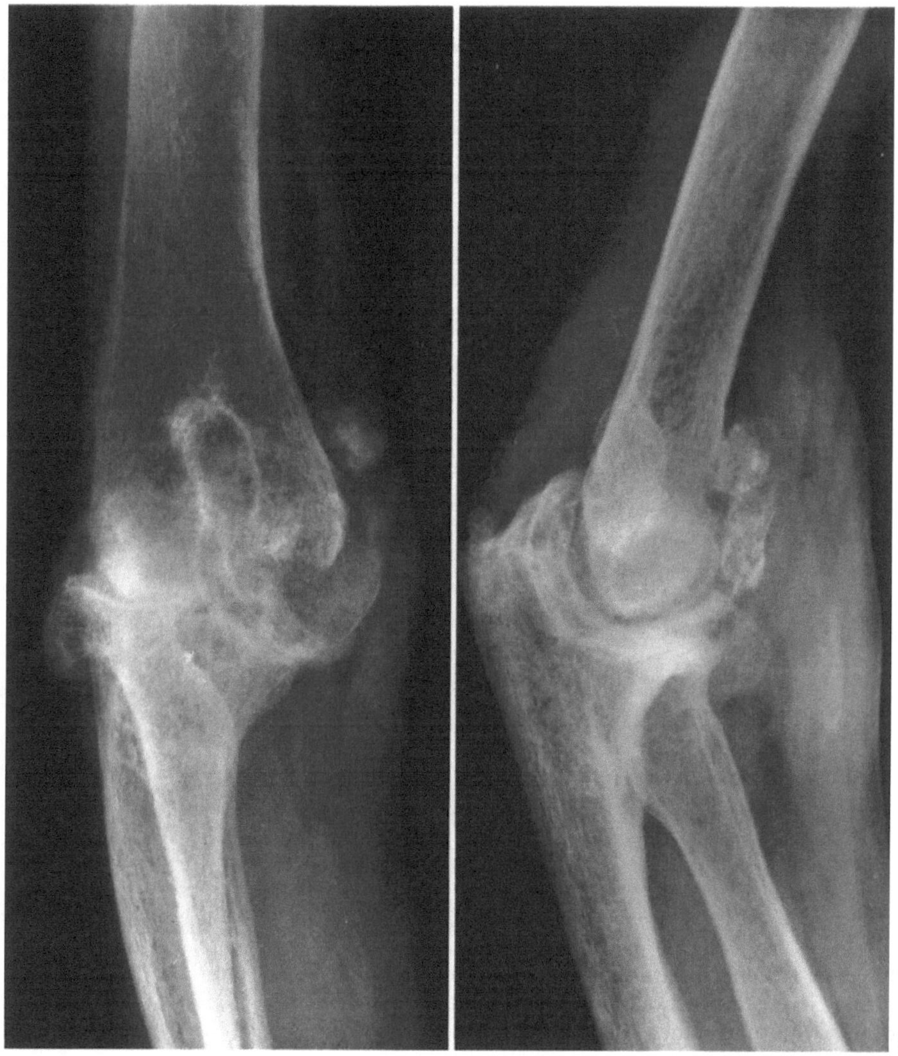

a b

Fig. 53 a, b. Long-standing tuberculosis of the elbow joint. Woman, 76 years old. Positive culture for *M. tuberculosis*. Fifty years previously, tuberculous pleuritis and active tuberculous affection of the right shoulder joint. Moderate destruction of the joint especially in the lateral condyle of the humerus. Osteosclerosis, secondary osteoarthrosis, and ossifications in the capsule and other soft tissues

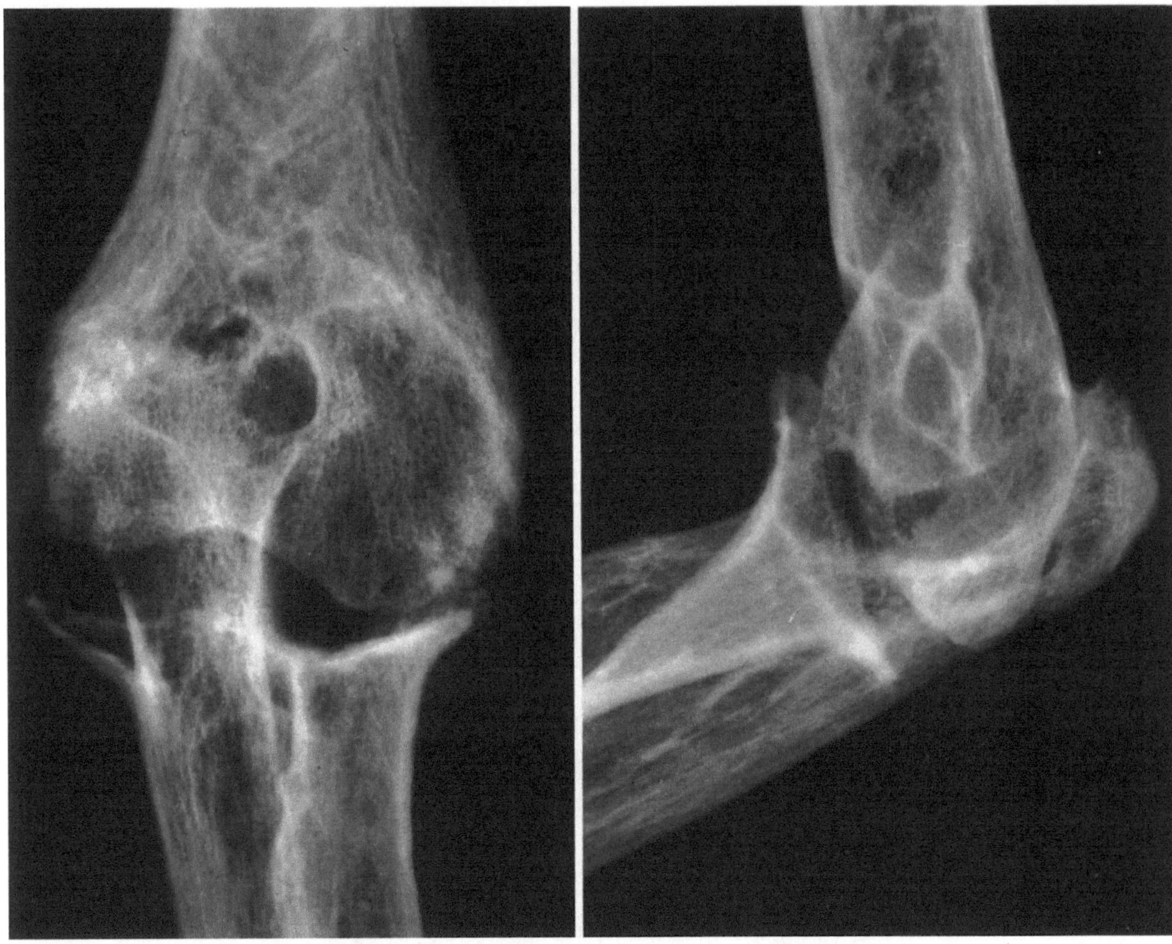

a b

Fig. 54a, b. Differential diagnosis: adult rheumatoid arthritis. Severe destruction of the elbow joint comparable to that with tuberculous affection

7.3 Wrist and Hand

Involvement of the wrist and hand is reported in 2.2%–6.9% of cases with skeletal tuberculosis [12, 79, 93, 109, 146, 147, 151, 163]. We collected 15 patients (3.3%) in the Beatrixoord Hospital and 12 patients from other hospitals. In one of the patients from our hospital another osseous focus was present (knee). Of the 27 patients 21 were adults. In these 27 patients, 28 cases of tuberculous involvement were found: 3 in carpal bones and radiocarpal joints, 10 in carpal bones, 7 in metacarpal bones, (1 in metacarpal 1, 5 in metacarpal 2, 1 in metacarpal 4), and 8 in phalanges (4 in proximal phalanges). This pattern of tuberculous infection accords well with others reported in literature [12, 147].

In children the tubular bones are usually involved, probably because the ossification centers in young children are not yet well developed, and the tubular bones contain cancellous bone. In adults the carpal bones, with or without the radiocarpal joint, are predominantly affected; sometimes only one carpal bone is abnormal (Fig. 56). In the majority of cases sites of tuberculous bone disease are encountered in other bones of the body, and pulmonary tuberculosis or pleuritis is also present [147]. Although most infections are caused by the *M. tuberculosis* and *M. bovis*, bone lesions are also described in infections caused by atypical mycobacteria such as *M. marinum* [34, 179], *M. avium*, and *M. kansasii* [85].

7.3.1 Pathology

Initial synovitis as well as an initial osseous focus may be the first abnormality, but in many cases this discrimination is not possible.

7.3.1.1 Wrist

Tuberculous affection of the wrist results from either initial synovitis or osseous foci and secondary infection of the wrist from adjacent tenosynovitis [109]. Initial synovitis may lead to a more serious form of synovitis, with panarthritis, disturbed nutrition of the carpal bones, and necrosis. In adult patients initial osteitis occurs usually in one of the carpal bones, mostly in the navicular or lunate bones, evolving into a secondary synovitis of the intercarpal, radiocarpal, or carpometacarpal joints. Abscesses and sinuses, if present, are most often found on the dorsal side of the wrist. As a consequence of this involvement, destruction of the finger tendons may occur. During healing a bony fusion of the wrist may be formed.

7.3.1.2 Small Tubular Bones

Affection of the small tubular bones in childhood is usually diaphyseal, as the epiphyseal plate may prevent epiphyseal spread and subsequent joint infection. Tuberculous dactylitis is rarely encountered [170], especially in adults. Tuberculous involvement of the metacarpophalangeal and interphalangeal joints is mentioned by some as being frequent [12]; others describe it as a rare localization [48, 109]. In only one of our patients was metacarpophalangeal arthritis found. In the other cases diaphyseal tuberculous osteomyelitis was present (Figs. 59–63).

In children destruction of cortical bone caused by thrombosis of the osseous arteries, continuing growth, and periosteal bone formation results in the formation of a so-called spina ventosa [109]. This extensive periosteal bone formation is uncommon in adults [12, 29, 48] (Figs. 59–61). Spontaneous bony fusion is more frequently encountered after the use of chemotherapy but is not commonly found in the finger joints [109].

7.3.2 Radiologic Findings

7.3.2.1 Wrist/Carpal Bones (Figs. 55–58)

Synovitis
- Demineralization/osteoporosis.
- Soft tissue swelling.
- Marginal erosions.
- Narrowing of joint space(s).
- Joint destruction.

a b c d

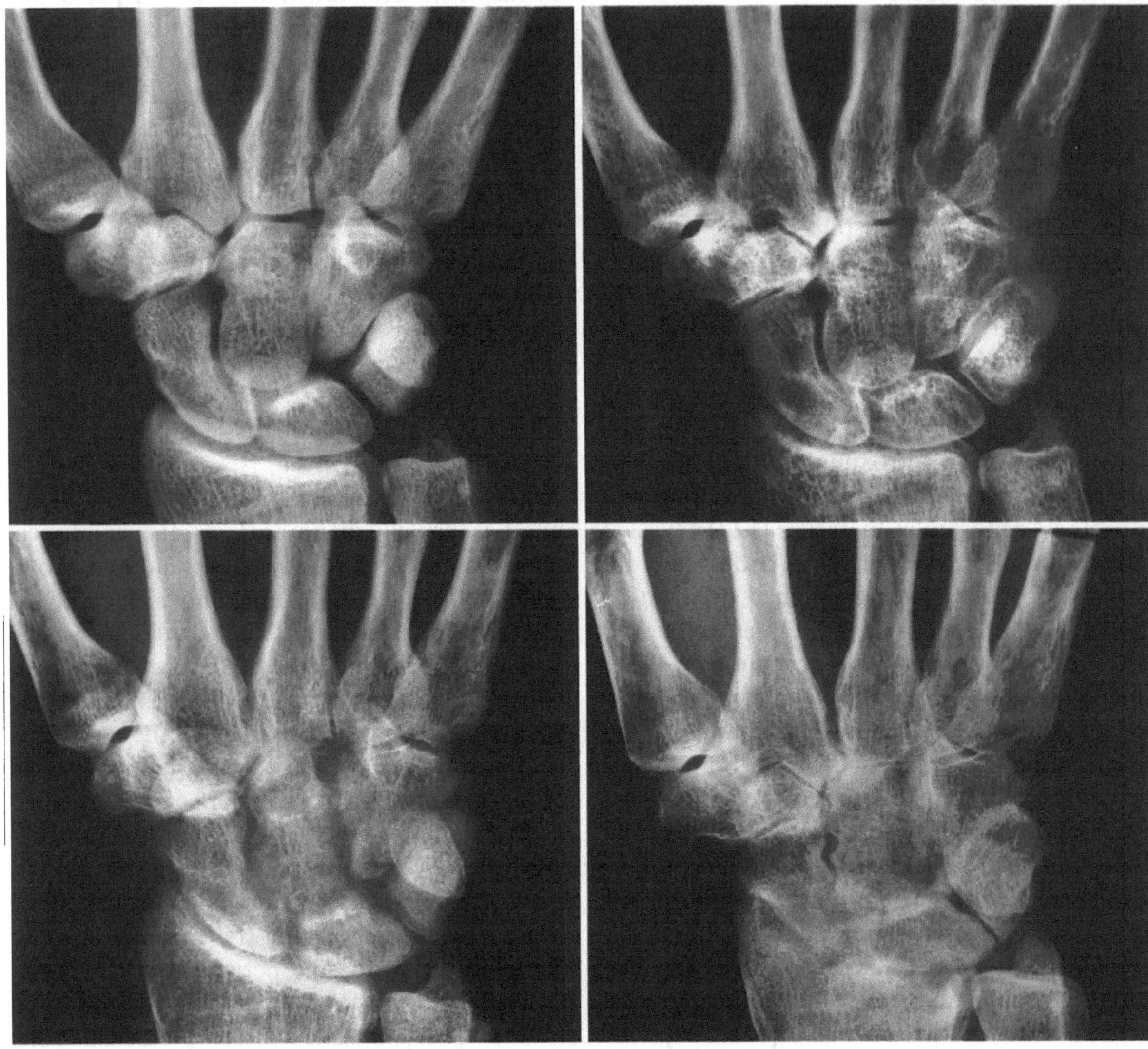

Fig. 55 a–d. Tuberculosis of the wrist and intercarpal joints. Man, 22 years old. Active tuberculous pleuritis. **a** No abnormalities. **b** Demineralization and slight narrowing of the joint spaces. **c** Two years after **a**: hazy aspect of the carpal bones and small defect in the scaphoid. Demineralization and destruction of intercarpal joint spaces. **d** Three years after **a**, after chemotherapy: healing of the tuberculous process with spontaneous bony fusion between the radius and the proximal carpal bones. Remineralization and some restoration of the bony contours

Osseous Focus

- Bone cavities.
- Demineralization/osteoporosis: either localized or diffuse.
- Cortical erosions, bone destruction.
- Sequestra.

Accelerated Skeletal Maturation

Abscesses and Sinuses

Healing and Healed Stages

- Osteosclerosis.
- Bony fusion: especially in the carpal and radiocarpal areas.

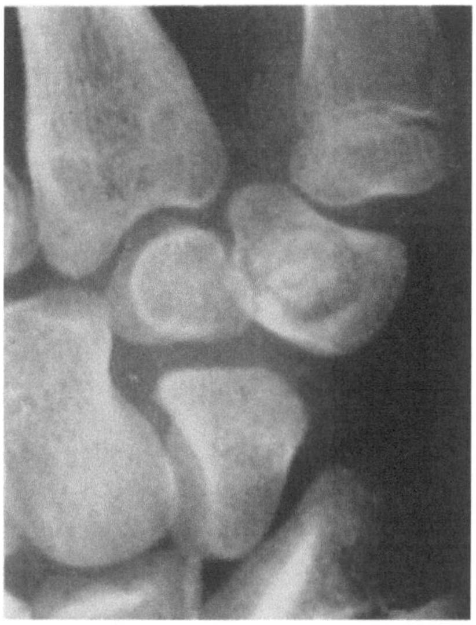

Fig. 56. Tuberculosis of the os trapezium. Well-defined bone cavern with large sequestrum

Fig. 57a, b. Tuberculosis of the wrist, intercarpal joints, and carpometacarpal joints. Man, 57 years old. Forty years earlier, tuberculous tendovaginitis of the flexor tendon sheath. Severe destruction of the carpal bones and intercarpal joint spaces. Erosions of the carpal bones and radiocarpal joint. Probably some sequestra
▼

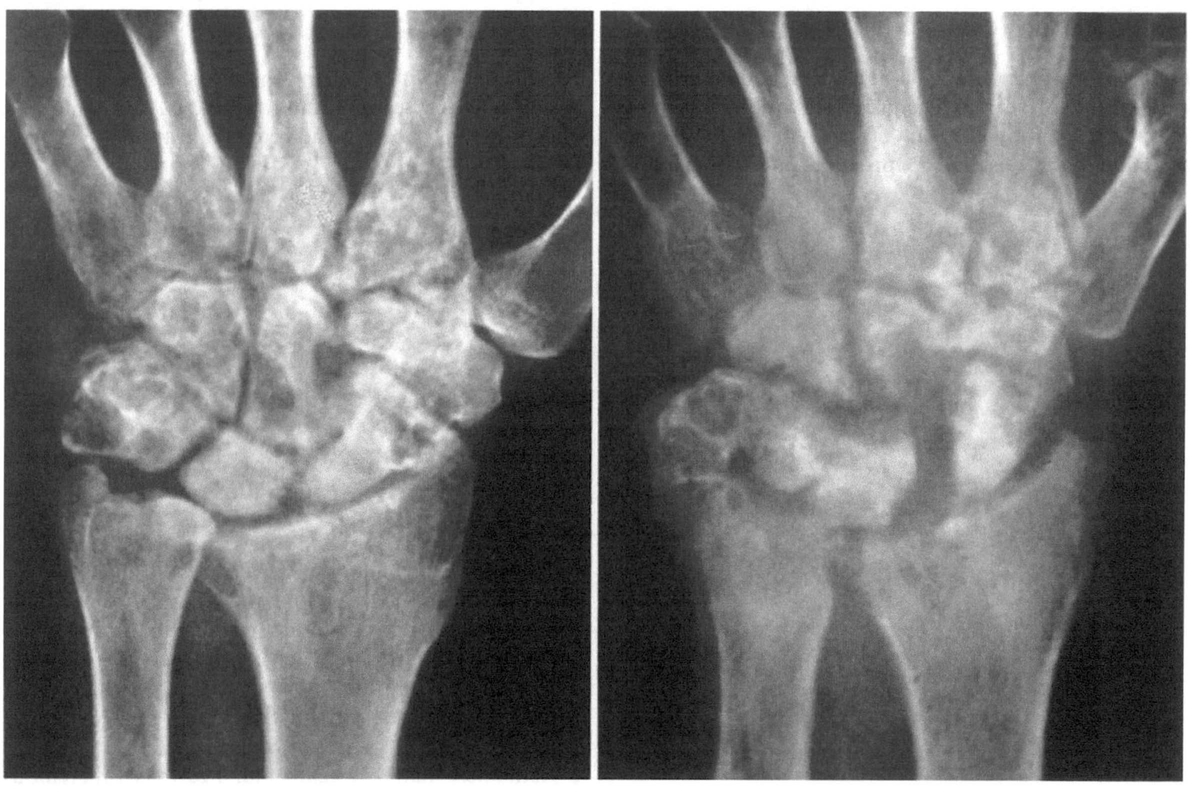

a b

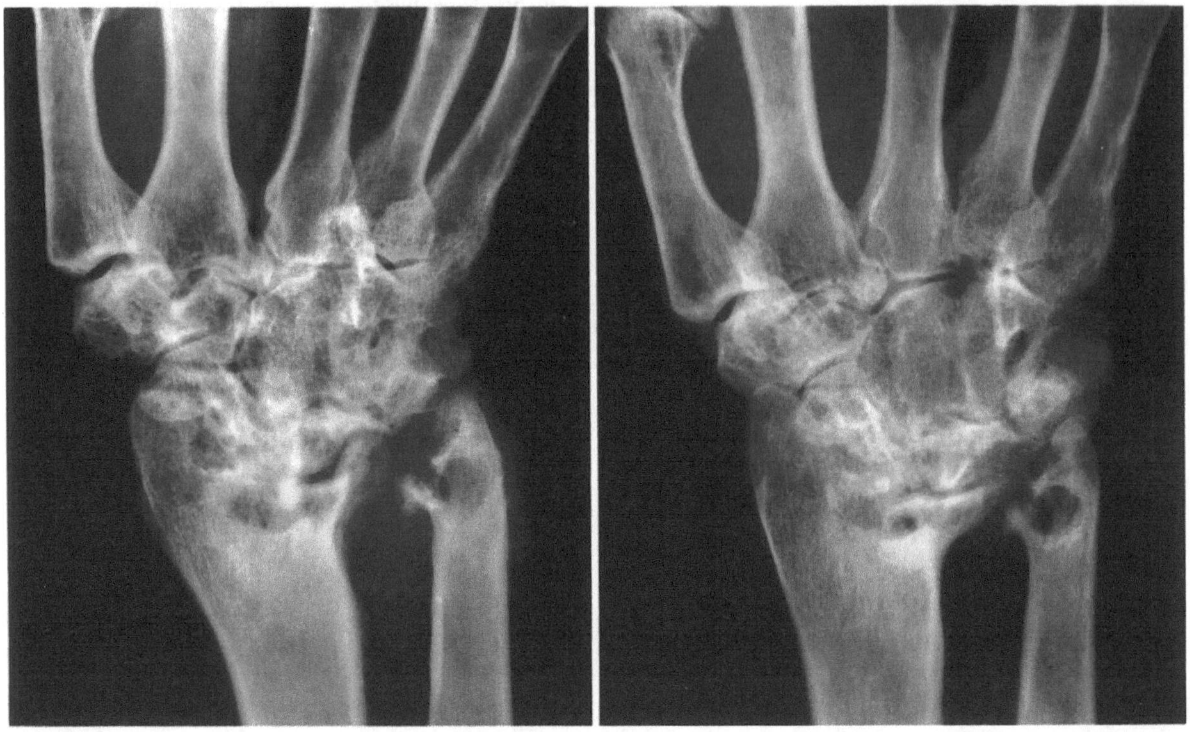

a b

Fig. 58 a, b. Tuberculosis of the wrist and intercarpal joints. Man, 55 years old. Third reactivation in 17 years of tuberculous involvement of the wrist. **a** Severe destruction of the wrist and the proximal intercarpal joints. Small bone cavities and marginal osteosclerosis. Bony fusion between scaphoid and radius. **b** After 9 months, chemotherapy: healing and remineralization

Fig. 59 a–d. Tuberculous involvement of small tubular ▶ bones. Woman, 18 years old (**a, b**). **a** Periosteal bone formation and abnormal bone structure in the first metacarpal bone. Spotty bone density. **b** Dactylitis of proximal phalanx, abnormal bone structure, periosteal bone formation and well circumscribed marginal osteolytic defect.

c Vietnamese man, 32 years old. Previous tuberculous pleuritis. Tuberculous infection of the hand with multiple sinuses on the dorsum of the hand. The second metacarpal bone presents a localized bone cavern with extensive marginal osteosclerosis and cortical thickening. **d** Tuberculous infection of the proximal phalanx. Centrally located bone cavern with marginal osteosclerosis and tendency to spina ventosa

7.3.2.2 ***Metacarpal Bones, Phalanges*** (Figs. 59–63).

Soft Tissue Swelling
Soft tissue swelling is sometimes an isolated feature for a long time.

Osseous Focus
- Bone cavities or honeycombing [12, 170].
- Demineralization/osteoporosis: sometimes very extensive.
- Marginal osteosclerosis.
- Sequestra.
- Periosteal bone formation.
- Spina ventosa.

Accelerated Skeletal Maturation

Cortical Destruction [12, 170]

Abscesses and Sinuses at the Dorsal Surface of the Fingers

Joint Involvement with Soft Tissue Swelling, Joint Space Narrowing, Marginal Erosions, and Fibrous or Bony Fusion

Subluxation

Pathologic Fracture

Healing and Healed Stages
- Osteosclerosis.
- Deformation of fingers by affection of the epiphyseal plates.
- Bony fusion.

7.3.3 Differential Diagnosis

- Osteomyelitis.
- Pyogenic arthritis.
- Adult rheumatoid arthritis.
- Juvenile rheumatoid arthritis.
- Sympathic reflex dystrophy.
- Primary bone tumor.
- Sarcoidosis.
- Villonodular synovitis.
- Gout.
- Renal osteodystrophy.
- Metastatic disease.

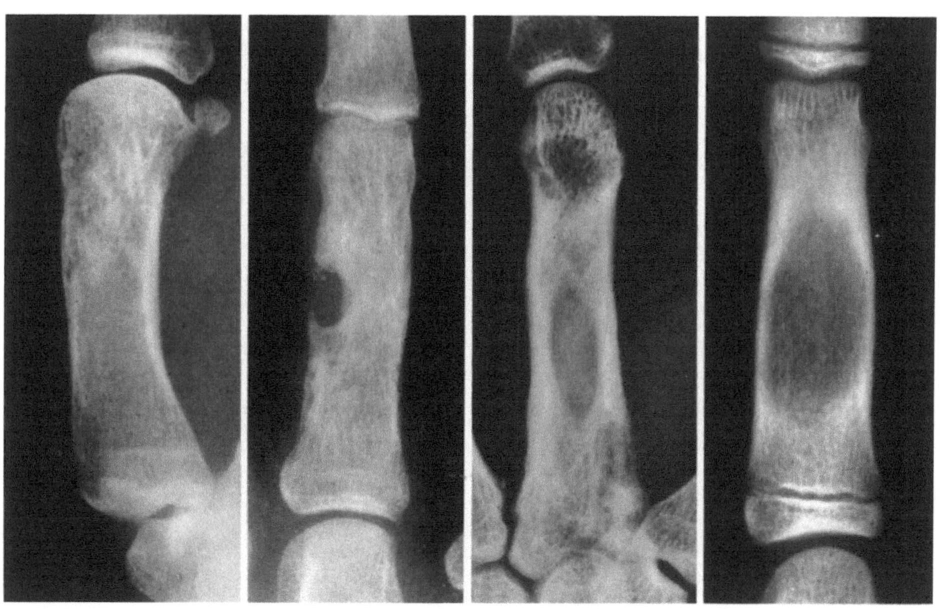

a–d

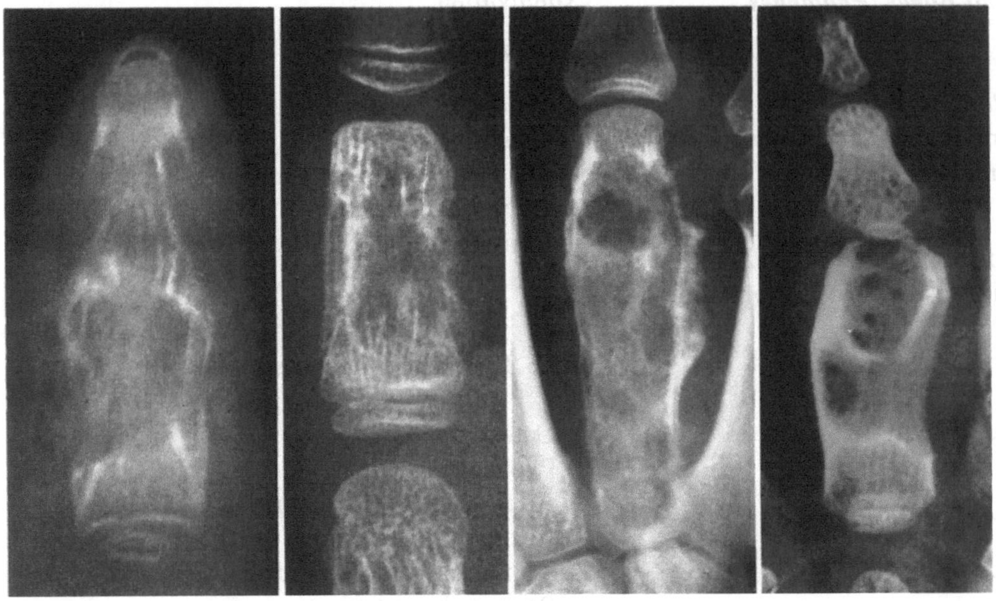

a–d

Fig. 60 a–d. Tuberculous dactylitis (spina ventosa). Four different patients. **a** Dactylitis of the index finger. Cystic tuberculous lesion in the proximal phalanx, with soft tissue swelling and affection of the proximal interphalangeal joint. (By courtesy of Dr. S.P. Bohrer, Winston-Salem) N.C., U.S.A.) **b** Dactylitis of proximal phalanx. Boy, 5 years old. Destructive diaphyseal lesion with periosteal bone formation and spina ventosa. Adjacent joints are normal. **c** Tuberculous affection of fourth metacarpal. Adult man, significant spina ventosa with centrally located bone caverns and periosteal bone formation. Metacarpophalangeal joint not affected. **d** Tuberculous dactylitis in the proximal phalanx of the fourth finger. Extensive widening of the shaft with cystlike lesions and marginal osteosclerosis. (By courtesy of Prof. B.J. Cremin, Cape Town, South Africa.)

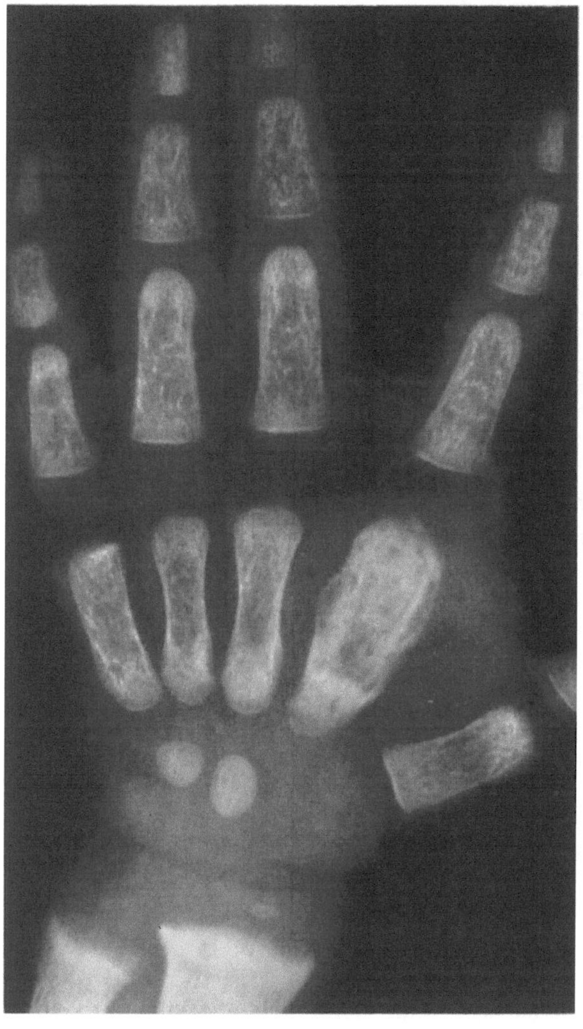

Fig. 61. Tuberculous involvement of the second metacarpal bone. The child also suffers from rickets. Extensive widening of the metacarpal bone with periosteal bone formation. Spina ventosa. (By courtesy of Prof. B.J. Cremin, Cape Town, South Africa.)

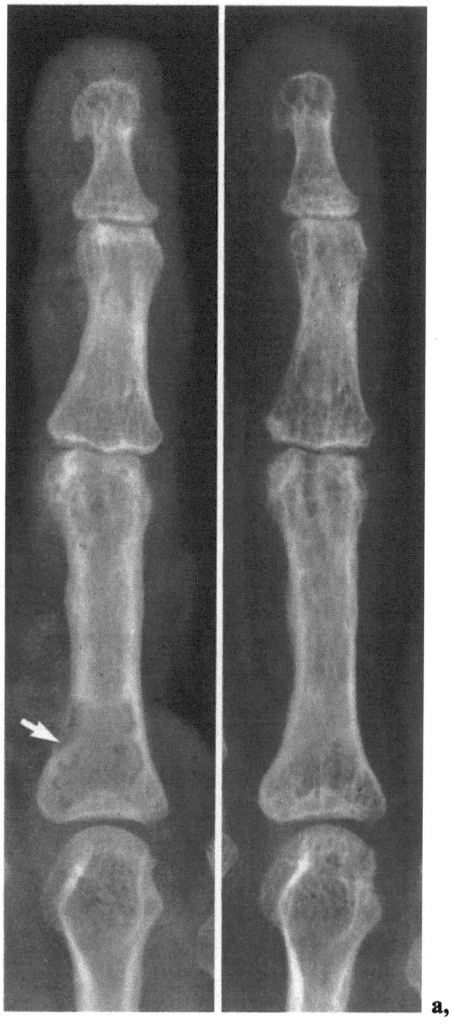

a, b

Fig. 62a, b. Tuberculous osteomyelitis of the fourth finger. Woman of Asian origin, 52 years old. Old pulmonary tuberculosis. On admission, also active retroperitoneal tuberculous lymphadenitis and sinuses. **a** Circumscribed osseous defect in the proximal phalanx of the fourth finger and cortical erosion (*arrow*). Metacarpophalangeal joint intact. **b** After 8 months: reconstruction of the cortex and completely healed tuberculous focus

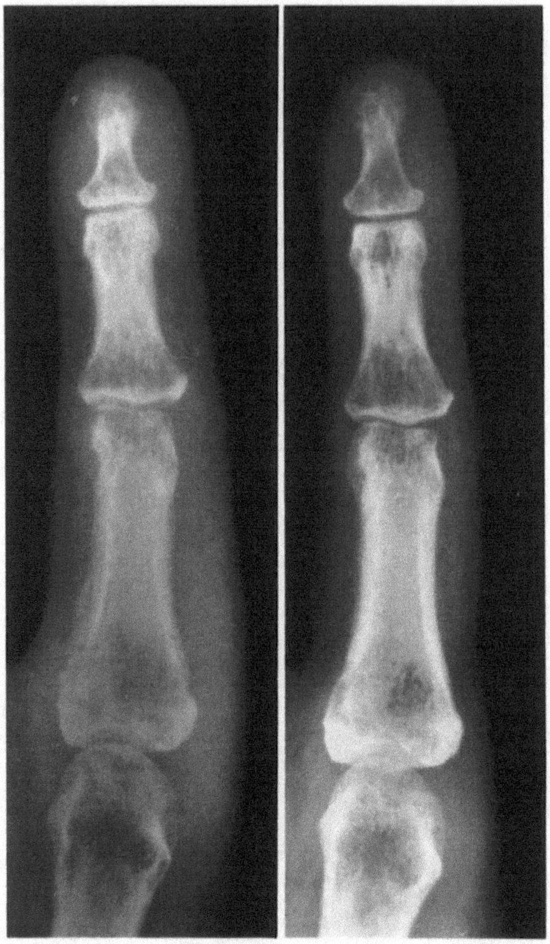

a b

Fig. 63a, b. Tuberculosis of the index finger. Female asian immigrant, 35 years old. Active cavernous pulmonary tuberculosis and fistulas on the back of the thorax presumably from tuberculous lymphadenitis. Positive cultures for M. tuberculosis from all locations. **a** Soft tissue swelling around the second metacarpophalangeal joint and demineralization. Periosteal bone formation on the base of the proximal phalanx. The joint is not significantly affected. **b** After 3 months, antituberculous therapy: well-defined cortical contours and reconstruction of spongiosal bone. Normal joint space of the metacarpophalangeal joint

8 Tuberculous Affection of the Lower Limb Joints

8.1 Hip

In tuberculosis of the large joints, the hip is the second or the third most commonly affected joint [96, 110, 158] (Table 1, see p. 11). The advent of chemotherapy has substantially decreased the frequency of tuberculous coxitis; the rate may be lower than that of tuberculosis of the knee joint [109]. Most tuberculous infections of the hip are caused by *M. tuberculosis*; coxitis caused by atypical mycobacteria is uncommon [52, 53]. BCG coxitis has been described [145, 155]. Usually only one hip joint is affected; in patients with bilateral affection involvement often occurs at the same time [147]. Besides the tuberculous process in one or both joints, affection of the other bones in the body may be present. Especially in earlier days but still today in patients from tropical areas, the onset of the tuberculous process has been reported to be below the age of 20 years [81, 147]. Nowadays in low-prevalence countries most patients are adults. In our material 58 patients (57 adults, 1 child) with tuberculosis of the hip were studied. In 11 of these patients multifocal lesions were encountered (spine in five, greater trochanter in five, contralateral hip in one, knee in one). A history of active pulmonary tuberculosis can be found in about one-third of patients. Even more show sequelae of pleuritis as a result of previous hematogenous spread of mycobacteria. Relatively higher rates of active pulmonary tuberculosis are encountered in patients with relatively short history of disease. Initial negative radiologic findings do not exclude a beginning tuberculous coxitis. Suspicion is enough to start treatment!

8.1.1 Pathology

As involvement of the hip may originate either from primary synovitis or a nearby osseous focus, the clinical and radiologic course of the disease is variable (Chap. 6).

8.1.1.1 Initial Synovitis

Initial synovitis seems to be less frequent than osseous tuberculous foci [147]. Depending on the immunologic condition of the patient, synovitis causes some degree of hydrops and demineralization of the periarticular osseous structures by hyperemia (Fig. 65). The altered composition of the synovial fluid and the raised intra-articular pressure cause impaired nutrition of femoral head, femoral neck, and joint cartilage, and a rapid necrosis of the femoral head may occur. In the hip joint stress is provoked by gravity and muscular activity. In tuberculous hip infection these factors may also lead to a rapid destruction of the joint. In cases with caseous synovitis the joint cavity is covered with caseous granulation tissue. This leads to cartilage destruction, and loosened parts of cartilage and capsule fragments can be found intra-articularly. The bony structures are no longer covered by cartilage, which results in a caseous osteitis with rapid destruction of the whole joint. Progressive destruction of subarticular bone on both sides of the joint may lead to protrusio acetabuli and ballooning of the acetabulum (Figs. 65, 66). Adequate treatment of a tuberculous synovitis, including immediate decompression in the joint cavity, may lead to total cure or only slight sequelae, as altered bone texture and, in children, enlargement of the capital epiphysis may be found. A long delay by patient or physician, however, often results today in less favorable status of the joint.

8.1.1.2 Osseous Focus

Osseous foci can be divided according to their relation to the insertion of the joint capsule. Involvement of the joint cavity occurs more often if the foci are intra-articular. Most femoral foci are of the intracapsular type and are situated in the epiphysis or the metaphysis (Figs. 67, 68). An extracapsular osseous focus may extend to the soft tissues and secondarily infect the joint cavity. This extension, however, is rather uncommon except for foci originating in the greater trochanter; it was seen in five of our patients. In such cases the occurrence of bursitis of the overlying bursa and abscesses in the region above the capsule may induce tuberculous arthritis (Figs. 65, 66). Because of the deep-seated location of the hip joint, abscesses present rather late in the course of the disease. Spread of the abscesses may be anteriorly, posteriorly, medially, or in the direction of the pelvis (Fig. 69). Sinuses rarely occur [109]. Iliac osseous foci are almost always situated in the vicinity of the joint space (Fig. 70). Pubic and ischial foci rarely cause tuberculous arthritis of the hip joint by extension of their infectious processes (Figs. 107, 111).

8.1.2 Radiologic Findings (Figs. 64–71)

8.1.2.1 Synovitis

- Demineralization/osteoporosis: The degree of both these features depends on the seriousness of the joint involvement and duration of the infection before admittance.
- Soft tissue swelling: Increased density around the hip (haziness) is caused by synovitis, intra-articular exudate, infected periarticular bursa(e), and edema.
- Erosions of joint margins: at the sites of capsular insertion.
- Joint space narrowing: usually a relatively late feature.
- Joint destruction.

8.1.2.2 Osseous Focus

- Bone cavities: either in the epi/metaphyseal region of the femur or in the acetabulum. The lesions may be difficult to detect, especially the acetabular lesions. Tomography is often necessary. A single cystic lesion, with or without a sclerotic margin, may be hardly distinguishable from a benign bone tumor.
- Demineralization/osteoporosis.
- Marginal osteosclerosis.
- Necrosis of femoral head: Depending on the degree of this, necrotic fragments (sequestra) are more or less numerous.

8.1.2.3 Abscesses und Sinuses

Abscesses and sinuses appear relatively late in the course of the disease. The site of capsular penetration of the tuberculous process either superiorly, inferiorly, or posteriorly determines the position of the abscess(es). Extension into the pelvis through the acetabulum is only rarely found. Extra-articular acetabular foci, nor penetrating into the joint space, may produce abscesses in the gluteal and adductor regions. Ascending and secondary infection of sinuses may lead to secondary joint involvement and ankylosis. Sinography, ultrasonography, CT, and MRI can be helpful in detecting abscesses.

8.1.2.4 Disturbances in Growth

A long-lasting synovitis in infancy may lead to chronic hyperemia, with overgrowth of the femoral epiphysis. A significant and disproportional enlargement of the femoral head in relation to the acetabulum and subluxation may result.

8.1.2.5 Osseous Deformities

In young patients epiphysiolysis of the femoral head is rare but is possible either by loss of cohesion between metaphysis and epiphysis or following a rapid necrosis of the femoral head. Coxa vara may follow a period of marked demineralization in the joint with decreased mechanical resistance, and/or it may occur as a sequela after long-standing and severe joint involvement.

8.1.2.6 Healing and Healed Stages

- Osteosclerosis: a rather late feature and usually related to the healing stages of tuberculous bone affection. Marginal osteosclerosis can be found around osseous foci, and more diffuse osteosclerosis occurs in former tuberculous bone lesions.
- Calcifications and/or ossifications in the soft tissues.
- Bone fusion: either spontaneous during the healing process (fibrous or osseous) or osseous fusion following surgical treatment.
- Secondary osteoarthrosis.

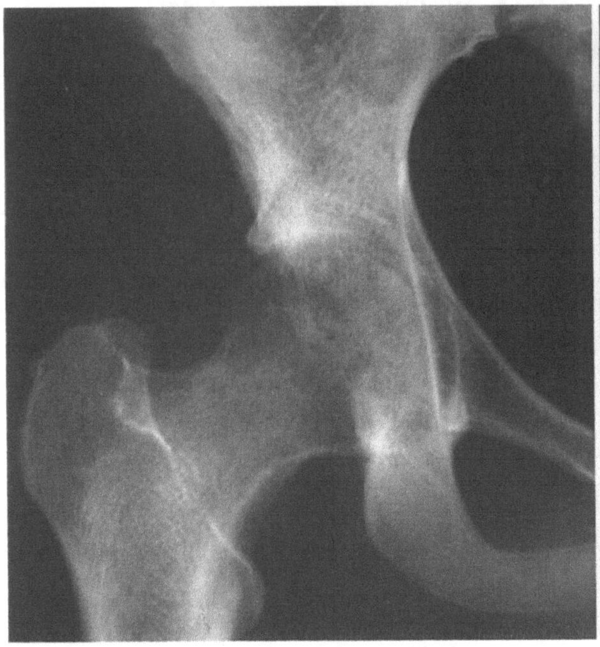

a

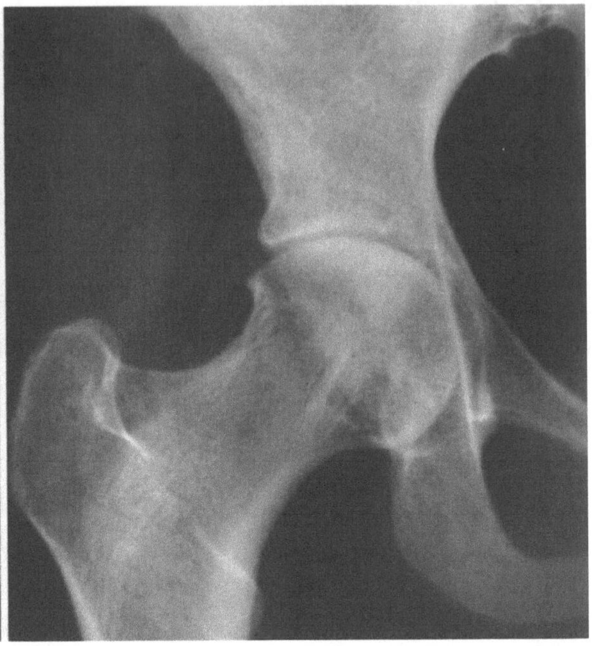

b

Fig. 64a, b. Tuberculosis of the hip. Woman, 21 years old. Positive bacteriological findings of tuberculosis. **a** (1930) Probably initial synovitis of the hip joint with extensive demineralization and blurred joint margins. Narrowing of the joint space. **b** After 1 year immobilization, healing of the tuberculous process and residual narrowing of the joint space. Restoration of bone trabeculation. (Medicamentous treatment at that time was not yet available.)

Fig. 65a–d. Tuberculosis of the left hip. Woman, 60 years old. As a child, tuberculous coxitis of the right hip and tuberculous affection of the greater trochanter on the left side. At the age of 4–10 years, also tuberculous affection of the carpal bones with intermittent draining sinuses. **a** Reactivation of tuberculous affection of the left greater trochanter. Ossifications in the soft tissues. Impaired function of the hip. Femoral head still intact. **b** After 1 year: secondary affection of the hip joint, with demineralization, joint space narrowing, marginal erosions, and destruction of the femoral head and the acetabulum. **c** Three months after **b**: further destruction probably because the patient was not yet immobilized. In the meantime beginning osteosclerosis. **d** Four years after **c**: ballooning of the acetabulum, with significant deformation of the femoral head after removal of destructed bone tissue. Fibrous ankylosis and secondary osteoarthrosis ▶

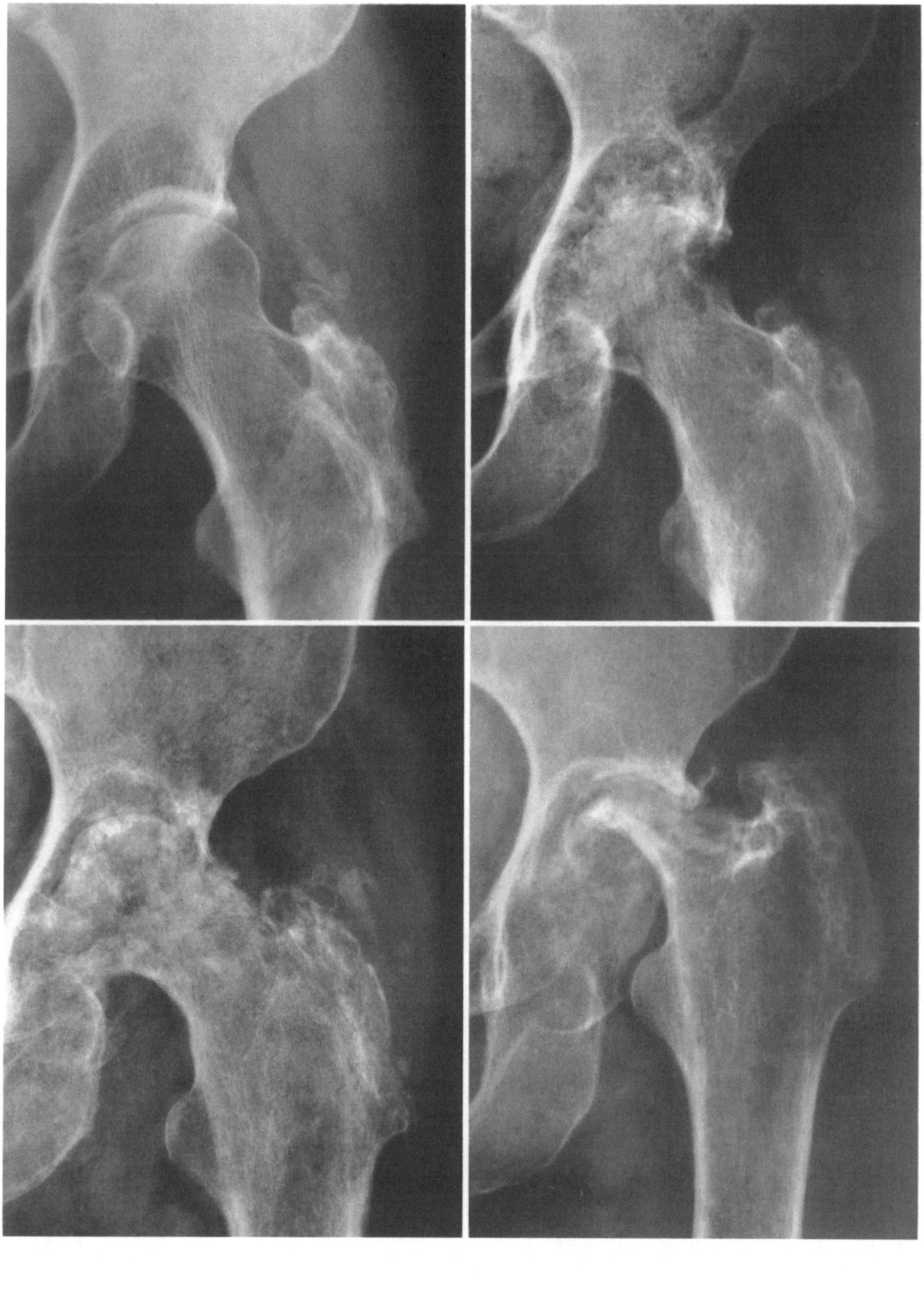

a b c d

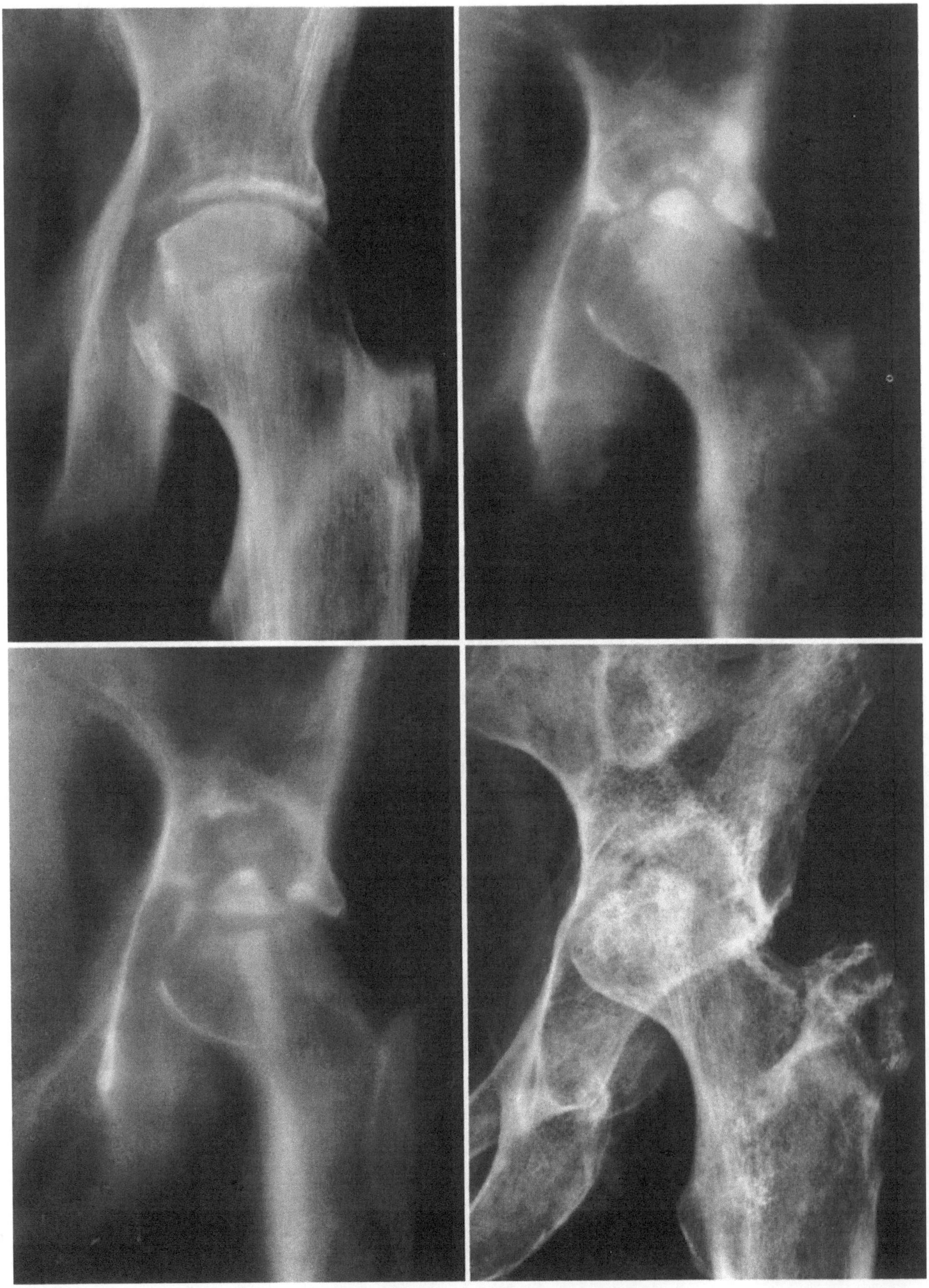

a b c d

◀ **Fig. 66a–d.** Tuberculosis of the left hip. Woman, 68 years old. At the age of 17 years, bilateral pulmonary tuberculosis and spina ventosa. Probably at that age also tuberculosis of the greater trochanter with a sinus. **a** Tomography: residua of tuberculous affection of the greater trochanter. Femoral head normal. **b, c** Tomography: destruction of acetabulum and femoral head. **d** After explorative and decompressive operation immobilization and chemotherapy: remineralization and healing of the tuberculous process

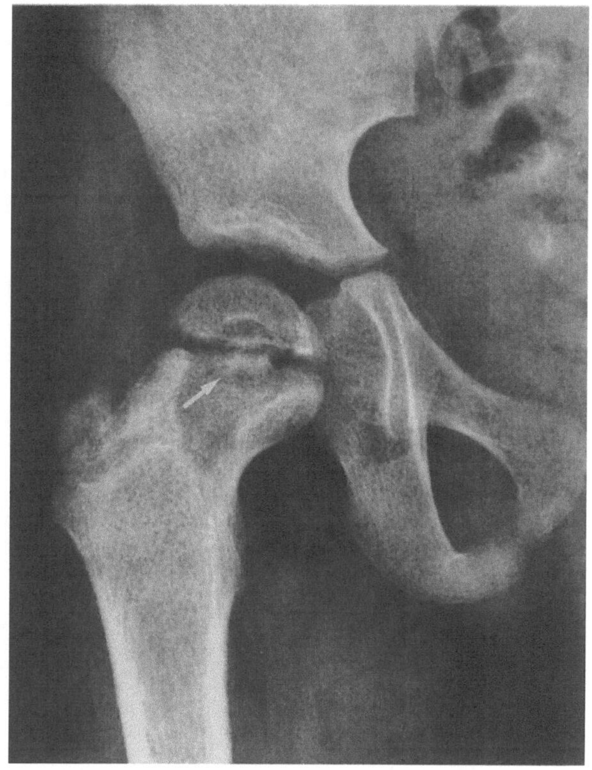

Fig. 67. Tuberculosis of the hip. Epi/metaphyseal focus, with some marginal osteosclerosis and centrally located sequestrum (*arrow*). Widening of the joint space and somewhat cloudy aspect of the greater trochanter. (By courtesy of Prof. B.J. Cremin, Cape Town, South Africa.)

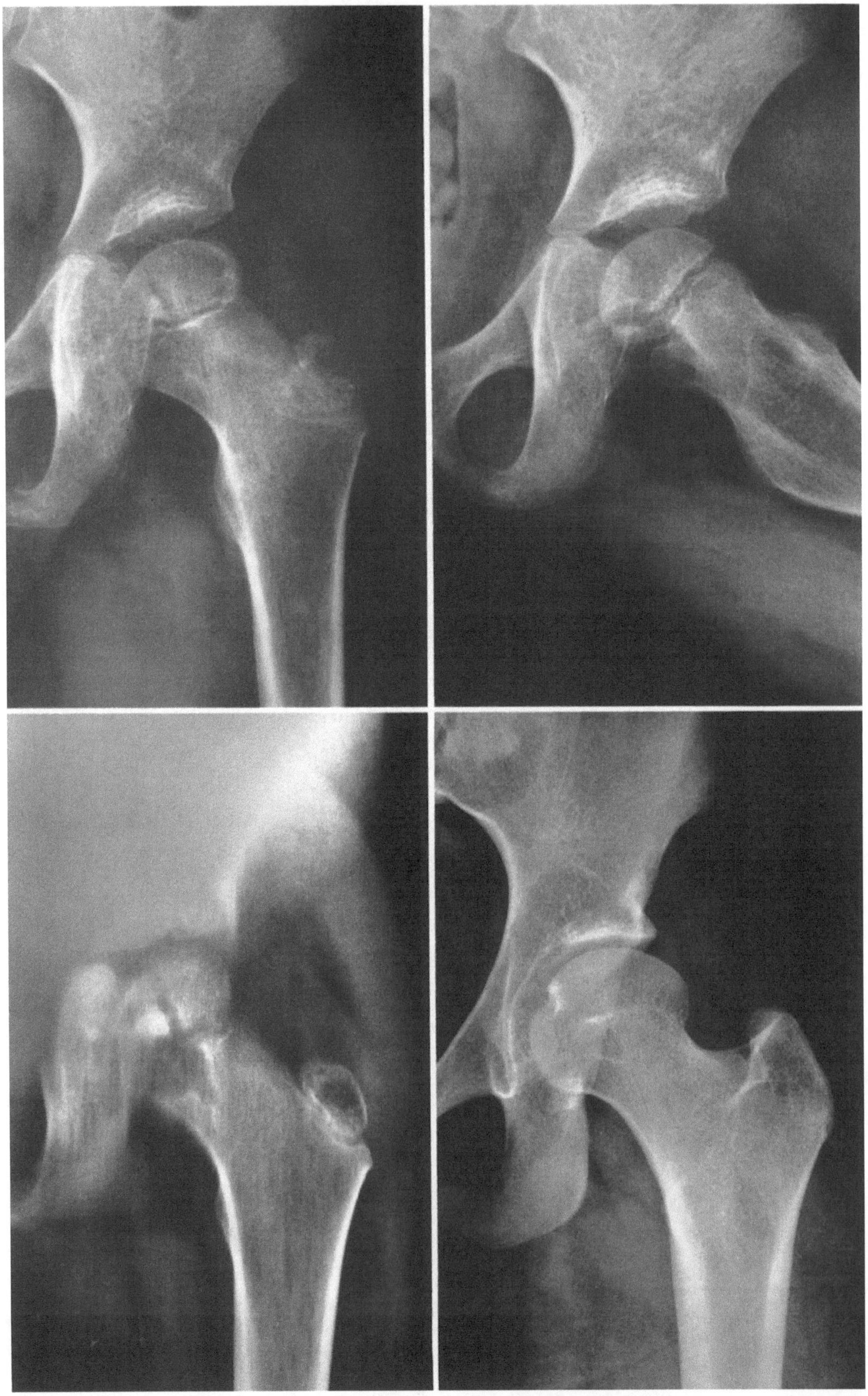

a b c d

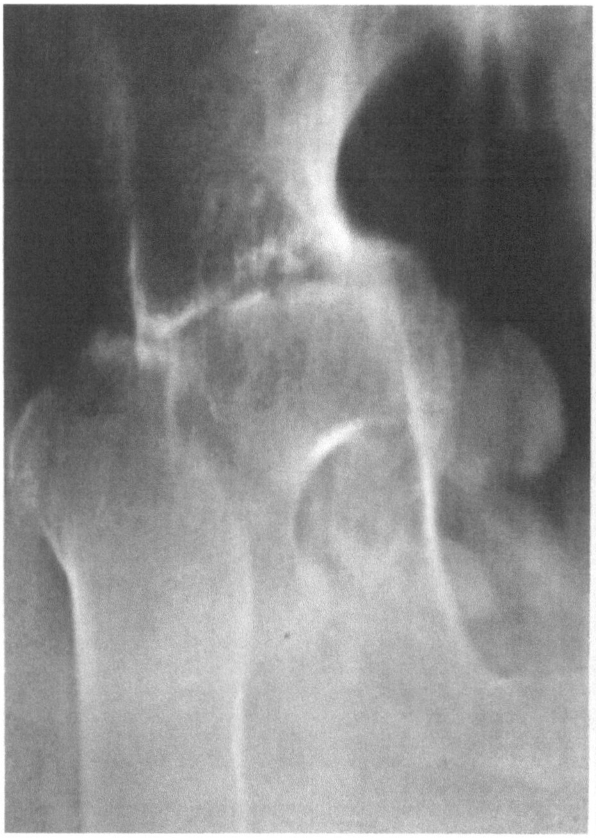

a

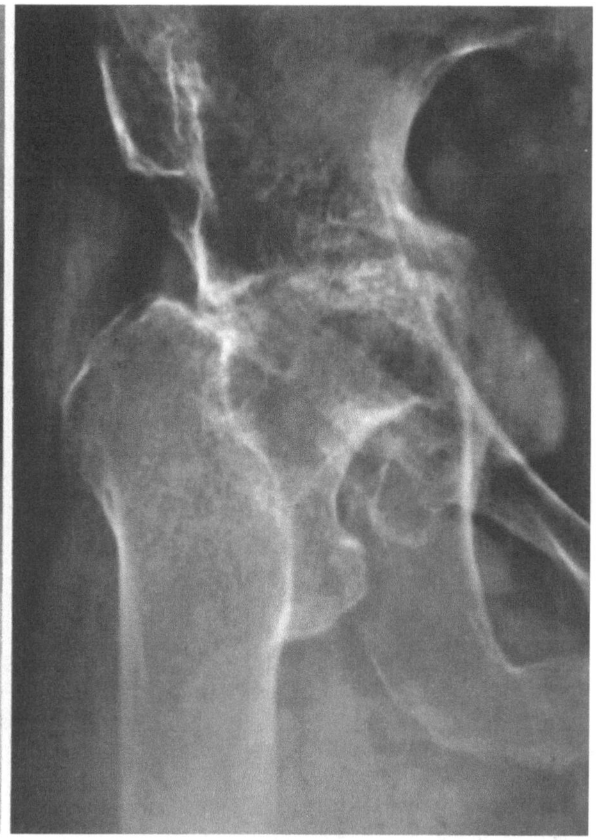

b

◀ **Fig. 68a–d.** Tuberculosis of the hip. Girl, 5 years old. Posttraumatic complaints of the left hip. Positive culture of *M. tuberculosis* from the biopsied synovial membrane. Immediate decompression of the joint cavity was performed, with local treatment with antituberculous drugs in addition to oral therapy. **a** Osseous abnormalities on the medial side of the femoral head and slight widening of the joint space in comparison with the right hip joint. **b** In abduction, epi/metaphyseal focus. **c** Tomography: significant osseous focus in the epi/metaphyseal area. **d** After 10 years: complete restoration of bone structures. Normal joint space

Fig. 69a, b. Tuberculosis of the hip. Woman, 80 years old. Previous bilateral pulmonary tuberculosis with reactivation of hip affection. Severe destruction of the hip joint with central luxation of the femoral head and intrapelvic abscesses

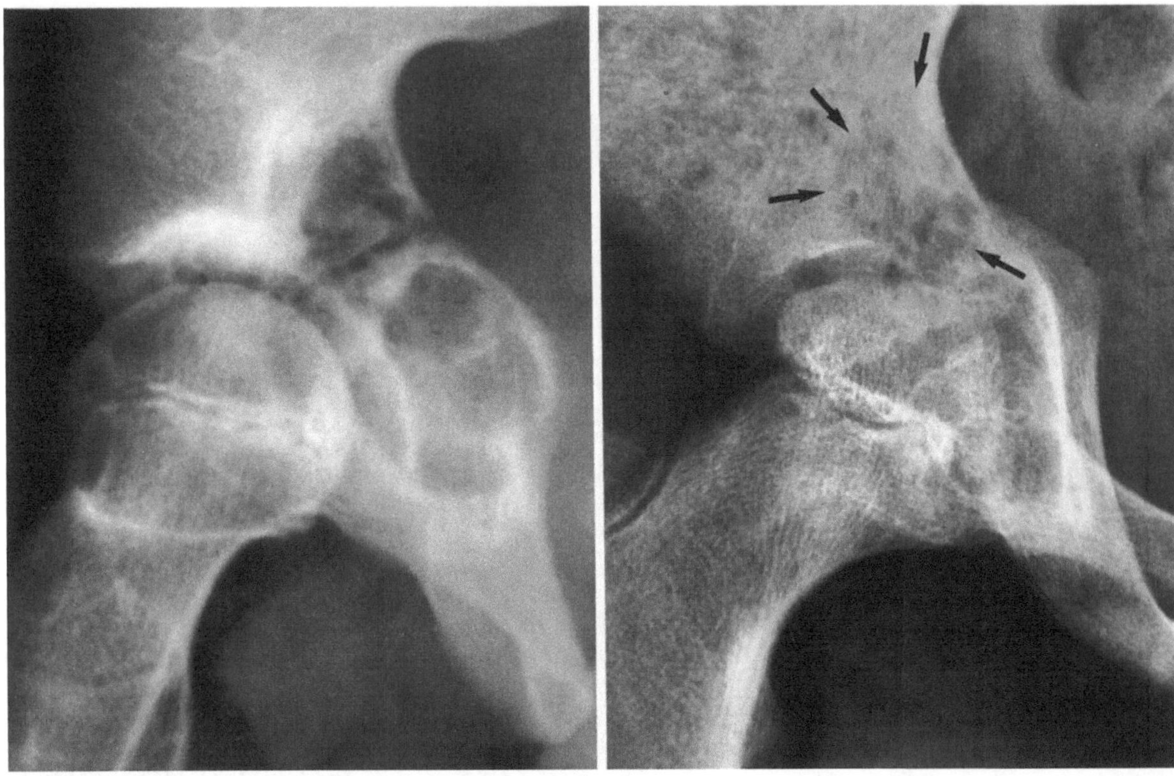

a b

Fig. 70a, b. Tuberculosis of the hip. Iliac osseous foci. **a** Cystlike focus in the right iliac bone in the vicinity of the hip joint. Expansion of bone and marginal osteosclerosis. (By courtesy of Dr. W.P. Cockshott, Hamilton, Ont., Canada.) **b** Large osseous focus in the ilium adjacent to the hip joint. Somewhat triangle-shaped femoral head and slightly blurred contour of the femoral head on the mediocaudal contour (*arrows*). (By courtesy of Prof. B.J. Cremin, Cape Town, South Africa.)

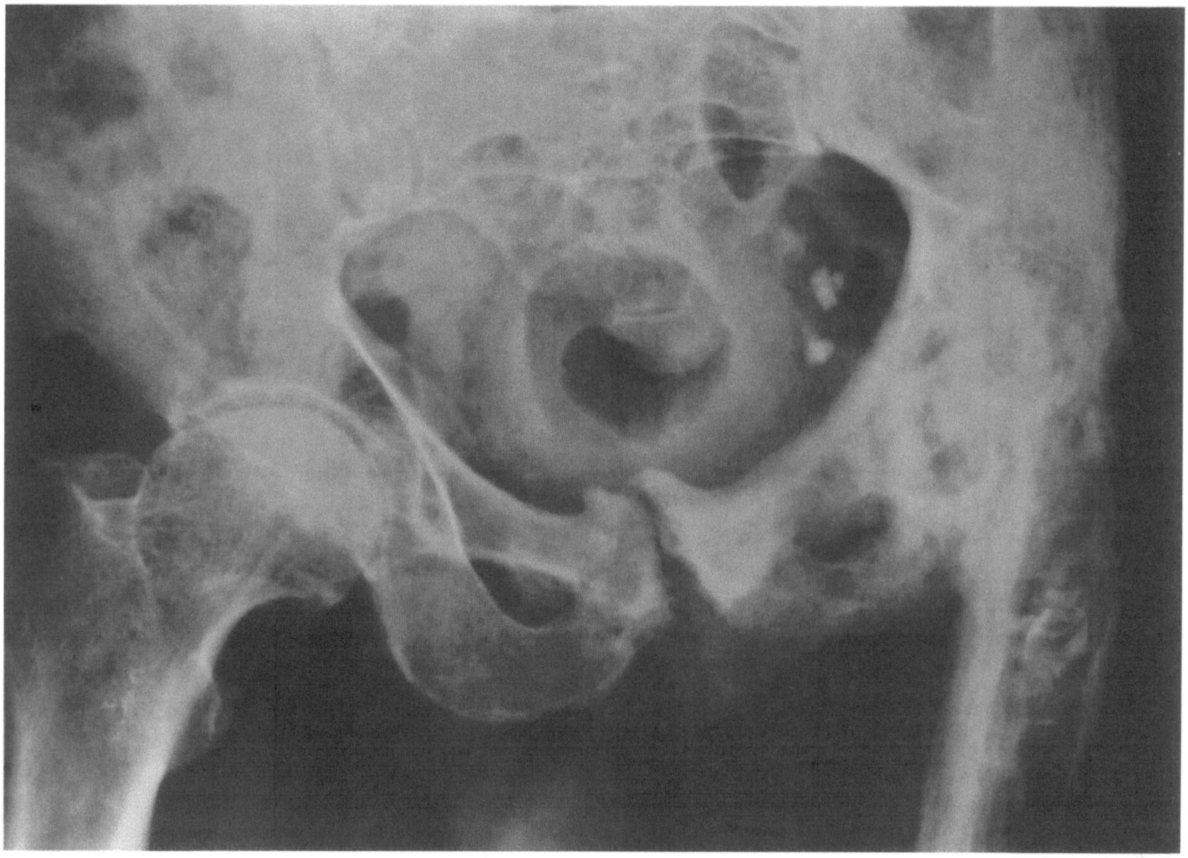

Fig. 71. Tuberculosis of the left hemipelvis. Woman, 63 years old. At the age of 4 years, tuberculosis of the left hip with intermittent draining sinuses; in puberty, bilateral tuberculous pleuritis. Fifty years later, reactivation of coxitis with draining sinus medially and urogenital tuberculosis. Spontaneous bony fusion of the hip and extensive old tuberculous lesions as well as active lesions in the symphysis and ischium, with draining sinuses medial in the left thigh. The radiograph presents extensive changes in anatomy and bone structures. Spontaneous bony fusion. The symphysis is also affected

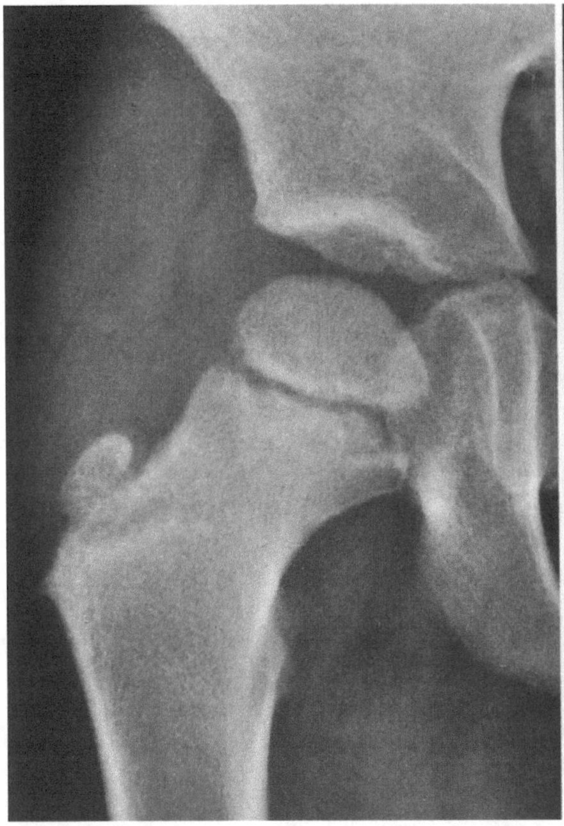

a

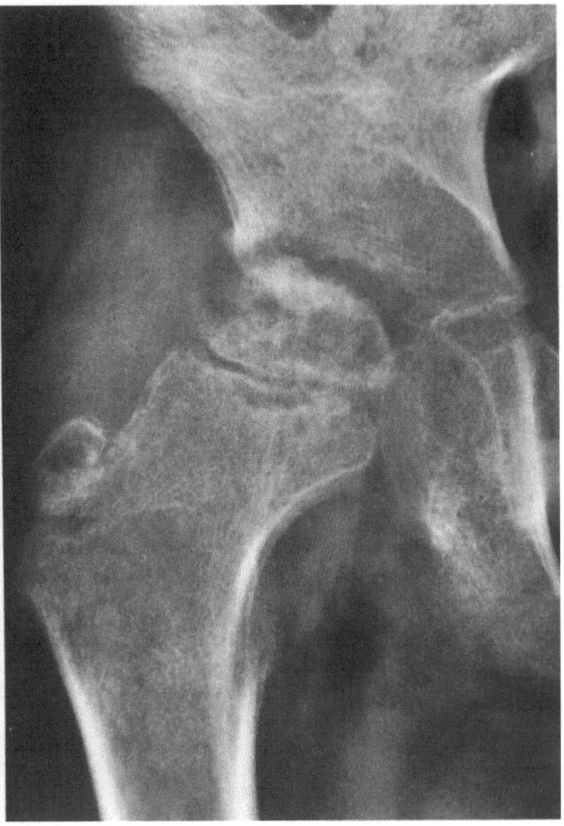

b

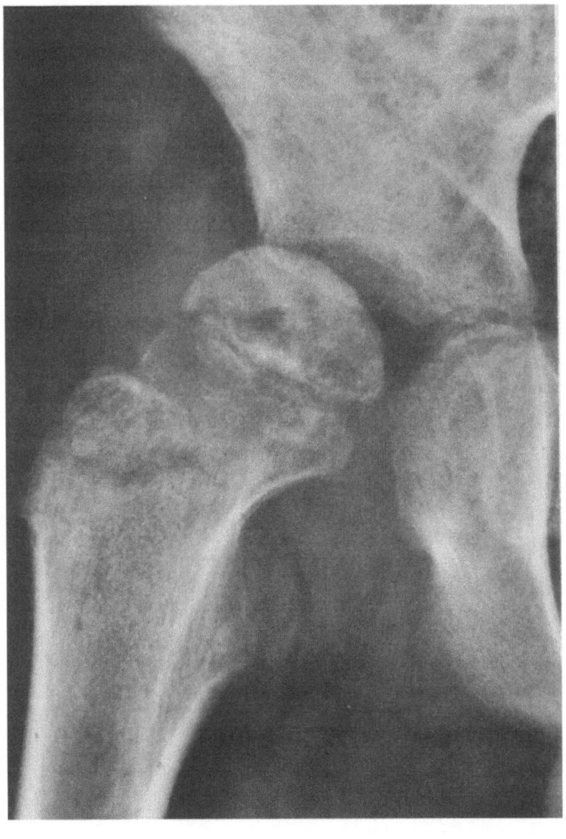

c

Fig. 72a–c. Differential diagnosis: pyogenic arthritis. Boy, 6 years old. **a** Soft tissue swelling. Possibly slight blurring at the medial edge of the metaphysis and widening of the joint space. **b** Two months after **a**: demineralization and destruction of the hip joint, with narrowing of the joint space and irregular joint contours. **c** Three and a half months after **a**, after immobilization and chemotherapy: restoration of the bony contours and still patchy demineralization around the epiphyseal plate. Hydrops of the joint and narrowing of the joint space cranially caused by destruction of joint cartilage

8.1.3 Differential Diagnosis

In infancy:
- Perthes' disease.
- Juvenile rheumatoid arthritis.
- Coxitis fugax.
- Pyogenic arthritis (Fig. 72).
- Primary bone tumor.

In adulthood:
- Rheumatoid arthritis.
- Pyogenic arthritis.
- Osteoarthrosis (Fig. 74).
- Osteonecrosis.
- Metastatic disease.
- Neuropathic joint disease.
- Primary bone tumor (Fig. 73).
- Villonodular synovitis.

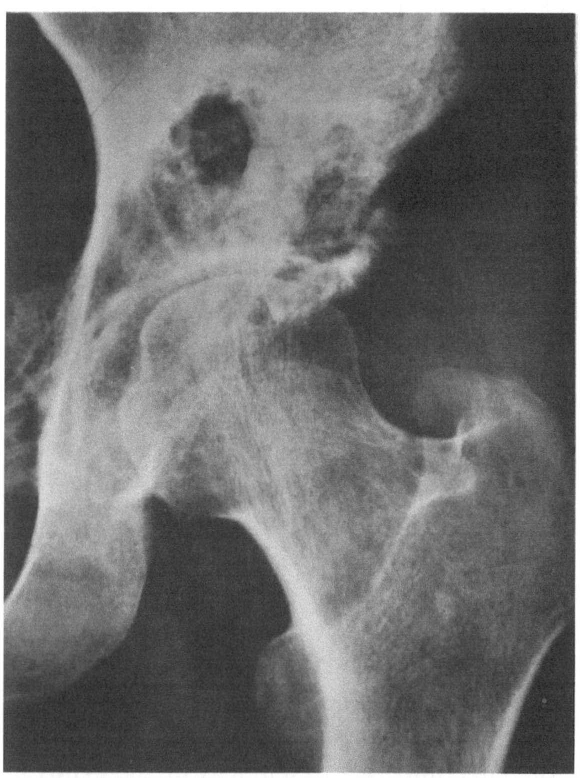

Fig. 73. Differential diagnosis: eosinophilic granuloma of the acetabulum. Woman, 26 years old. The abnormalities adjacent to the joint space may simulate an osseous lesion caused by tuberculosis

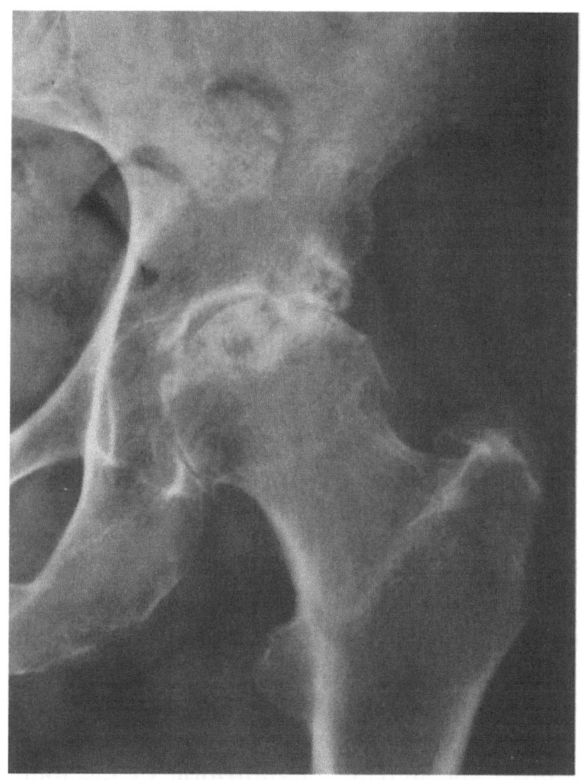

Fig. 74. Differential diagnosis: osteoarthrosis of the hip. Woman, 70 years old. Joint space narrowing, osteosclerosis, small osteophytes, and pseudocysts are present

8.2 Knee

The knee joint is generally reported to be the second or the third most common joint to be involved in tuberculosis [109, 110] (Table 1, see p. 11). Before the era of chemotherapy, the age at onset (admission) was usually below 20 years [31, 147]. Nowadays, most patients in our country are adults. In our material 50 cases (10.9%) with tuberculous affections of the knee were encountered. All patients except one were adults. Active or old pulmonary tuberculous lesions or pleuritis rests are frequently present; a family history of tuberculosis has been described in 30% of patients and multifocal lesions in 16% of those with tuberculous gonitis [147]. Five of our 50 cases (10%) had multifocal bone lesions: other knee (in two), hip (in two) and greater trochanter (in one). In BCG osteomyelitis about 50% of patients show affection of the knee [123].

8.2.1 Pathology

As in other joints, knee involvement originates either from an initial synovitis or an osseous bone lesion. Clinical and radiologic findings vary widely, depending on the site of infection and the degree of involvement (Chap. 6). The degree of residual joint destruction after tuberculous arthritis depends on the time of onset of the disease and the effects of growth [31].

8.2.1.1 Initial Synovitis

In the affection of the knee joint, initial synovitis seems to be more common than initial juxta-articular osseous foci. Hematogenous infection of the synovial membrane causes a granular synovitis, with the features of hyperemia, periarticular demineralization, and soft tissue swelling (Fig. 75). The composition of the synovial fluid changes and impairs the nutrition of the joint cartilage. Hyaline articular cartilage, however, may survive and/or be replaced by fibrocartilage [31]. At the sites of capsular attachment, invasion of the bone occurs and osseous lesions develop (Fig. 76). Progressive bone involvement leads to collapse of the articulating bone parts and destruction of the knee joint (Figs. 79, 80). If specifically tuberculous synovitis is accurately treated in the stages before bone destruction has occurred, only slight changes in bone texture may remain (Figs. 75, 77).

8.2.1.2 Osseous Focus

Initial juxta-articular osseous foci are usually found in the epi- and metaphyseal regions of femur and tibia (Figs. 78, 81, 82). Patellar lesions may occur, but these are less common [66]. The chance of perforation into the joint cavity and severe joint involvement by arthritis varies, depending on the distance of the osseous foci to the joint cavity. A nonbacterial perifocal inflammation of the synovial membrane is usually found in the presence of nearby osseous foci. Both tuberculous and nonbacterial synovitis may lead to acceleration of the process of ossification and growth. Abscesses are less frequent but occur during the disease, caused either by extension of tuberculous infection from a perforating osseous focus or by the spread of tuberculous arthritis to the adjacent soft tissues [31, 60, 147]. Sinuses are rarely encountered in children, but we have seen them in many of our adult patients [109]. Secondary infection of sinuses is usually responsible for increasing complaints of pain.

8.2.2 Radiologic Findings (Figs. 75–84)

8.2.2.1 Synovitis

- Demineralization in nonbacterial or specific synovitis: caused by hyperemia.
- Soft tissue swelling: caused by capsular thickening, exudate, and periarticular edema.
- Marginal erosions at the margins of articular cartilage and the attachment of the synovial membrane: These erosions may be ill-defined and obscured by the surrounding soft tissue swelling.
- Joint space narrowing or destruction.

- Widening of the intercondylar notch: involvement of bone arising from synovitis.

8.2.2.2 *Osseous Focus*

- Bone cavities: in the epi/metaphyseal region, either intracapsular or extracapsular.
- Demineralization/osteoporosis: sometimes severe demineralization and hardly visible initial infectious focus.
- Sequestra.
- Marginal osteosclerosis.

8.2.2.3 *Disturbances in Growth*

An increase in size and an altered modeling of epiphyseal nuclei of tibia and femur occur. Especially the medial femoral condyle appears larger. Chemotherapy may prevent affection of the growth plate and subsequent abnormalities.

8.2.2.4 *Posterior Subluxation of the Tibia*

Destruction of the cruciate ligaments leads to posterior subluxation of the tibia.

8.2.2.5 *Abscesses and Sinuses*

In children abscesses and sinuses are both uncommon [109]. Secondary infection of sinuses is an important cause of pain, but the major cause is bone destruction [31, 60].

8.2.2.6 *Collapse of Condyles and Necrotic Bone Fragments*

There may occur a collapse of condyles and necrotic bone fragments, often noticed first in the tibia.

8.2.2.7 *Healing and Healed Stages*

- Osteosclerosis.
- Bone fusion: either spontaneous or obtained by surgical treatment. Fibrous ankylosis is a frequently occurring sequela [109]. Sometimes partial fusion between epiphysis and metaphysis is found.
- Growth arrest lines in the growing child.
- Calcifications in the soft tissues.
- Congruous incongruity: joint space preserved but irregular in outline.
- Osteophytes: usually small.
- Osteoporosis.
- Abnormal patellae and small epiphyses: possible other residual findings especially in younger patients [31].

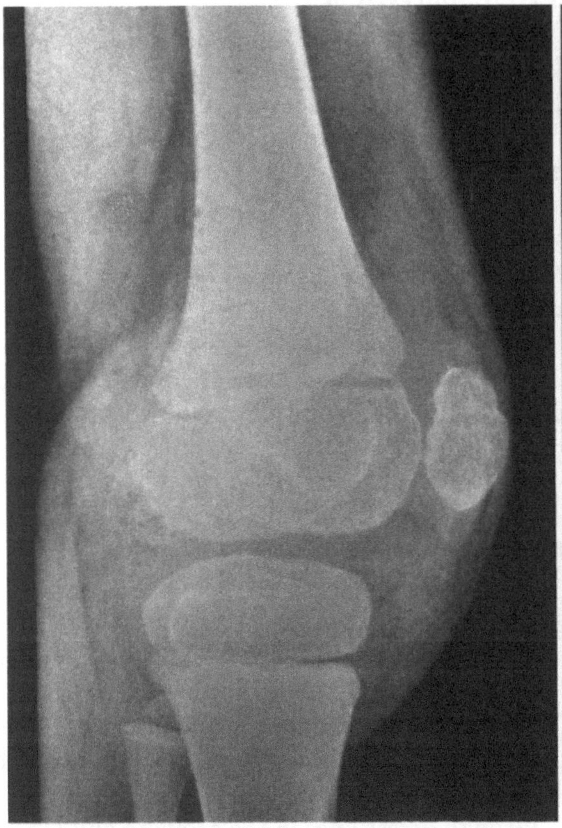

a

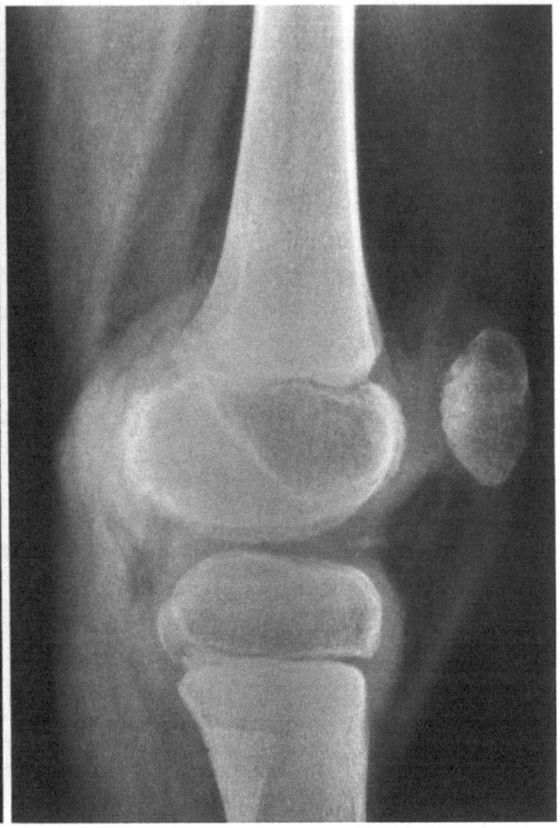

b

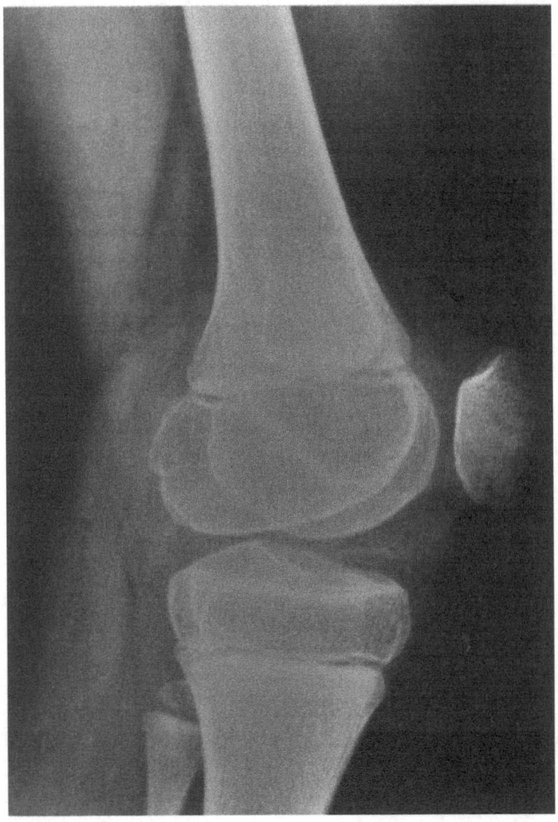

c

Fig. 75a–c. Tuberculous gonitis. Girl, 6 years old. Primary tuberculosis with hilar lymphadenitis. **a** Specific synovitis with soft tissue swelling. **b** After 8 months, antituberculous therapy: decrease in soft tissue swelling and better delineation of the bone contours. **c** Two years after **a:** healed tuberculous process. Normal bone structure and somewhat hypertrophic patella

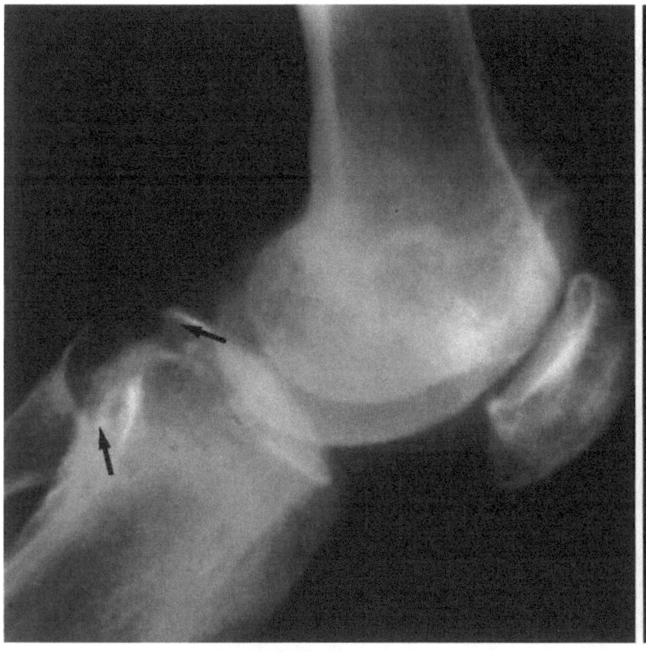

a

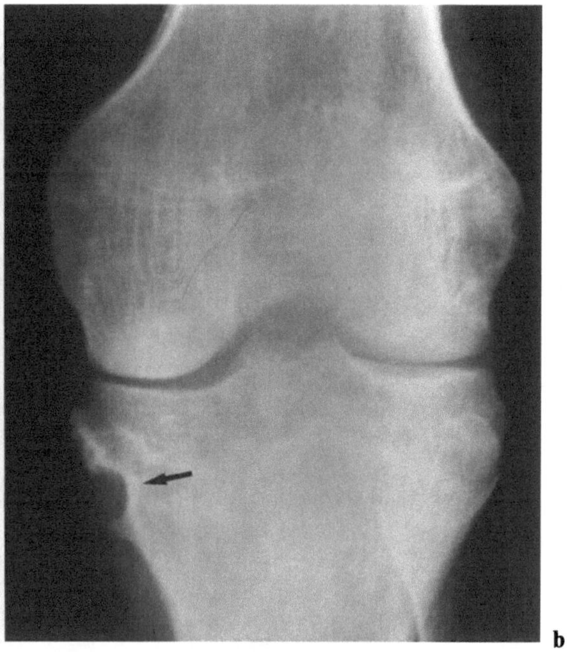

b

Fig. 76 a, b. Tuberculous gonitis. Man, 19 years old. Narrowing of the joint space and marginal erosions at the sites of attachment of the joint capsule to the tibia (*arrows*)

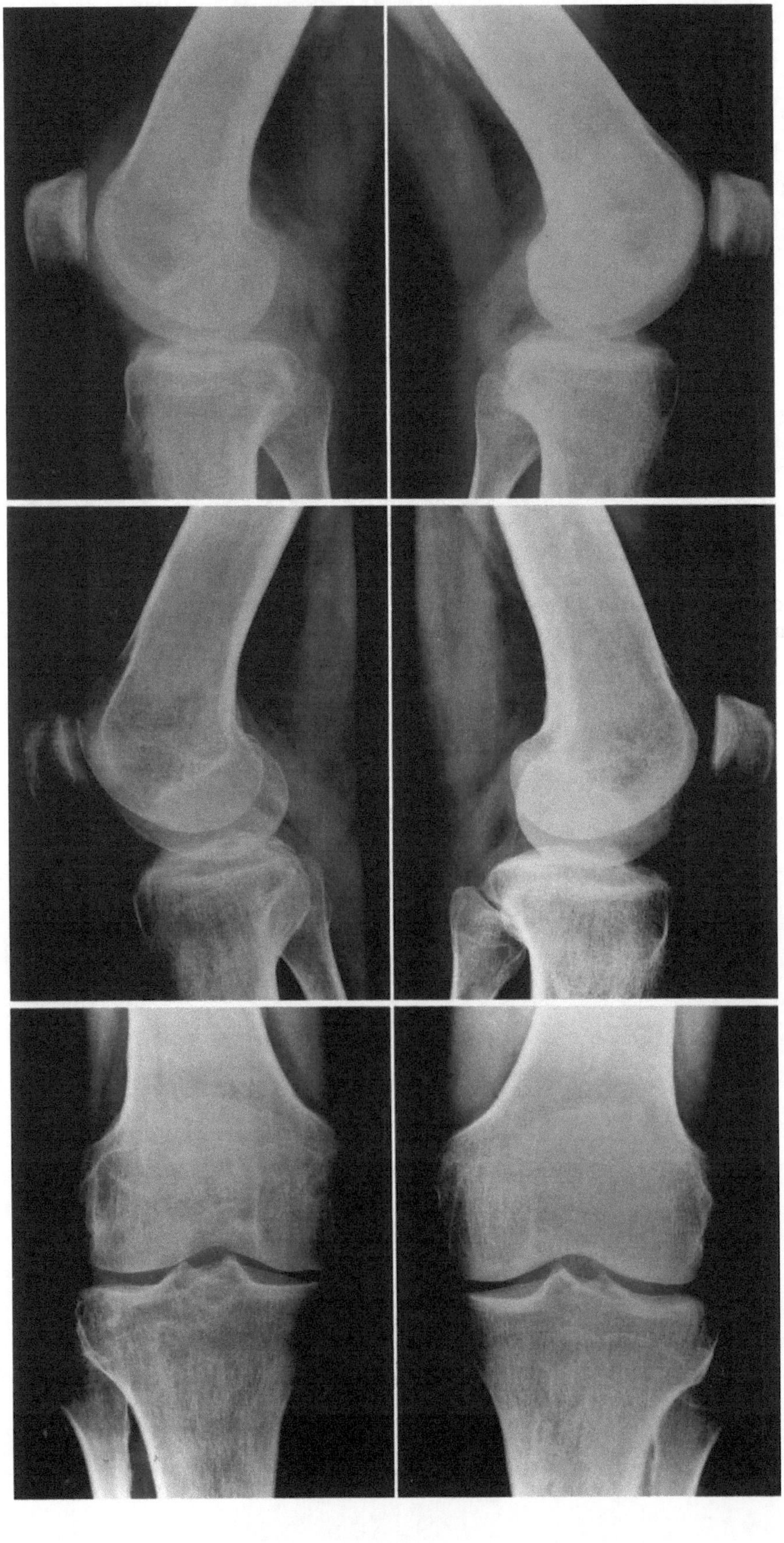
a
b
c

◀ **Fig. 77a–c.** Tuberculous gonitis. Man, 41 years old. Concomitant tuberculous empyema. **a** Soft tissue swelling of the right knee. **b, c** One and a half years after *a*: healed tuberculous process; osteoporosis is the only radiologic finding in the affected right knee

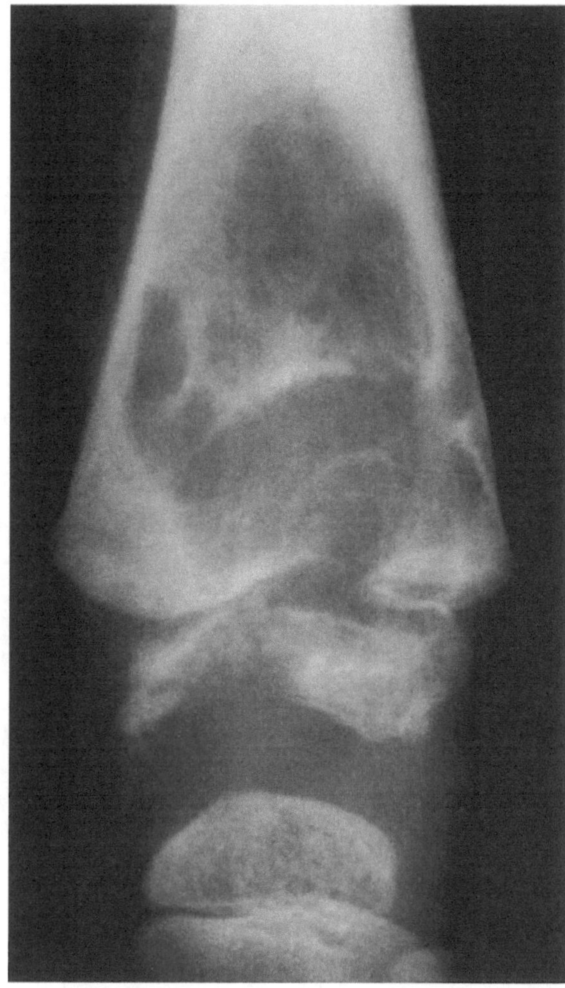

Fig. 78. Tuberculous gonitis. Large metaphyseal tuberculous focus, crossing the epiphyseal plate and affecting the epiphysis and the joint. By courtesy of Prof. B.J. Cremin, Cape Town, South Africa.)

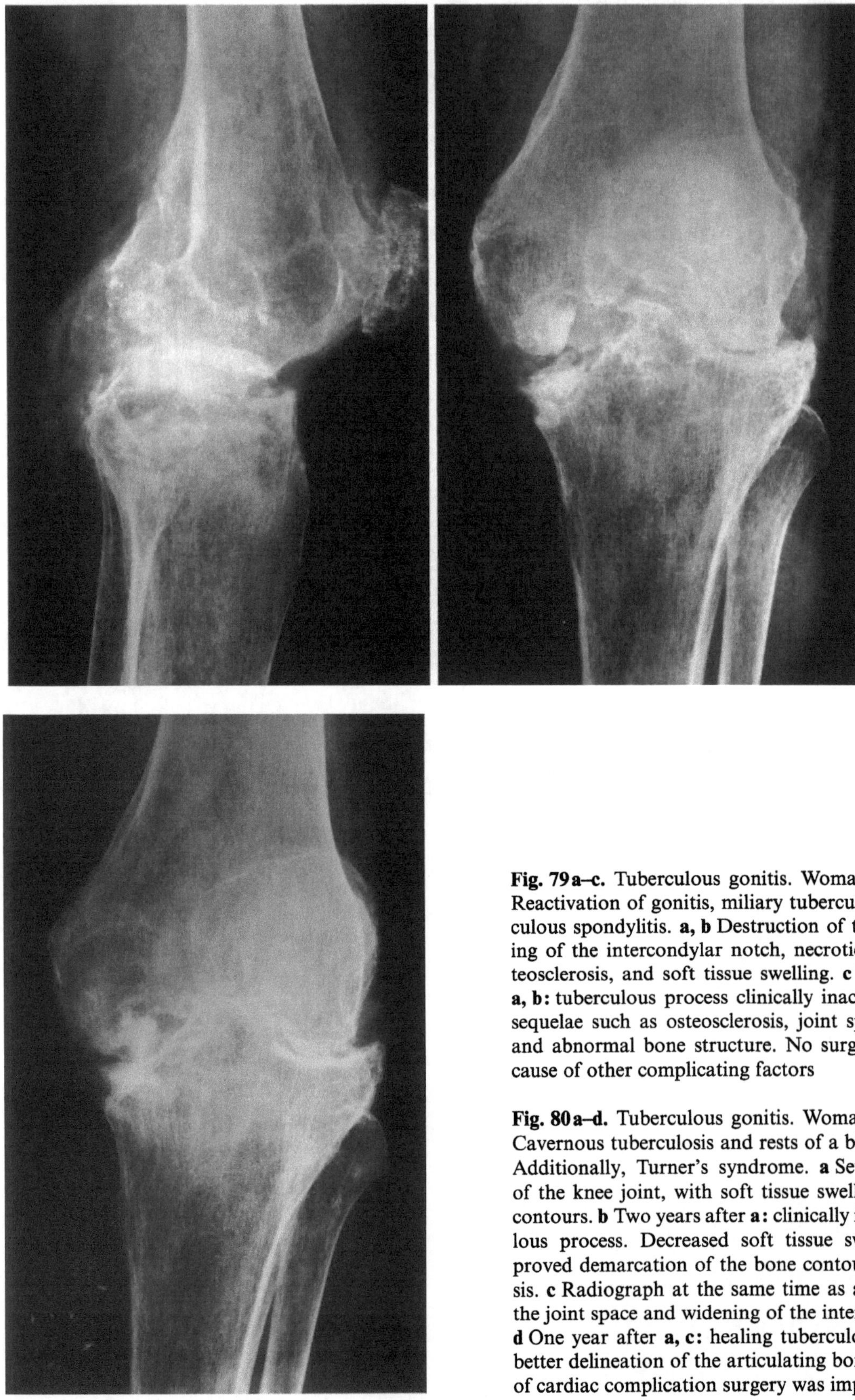

a b c

Fig. 79a–c. Tuberculous gonitis. Woman, 68 years old. Reactivation of gonitis, miliary tuberculosis, and tuberculous spondylitis. **a, b** Destruction of the joint, widening of the intercondylar notch, necrotic fragments, osteosclerosis, and soft tissue swelling. **c** Two years after **a, b**: tuberculous process clinically inactive. Radiologic sequelae such as osteosclerosis, joint space narrowing, and abnormal bone structure. No surgical therapy because of other complicating factors

Fig. 80a–d. Tuberculous gonitis. Woman, 58 years old. ▶ Cavernous tuberculosis and rests of a bilateral pleuritis. Additionally, Turner's syndrome. **a** Severe destruction of the knee joint, with soft tissue swelling and blurred contours. **b** Two years after **a**: clinically inactive tuberculous process. Decreased soft tissue swelling and improved demarcation of the bone contours. Osteosclerosis. **c** Radiograph at the same time as **a**: destruction of the joint space and widening of the intercondylar notch. **d** One year after **a, c**: healing tuberculous process with better delineation of the articulating bone ends. Because of cardiac complication surgery was impossible

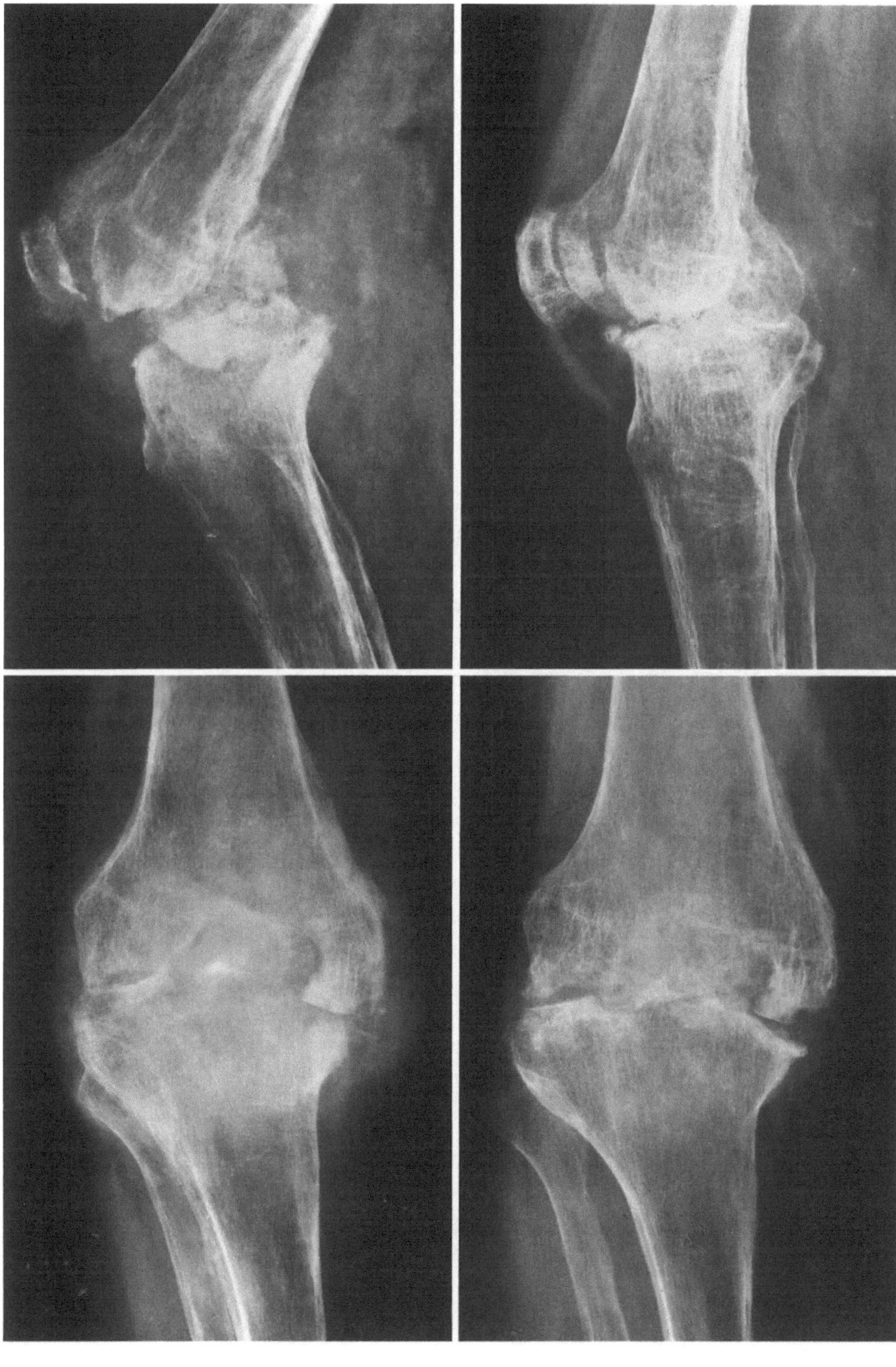

a b c d

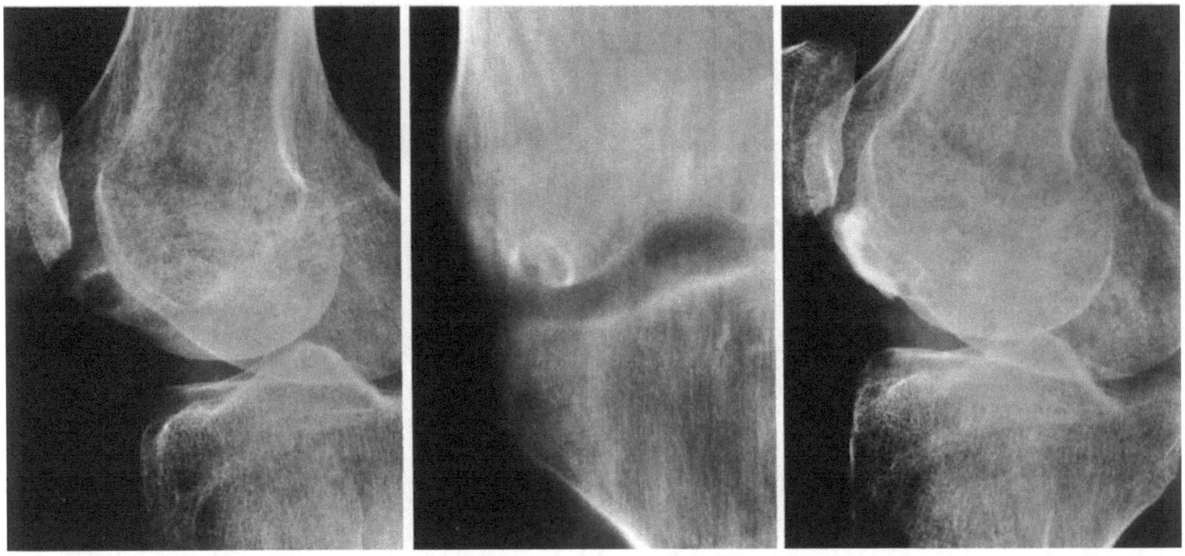

a–c

Fig. 81 a–c. Tuberculous gonitis. Woman, 20 years old. Inactive rests of tuberculosis in the right lung and active tuberculosis of the right kidney, ureter, and bladder. **a, b** Epiphyseal lesion of the lateral condyle with marginal osteosclerosis. **c** After 2 months, and surgery with excision of the affected synovia and excochleation of the bone lesion, filled up with bone chips of the tibia; only slightly impaired function of the joint

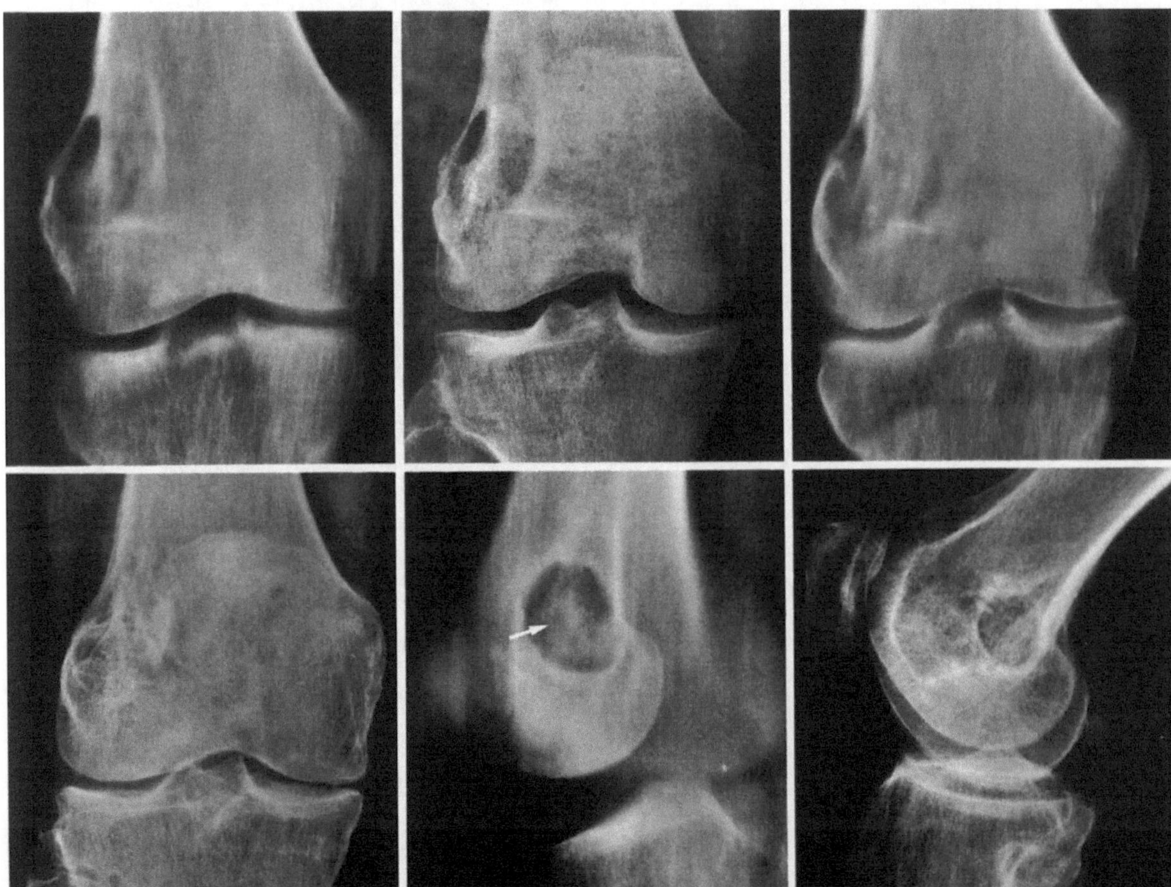

a–c

d–f

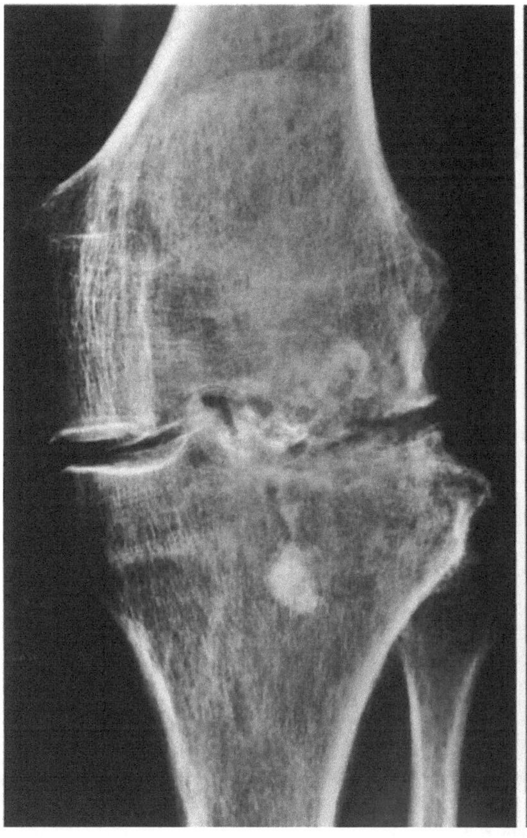

a

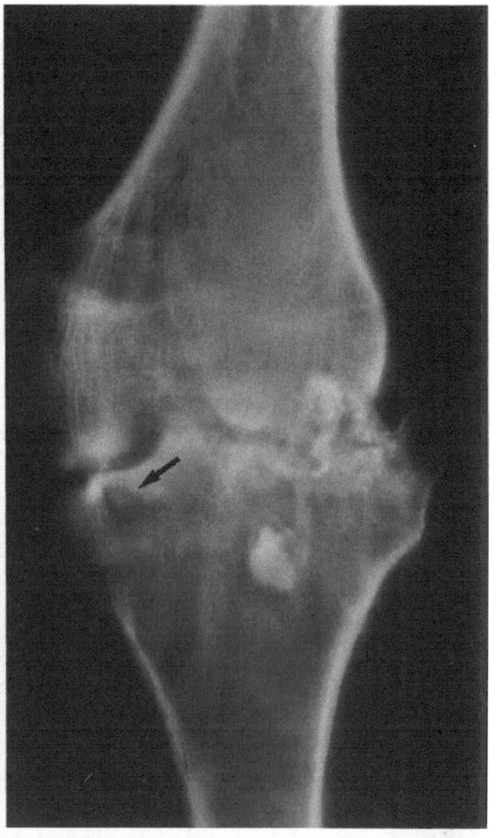

b

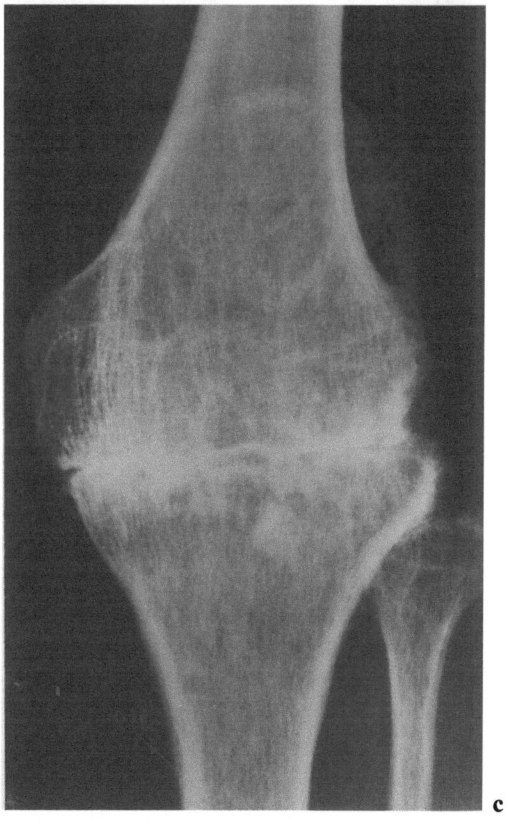

c

◀ **Fig. 82 a–f.** Tuberculous affection of the distal femur with draining sinus. Woman, 46 years old. Thirty years before admission, genital tuberculosis and peritonitis (*M. tuberculosis*). **a, b, e** Epi/metaphyseal bone lesion with sequestrum (*arrow*), marginal osteosclerosis, and somewhat patchy osteosclerosis of the lateral femoral condyle. No involvement of the knee joint. **c** One year after **a, b, e**: excochleation and removal of two sequestra and implantation of bone chips, new bone structures inside the osseous lesions. **d, f** Four years after **a, b, e**: healed tuberculous focus with complete incorporation of the bone chips

Fig. 83 a–c. Tuberculosis of the knee. Man, 59 years old. ▶ Thirty-two years after first tuberculous involvement of the knee joint, reactivation of the tuberculous process with draining sinus. **a, b** Destruction of the joint space with necrotic fragments. Irregular bone structures in the lateral side of the knee joint. Small bone lesion with sequestrum (*arrow*). **c** One year after **a**, after surgical treatment bony fusion of tibia and femur

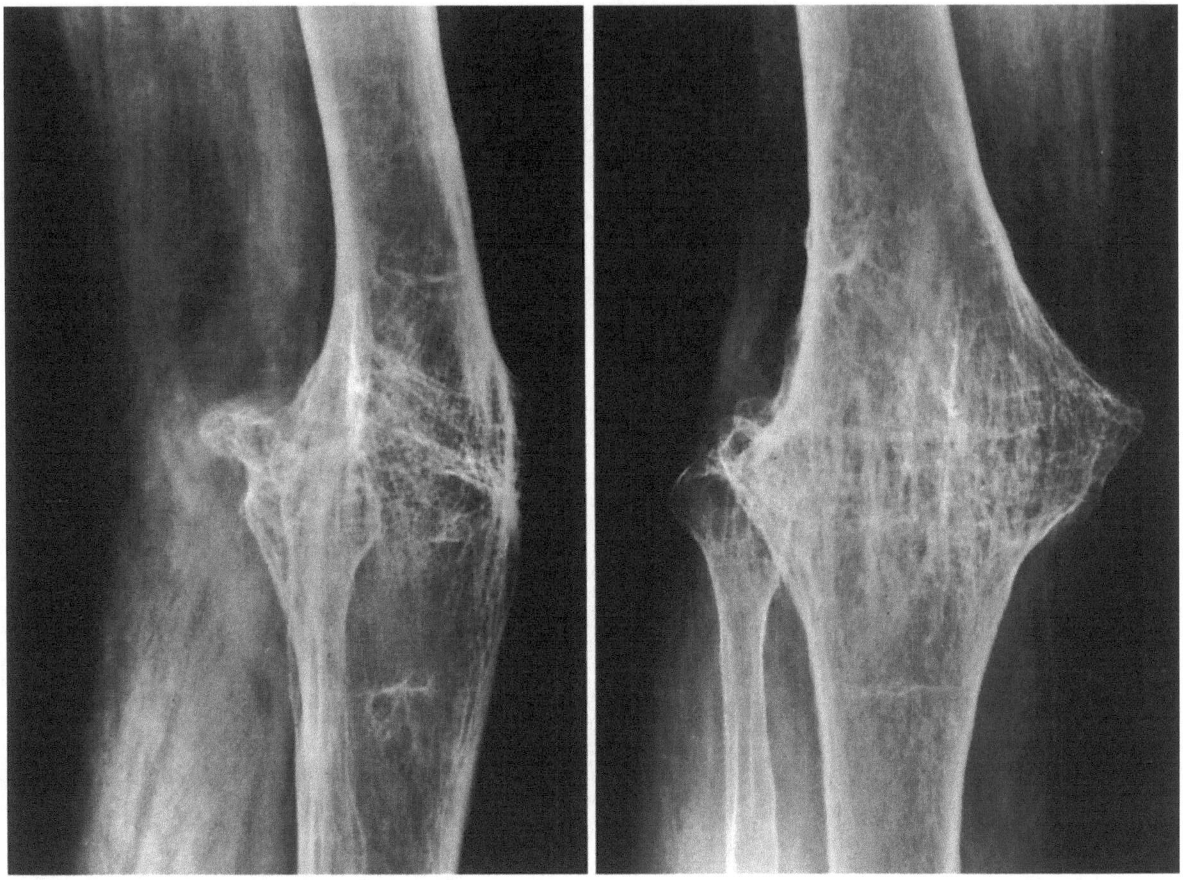

a b

Fig. 84a, b. Arthrodesis for tuberculous involvement of the knee joint. Woman, 65 years old

8.2.3 Differential Diagnosis (Figs. 85–87)

- Juvenile rheumatoid arthritis.
- Adult rheumatoid arthritis.
- Pyogenic arthritis/osteomyelitis (Fig. 86).
- Osteoarthrosis.
- Hemophilia.
- Metastatic disease (Fig. 85).
- Primary bone tumor (Fig. 87).
- Pigmented villonodular synovitis.
- Osteonecrosis (osteochondritis dissecans).
- Neuropathic joint.
- Para-articular soft tissue tumors.
- Pseudorheumatisme chronique tuberculeux [135].

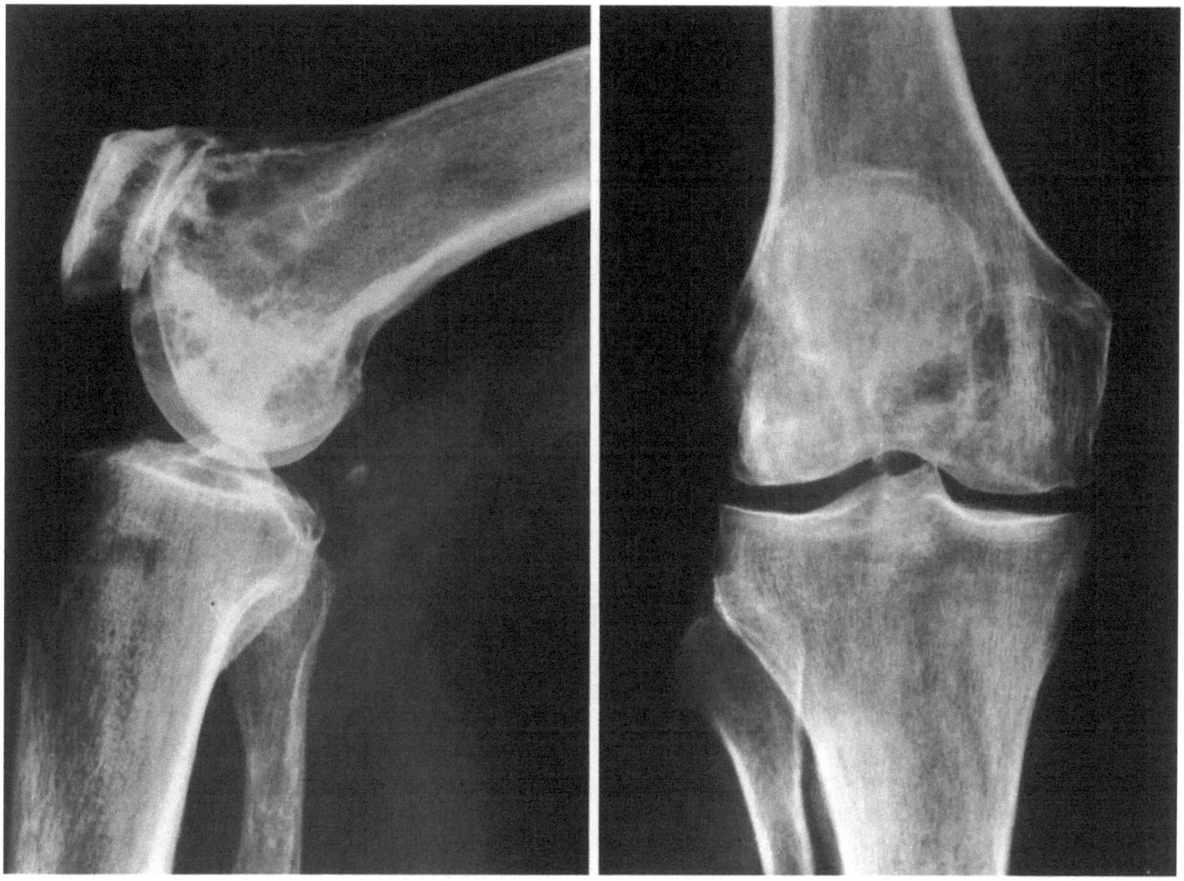

a b

Fig. 85a, b. Differential diagnosis: metastasis of breast carcinoma in the distal femur

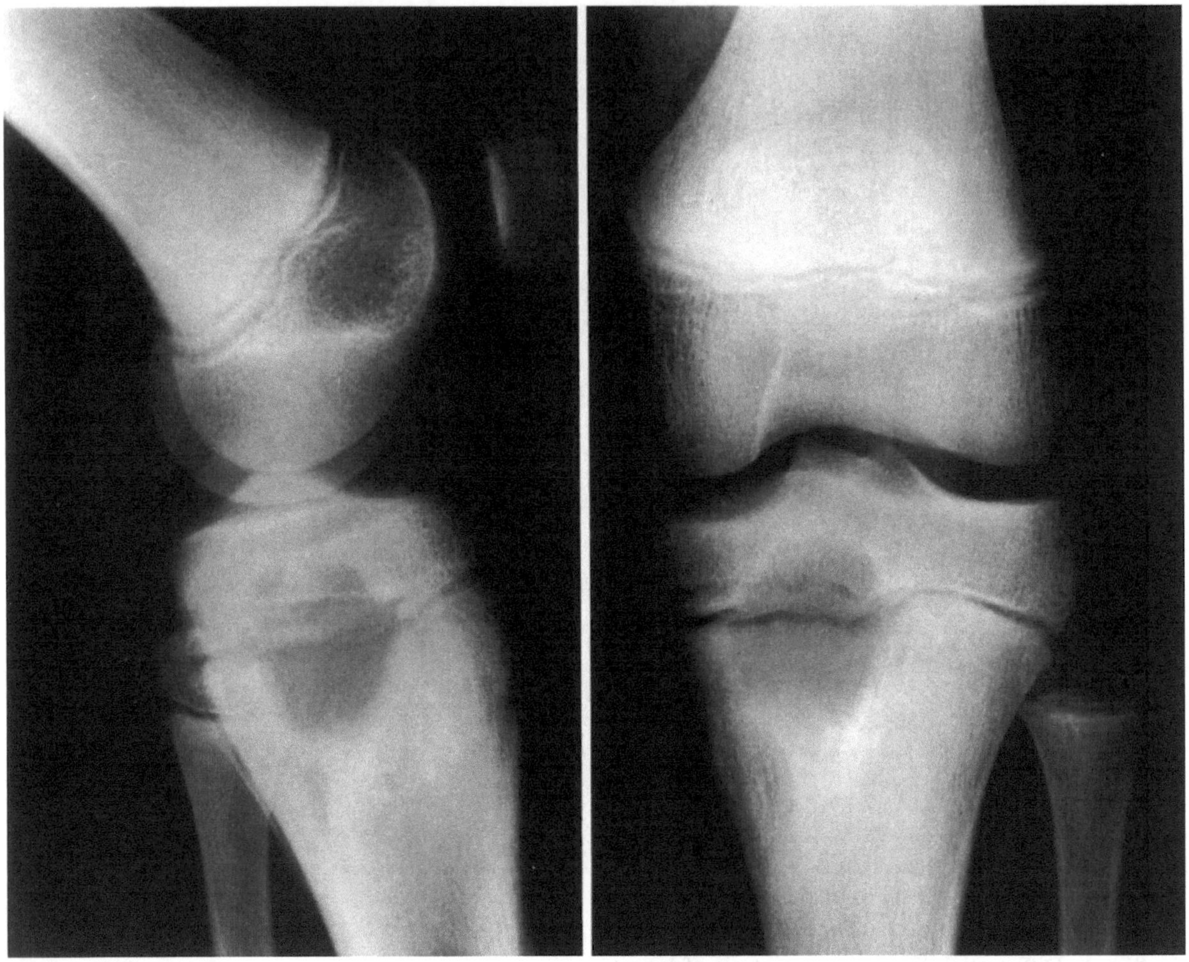

a b

Fig. 86a, b. Differential diagnosis: pyogenic abscess (Brodie's abscess) in the tibia. Usually pyogenic osteomyelitis does not penetrate the growth plate! Osteosclerosis and periosteal bone formation are present

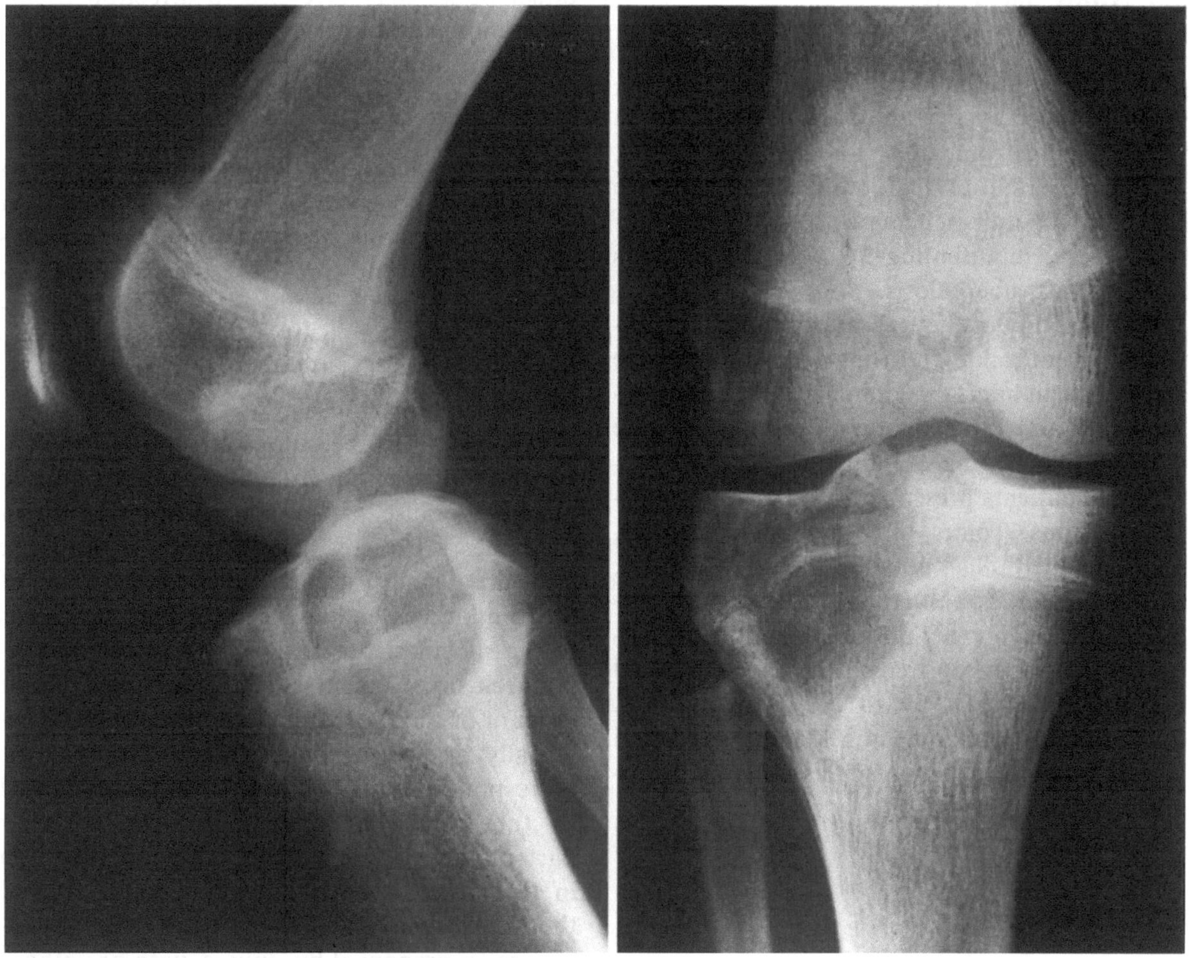

a b

Fig. 87 a, b. Differential diagnosis: chondroblastoma in the proximal tibia. Boy, 17 years old. Well-defined epi/metaphyseal bone lesion

8.3 Ankle and Foot

Involvement of the ankle and foot has been described especially in adults and is reported at rates ranging from 2.6% to 12% [32, 48, 64, 79, 88, 93, 109, 147] (Table 1, see p. 11). We collected 17 adult patients with involvement of these areas, representing 3.7% of the patients with osseous tuberculosis.

Localization of these cases of tuberculous involvement of ankle and foot were: Four in the ankle, nine in intertarsal joints, three in intertarsal joints and tarsometatarsal joints, and one in metatarsophalangeal joint I.

Three patients presented together four multifocal lesions (spine, hip, greater trochanter, knee). In the tarsus, possibly the talar, cuboid, and navicular bones are most frequently affected, although other authors mention the calcaneus as the most frequently affected tarsal bone [17, 48, 63, 87, 109, 141, 154]. Involvement of the first metatarsophalangeal joint was found in only one of our patients; this must be distinguished from gout [42, 56].

8.3.1 Pathology

As the majority of patients usually present rather late in the disease with severe destruction of the ankle joint, the initial focus of tuberculous affection frequently cannot be established [109]. This focus may be either synovial or osseous (Chap. 6).

Initial synovitis seems to be less common than osseous foci [147]. The chance of tuberculous arthritis of the ankle joint depends on localization more or less in the vicinity of the joint space. In children the extension of an initial metaphyseal focus may be withheld by the cartilaginous growth plates of the distal tibia and fibula. Perforation of a talar focus into the ankle joint is a dreaded complication and may lead to a destructive arthritis. Calcaneal foci seldom cause arthritis of the ankle joint but may spread to the talocalcaneal and calcaneocuboideal joint if the foci are located close to these intertarsal joints. Tuberculous involvement of the other tarsal bones may give rise to affection of the surrounding joint spaces, especially in adults. Spread of tuberculous affection from one tarsal bone to the others may also occur via the infected synovial membrane. In children, especially in early childhood, the ossification centers of the tarsal bones are still small, and the rather thick cartilaginous superficial layers of the tarsal bones prevent spread of the infection. Involvement of the metatarsal bones and phalanges is encountered mostly in infancy and usually presents with extensive periosteal bone formation and spina ventosa.

Abscesses of tuberculous affection of the ankle and foot are frequent and are usually noticed quickly because of the superficial location of the bones. Abscesses from arthritis of the ankle joint are usually situated on the lateral side of the joint and extend between the joint ligaments to the subcutaneous region. Abscesses from talar neck involvement spread over the anterior dorsum of the foot and extend internally or externally or present themselves in front of the corresponding malleoli [147]. Abscesses caused by tuberculous osteomyelitis of the posterior part of the talus spread in posterior direction in the space between the tibial epiphysis and the Achilles tendon. In many cases these abscesses are accompanied by sinuses, with or without secondary infection. Spontaneous bony fusion is more common since the use of chemotherapy and can be expected in about 60% of affections [110].

8.3.2 Radiologic Findings

8.3.2.1 Ankle Joint (Figs. 88, 89)

Synovitis
- Demineralization/osteoporosis.
- Soft tissue swelling.
- Hydrops.
- Marginal erosions.
- Joint space narrowing; usually relatively late in disease.

Osseous Focus
- Bony cavities: mostly hard to detect in cases with extensive demineralization.

- Demineralization/osteoporosis.
- Marginal osteosclerosis.
- Sequestra.

Periosteal Bone Formation

Bone Destruction

(Sub)luxation
(Sub)luxation occurs by anterior luxation of the talus [109].

Disturbances in Growth and Ossification During Childhood

Abscesses and Sinuses

Healing and Healed Stages
- Remineralization.
- Osteosclerosis.
- Bone fusion: Spontaneous osseous fusion and fibrous ankylosis may result after healing.

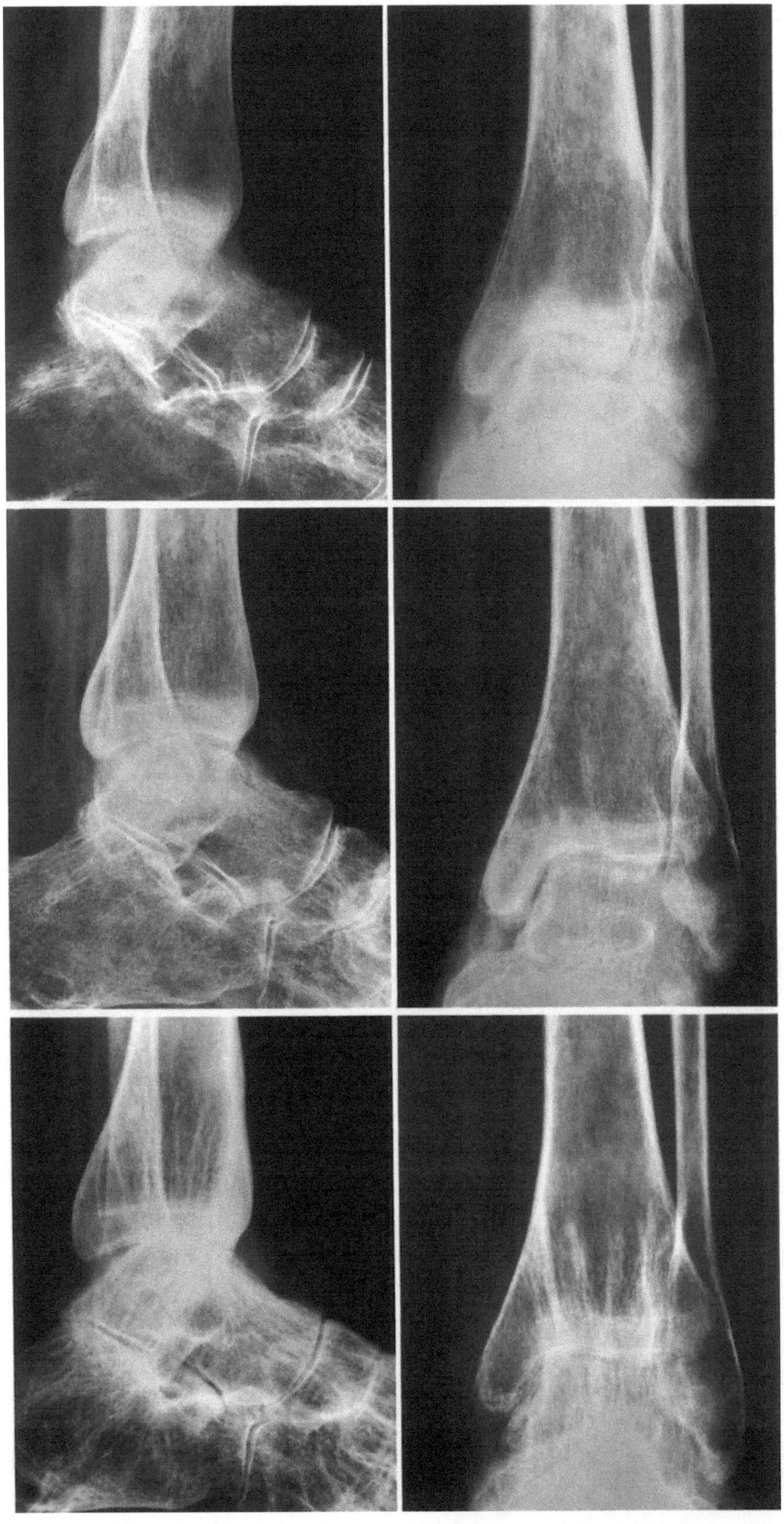

a

b

c

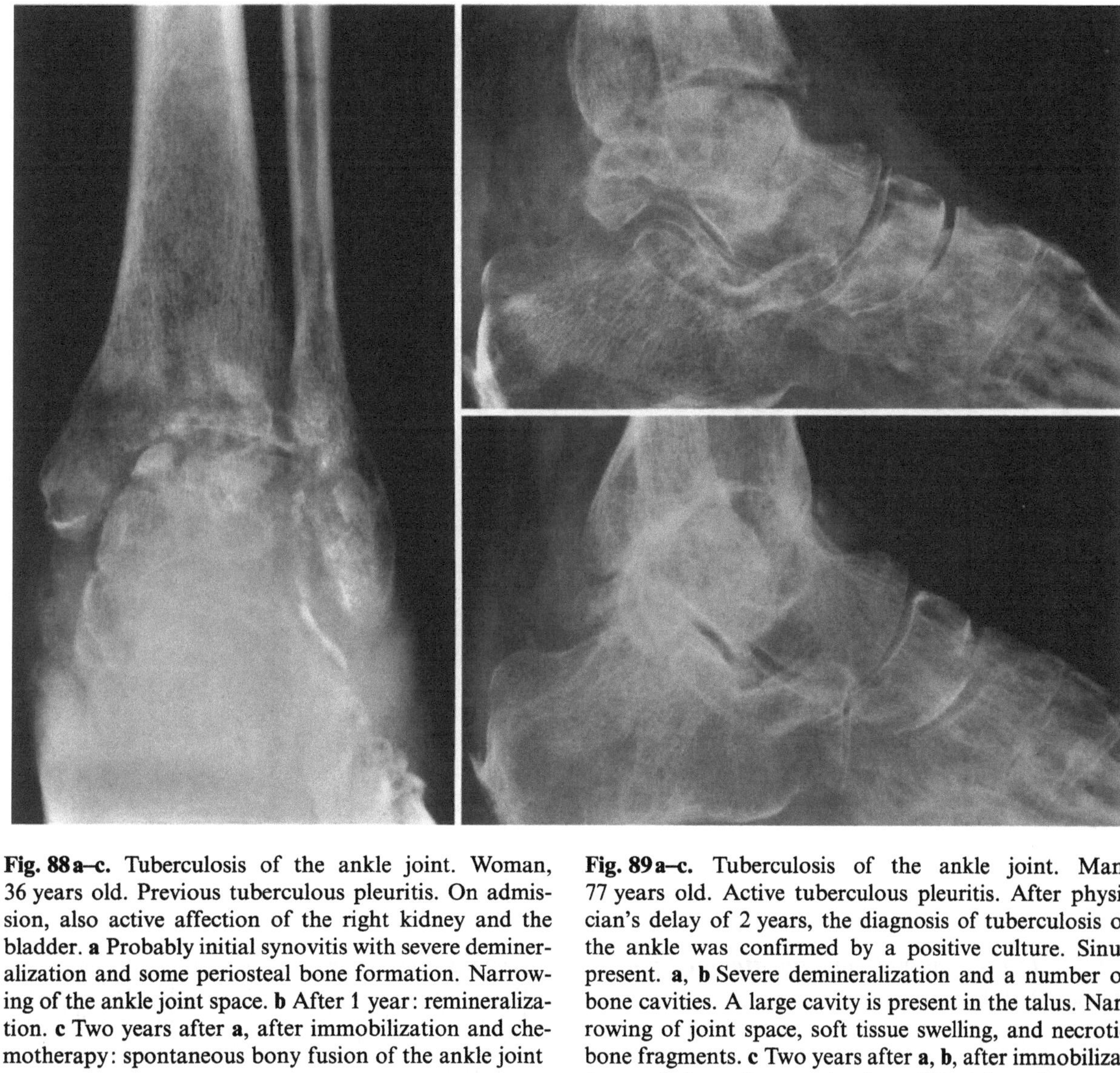

◄ **Fig. 88a–c.** Tuberculosis of the ankle joint. Woman, 36 years old. Previous tuberculous pleuritis. On admission, also active affection of the right kidney and the bladder. **a** Probably initial synovitis with severe demineralization and some periosteal bone formation. Narrowing of the ankle joint space. **b** After 1 year: remineralization. **c** Two years after **a**, after immobilization and chemotherapy: spontaneous bony fusion of the ankle joint

Fig. 89a–c. Tuberculosis of the ankle joint. Man, 77 years old. Active tuberculous pleuritis. After physician's delay of 2 years, the diagnosis of tuberculosis of the ankle was confirmed by a positive culture. Sinus present. **a**, **b** Severe demineralization and a number of bone cavities. A large cavity is present in the talus. Narrowing of joint space, soft tissue swelling, and necrotic bone fragments. **c** Two years after **a**, **b**, after immobilization and chemotherapy: healing of the tuberculous process with remineralization and spontaneous bony fusion of the ankle joint

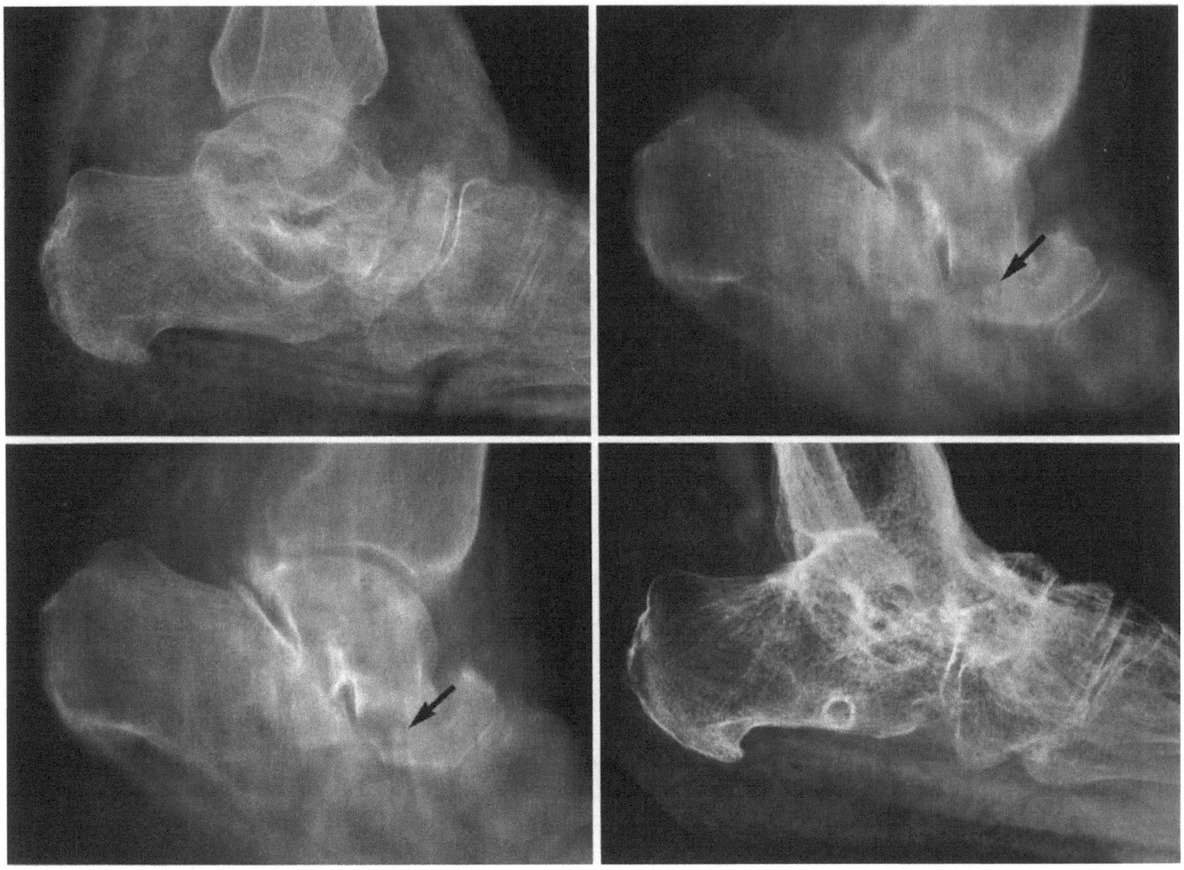

a b c d

8.3.2.2 Intertarsal and Tarsometatarsal Joints (Figs. 90–94)

Synovitis
- Demineralization/osteoporosis.
- Soft tissue swelling.
- Marginal erosions.
- Narrowing of joint space.

Osseous Focus
An osseous focus is generally difficult to detect. A sequestrum is possible.

Bone Destruction

Abscesses and Sinuses

Healing and Healed Stages
- Remineralization.
- Osteosclerosis.
- Bone fusion: spontaneous or surgical bony fusion or fibrous ankylosis.

Fig. 90 a–d. Tuberculosis of the intertarsal joints. Woman, 78 years old. Active pulmonary tuberculosis of the left lung. Fistula on the medial side of the ankle. **a–c** Affection of the talonavicular joint with demineralization, soft tissue swelling, marginal erosions, and destruction of the joint space. Small sequestrum in the talus (*arrow*). **d** After 1 year, chemotherapy and panarthrodesis: healing with remineralization of the tuberculous process

Fig. 91 a, b. Healed tuberculous affection of the subtalar joint. Man, 47 years old. Previous pulmonary tuberculosis, empyema, and tuberculous peritonitis. **a** Normal right ankle joint. **b** Situation after tuberculous synovitis of the left subtalar joint and spontaneous bony fusion ▶

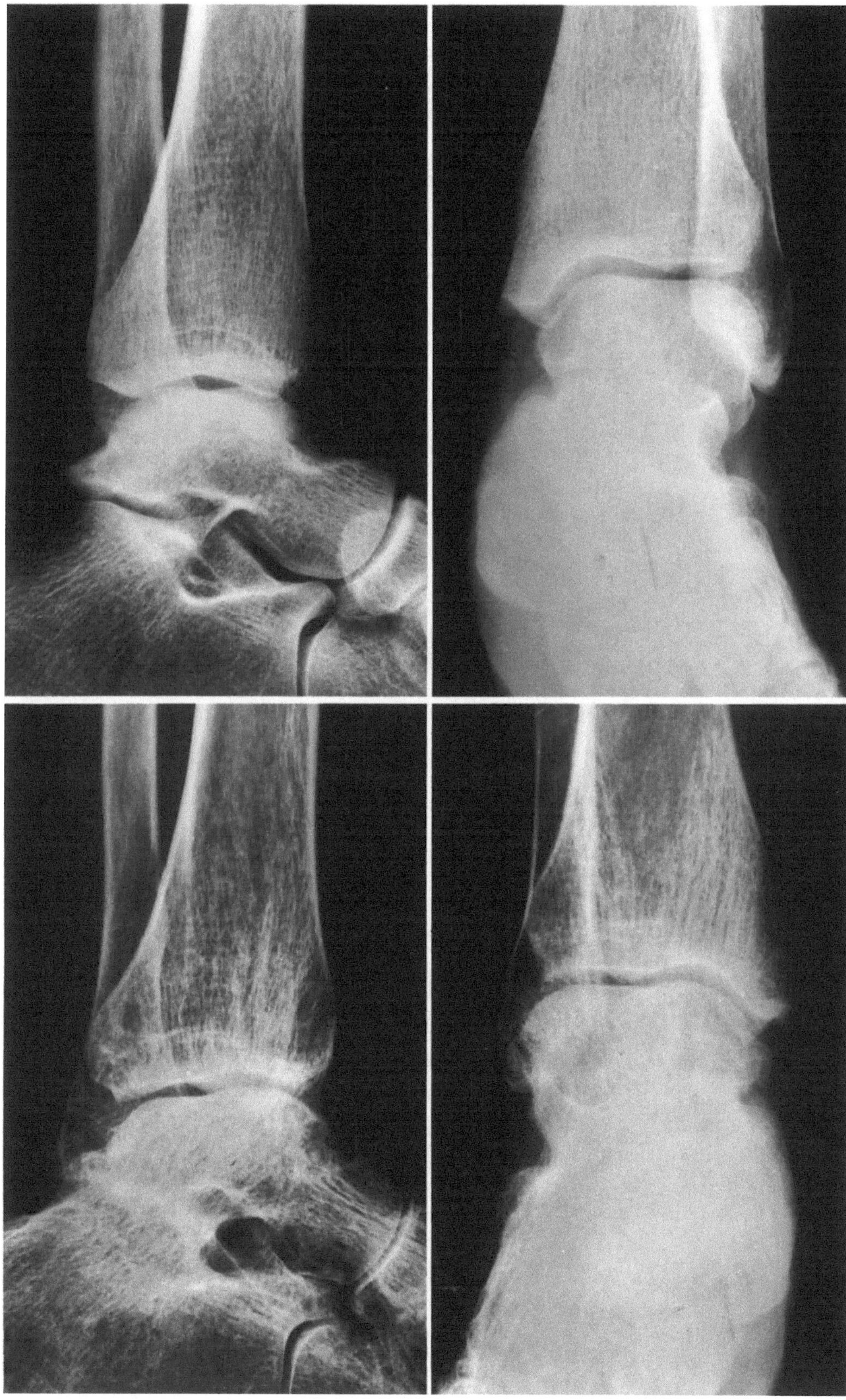

a

b

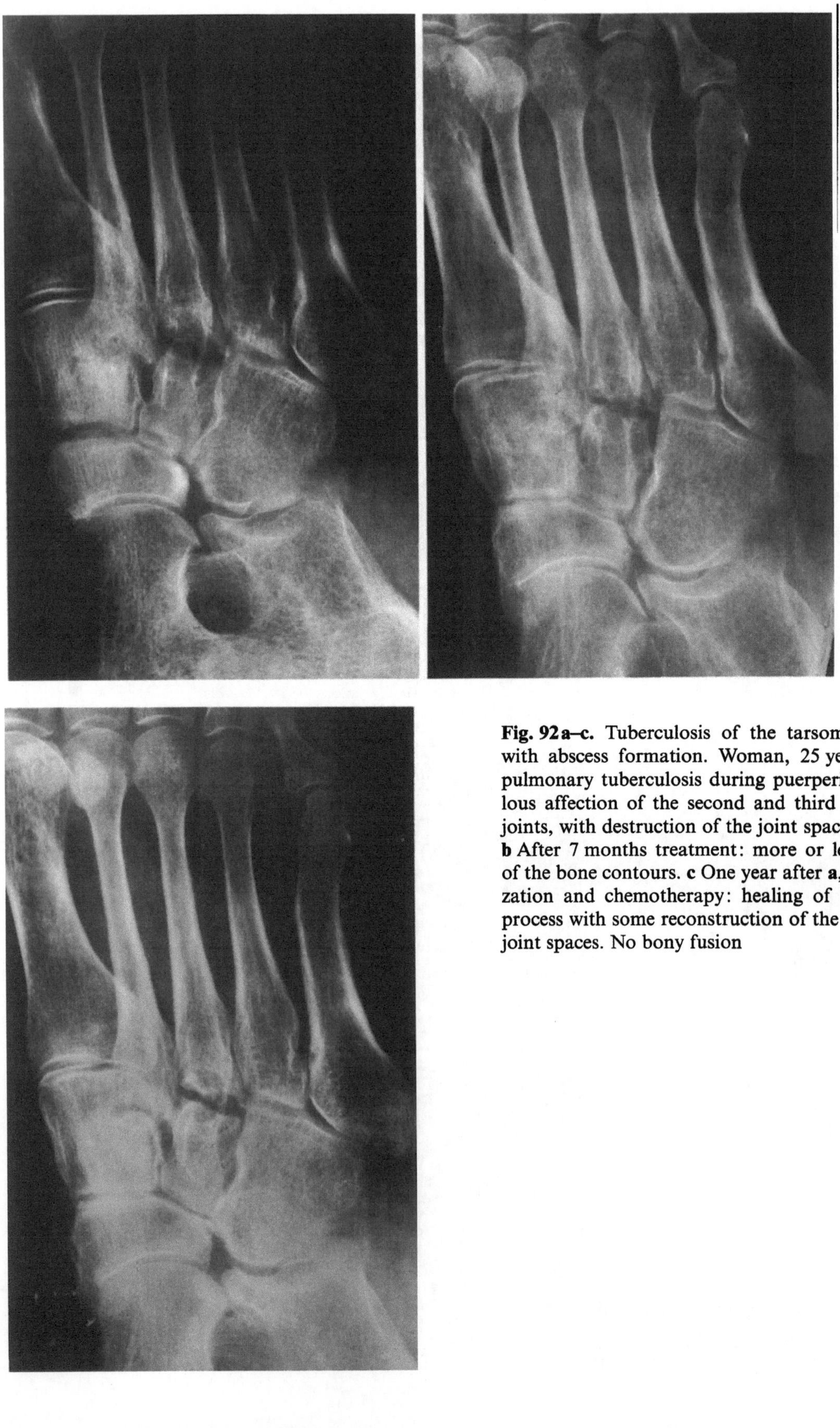

a b c

Fig. 92a–c. Tuberculosis of the tarsometatarsal joints with abscess formation. Woman, 25 years old. Active pulmonary tuberculosis during puerperium. **a** Tuberculous affection of the second and third tarsometatarsal joints, with destruction of the joint spaces and erosions. **b** After 7 months treatment: more or less demarcation of the bone contours. **c** One year after **a**, after immobilization and chemotherapy: healing of the tuberculous process with some reconstruction of the tarsometatarsal joint spaces. No bony fusion

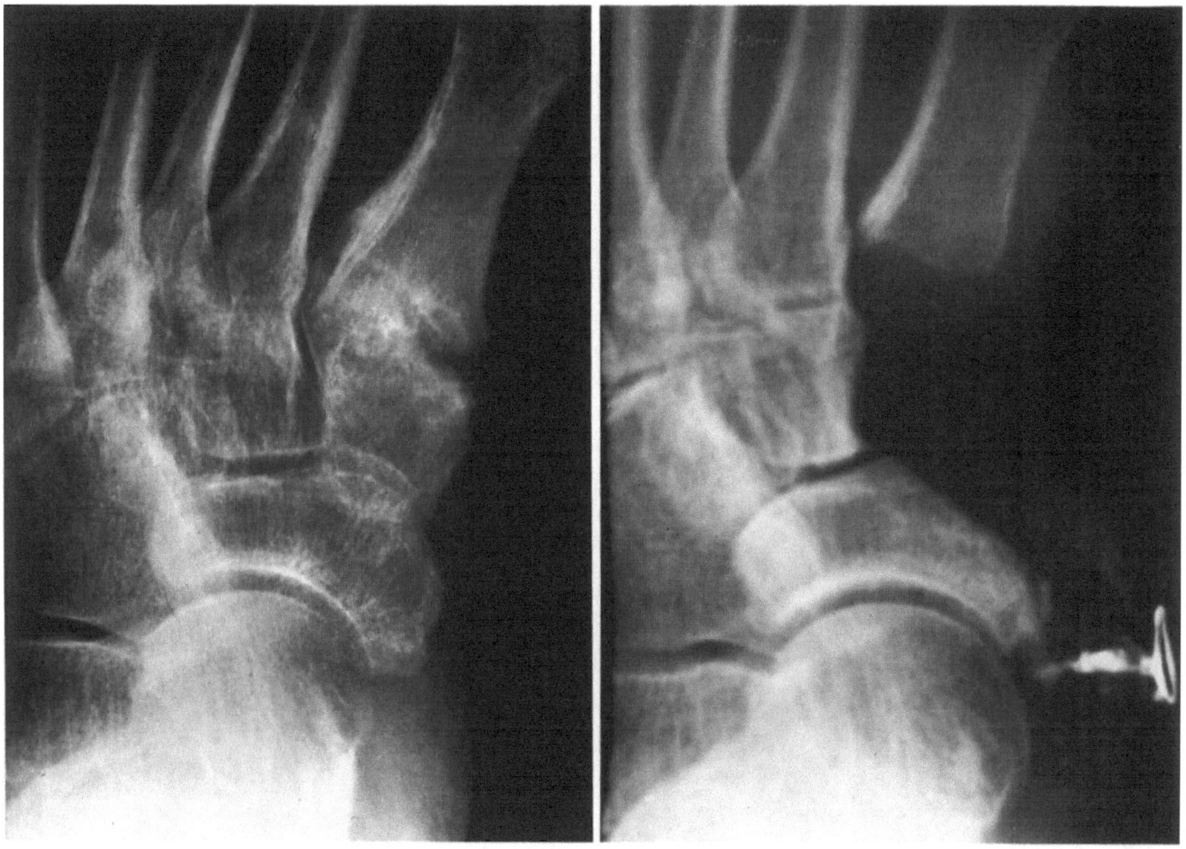

a b

Fig. 93a, b. Tuberculosis of the first tarsometatarsal joint. Adult man. Case history not available. **a** (1922) Synovitis with erosions, especially of the cuneiform bone. Destruction of the joint space and probably some periosteal bone formation on the lateral side of the first metatarsal bone. **b** After 1 year, and excision of the tuberculous process: residual sinus. The sinus may be the result of reactivation. (Antituberculous drugs were not available in the 1920s.)

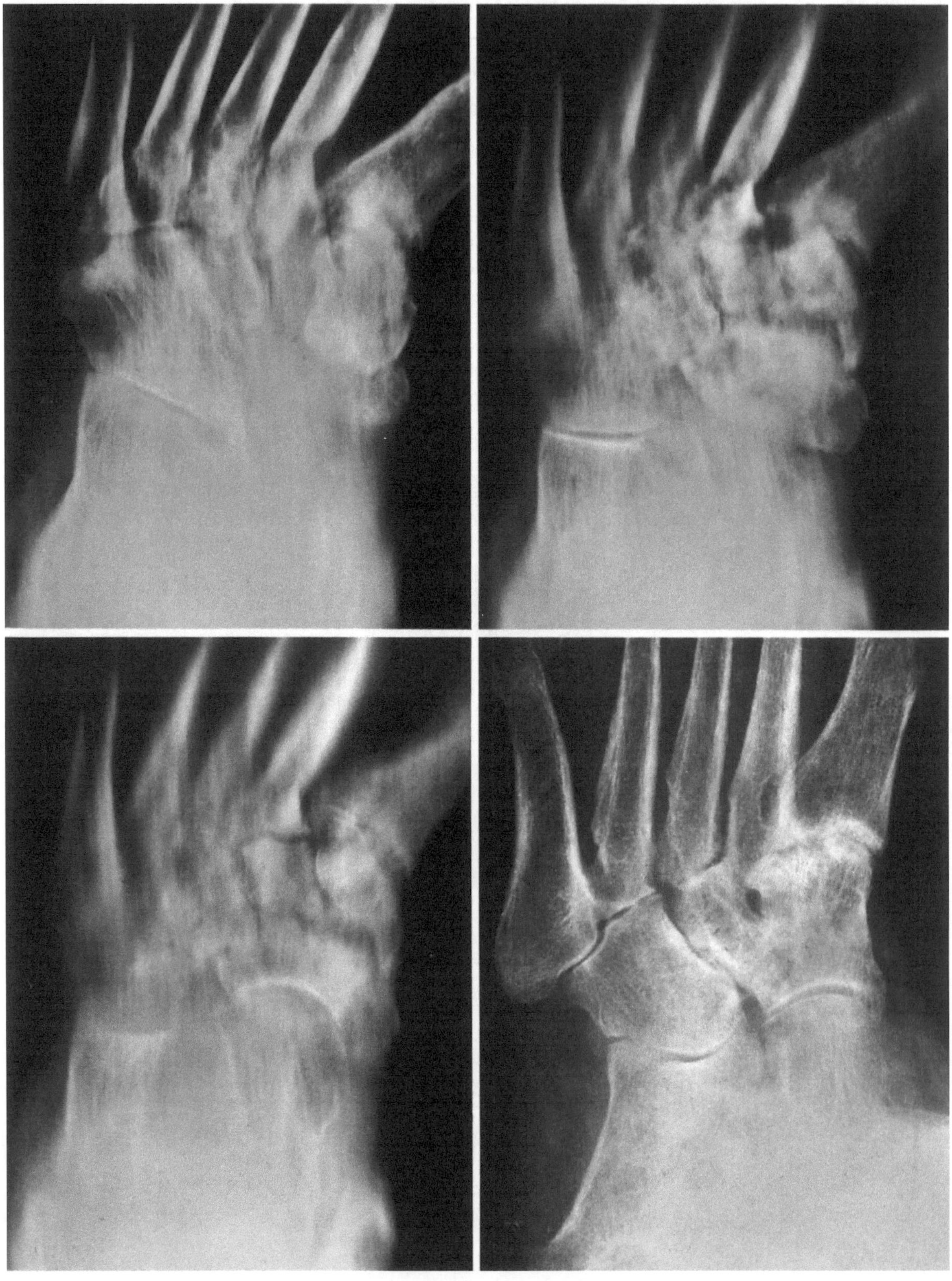

a b c d

◀ **Fig. 94 a–d.** Tuberculosis of the intertarsal and tarsometatarsal joints. Woman, 80 years old. Previous tuberculous pleuritis, tuberculous coxitis, and cervical lymphadenitis. **a, b, c** Tomography: extensive destruction of the intertarsal and tarsometatarsal joints. **d** After 2 years, chemotherapy, remineralization, some osteosclerosis, and spontaneous bony fusion between the cuneiforma and probably between the cuneiforma and several metatarsal bones

8.3.2.3 Metatarsal Bones, Phalanges and Metatarsophalangeal Joints (Fig. 95)

Synovitis
- Soft tissue swelling.
- Demineralization/osteoporosis.
- Marginal erosions.
- Joint space narrowing.

Abscesses and Sinuses

Osseous Focus
- Soft tissue swelling.
- Demineralization/osteoporosis.
- Periosteal bone formation.
- Spina ventosa.
- Sequestra.

Healing and Healed Stages
- Osteosclerosis.
- Remineralization.
- Shortening of tubular bones.
- Calcifications/ossifications in the soft tissues.
- Bone fusion (osseous or fibrous).

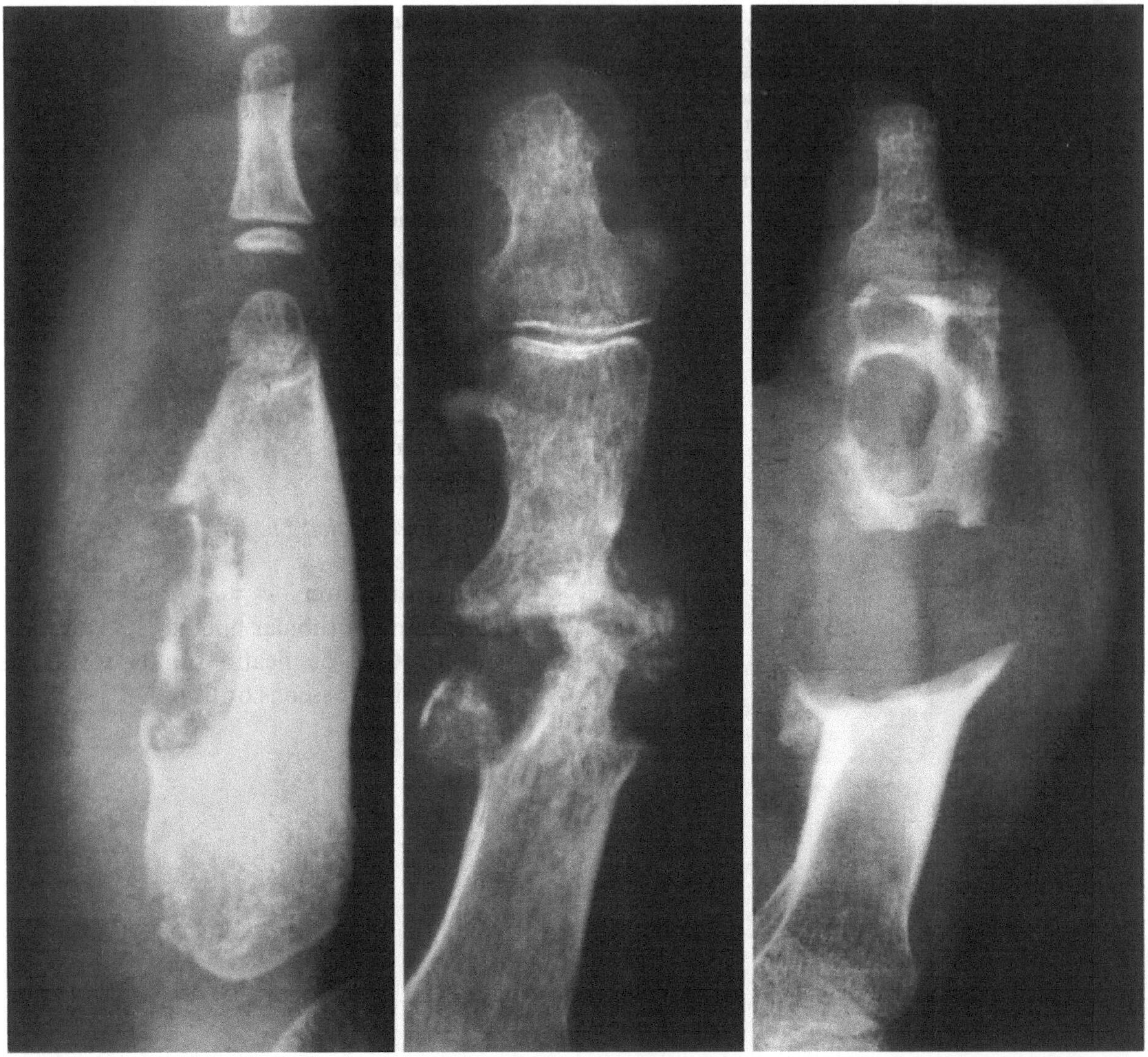

a–c

Fig. 95. a Tuberculosis of the fifth metatarsal bone. Thickening and extensive osteosclerosis. A number of sequestra are present. (By courtesy of Dr. W.P. Cockshott, Hamilton, Ont., Canada.) **b** Tuberculosis of the first metatarsophalangeal joint. Woman, 59 years old. Family history of tuberculosis. Three years physician's delay. Histology consistent with tuberculosis, positive culture for *M. bovis*. Synovitis with destruction of the joint space and the head of the first metatarsal bone. Marginal erosions and ossifications in the para-articular soft tissues. **c** Tuberculosis of the first metatarsophalangeal joint with severe destruction of bone and huge soft tissue swelling

8.3.3 **Differential Diagnosis** (Fig. 96)

8.3.3.1 Ankle Joint

- Pyogenic arthritis.
- Pyogenic osteomyelitis, localized as Brodie's abscess.
- Adult rheumatoid arthritis.
- Primary bone tumor.
- Metastatic disease.
- Osteoarthrosis.
- Neuropathic disease.
- Sympathic reflex dystrophy.
- Villonodular synovitis.
- Hemophilia.

8.3.3.2 Intertarsal and Tarsometatarsal Joints

- Pyogenic arthritis.
- Pyogenic osteomyelitis.
- Adult rheumatoid arthritis.
- Sympathic reflex dystrophy.
- Apophysitis of the calcaneus.
- Köhler's bone disease (navicular bone).
- Primary bone tumor.
- Metastatic disease.

8.3.3.3 Metatarsal Bones, Phalanges and Metatarsophalangeal Joints

- Pyogenic arthritis.
- Pyogenic osteomyelitis.
- Adult rheumatoid arthritis.
- Gout.
- Reiter's syndrome.
- Primary bone tumor.
- Metastatic disease.

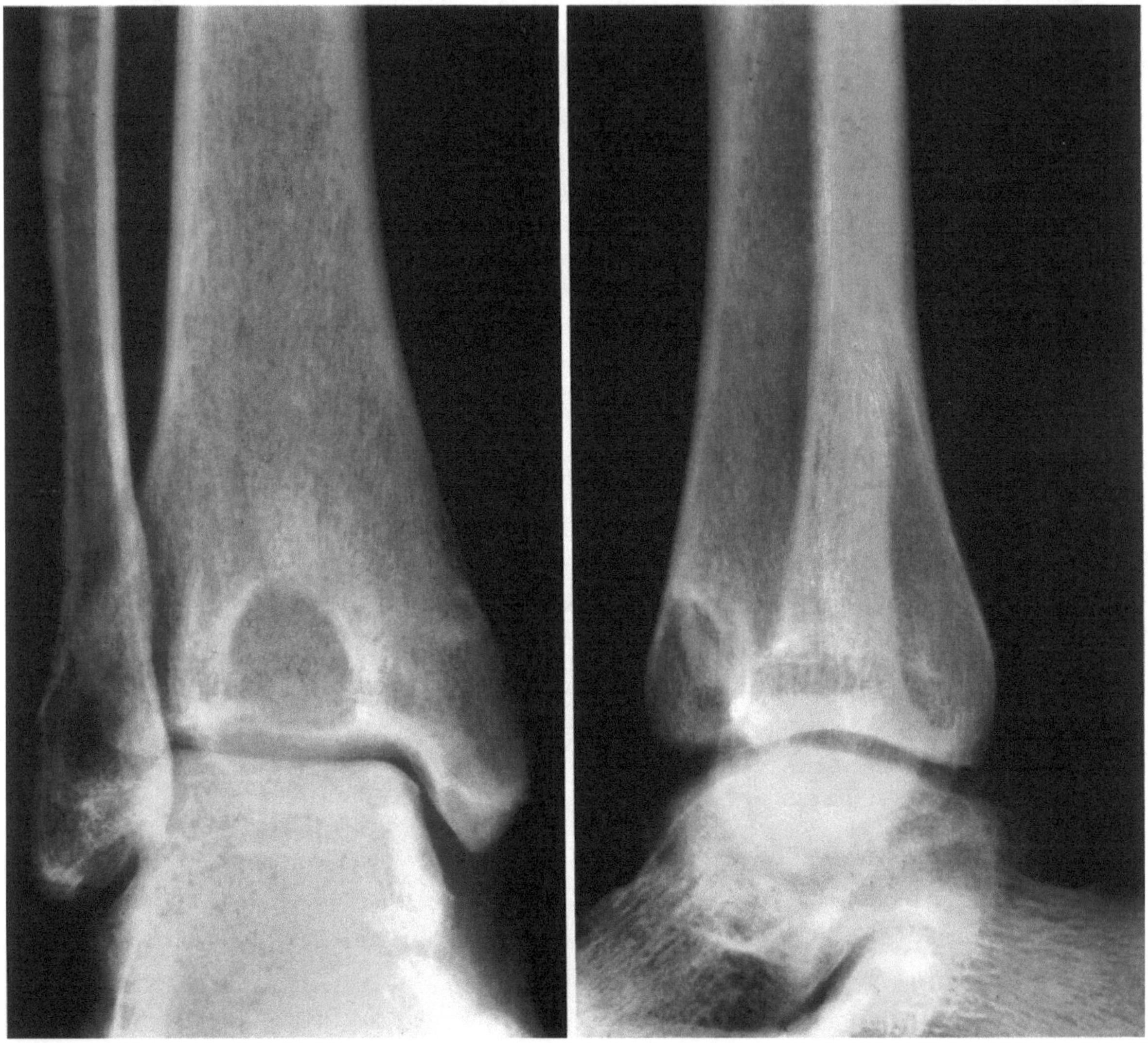

a b

Fig. 96 a, b. Differential diagnosis: pyogenic osteomyelitis, Brodie's abscess. Well-defined bone cavity with marginal osteosclerosis

9 Sacroiliac Joint

Tuberculous affection of the sacroiliac joints is a disease of adults and has been described at rates ranging from 0.5%–4.2% [64, 109, 147]. In our patients 12 cases (2.6%) of this type of osseous tuberculosis were found, all in adult patients. Multifocal lesions proved to be present in eight of these patients (Fig. 117). Localizations were: two in the shoulder, one in elbow, one in spine, two in greater trochanter, one in knee, and one in ankle. Although most patients present with unilateral involvement of the sacroiliac joints, bilateral affection may also occur; this is present in one of our patients. The initial stages of joint affection are usually difficult to detect because of the specific anatomy of the joint and the superimposion with intestinal shadows. Radioisotope scans may be of help (Fig. 97).

9.1 Pathology

Synovitis of the capsule and osseous foci in the vicinity of the joint as well as burrowing psoas abscesses are the initial lesions which are responsible for the involvement of the sacroiliac joint. The initial osseous foci are usually situated in the sacrum. After extension to the joint, destruction of joint cartilage and subcortical bone takes place. Abscesses are located mostly on the dorsal side of the joint; in other cases they may be situated anterior to the joint and in the perineal region [109]. Sinuses may be present.

9.2 Radiologic Findings (Figs. 97–101)

- Demineralization/osteoporosis.
- Erosions of the joint margins.
- Joint space widening.
- Bone cavities.
- Marginal osteosclerosis.
- Sequestra.
- Step formation in the symphysis in severe destruction of the sacroiliac joint [174].
- Healing and healed stages: spontaneous bony fusion, periarticular calcifications.

9.3 Differential Diagnosis

- Ankylosing spondylitis.
- Pyogenic arthritis.
- Psoriatic arthritis.
- Reiter's syndrome.
- Posttraumatic joint destruction.
- Primary bone tumor.
- Metastatic disease.

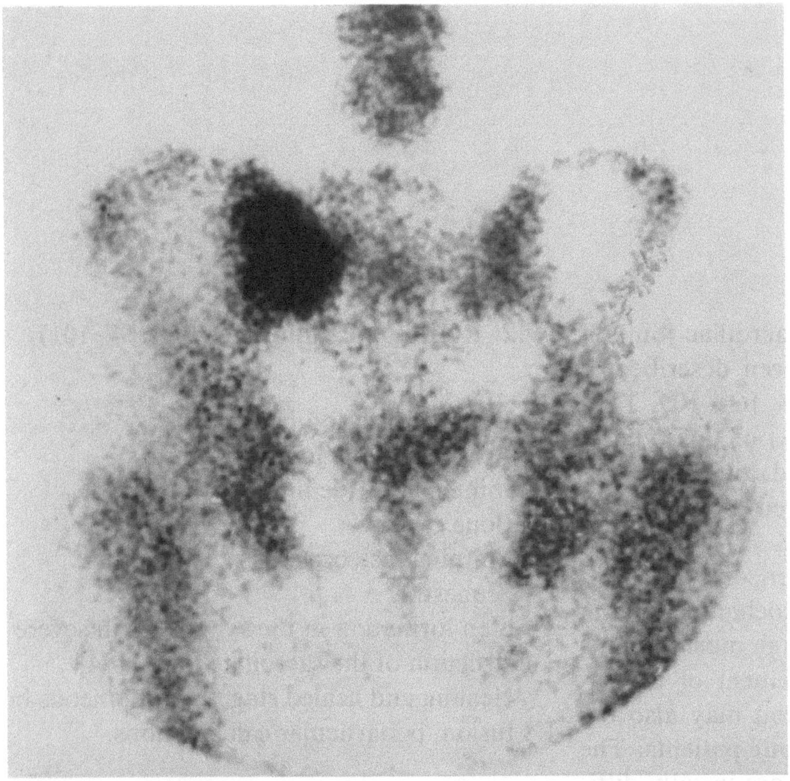

a

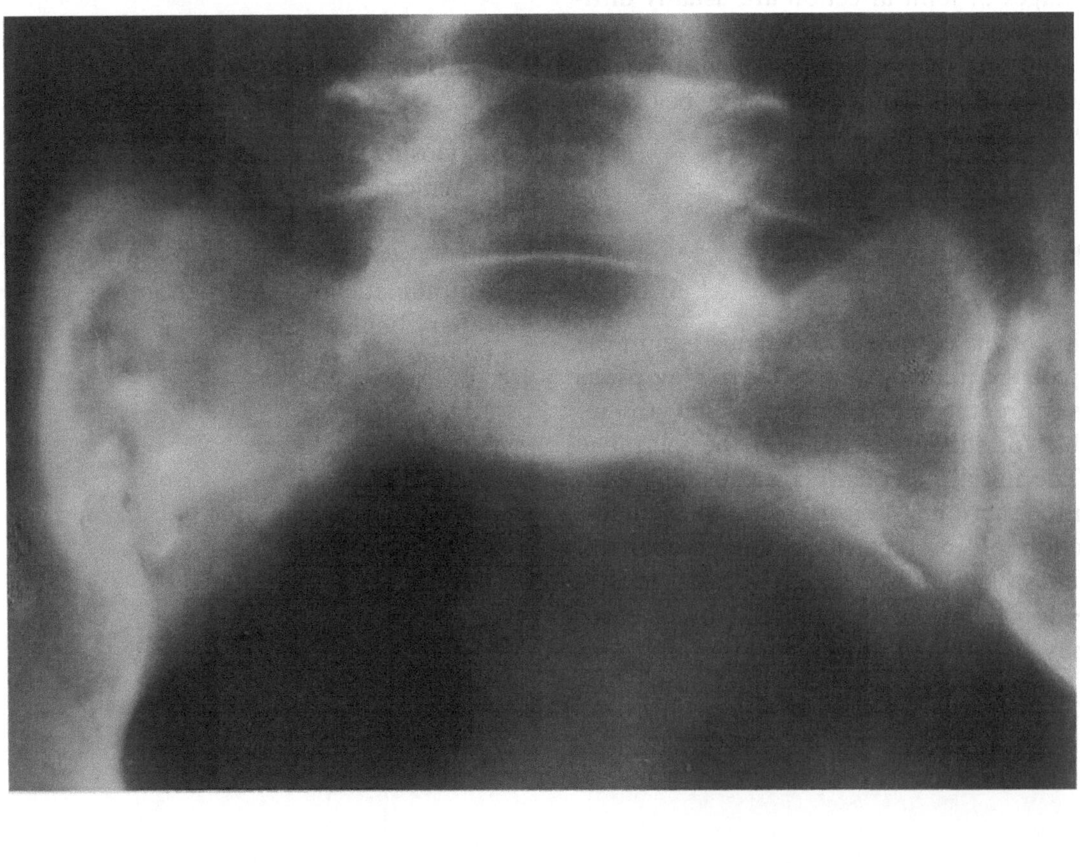

b

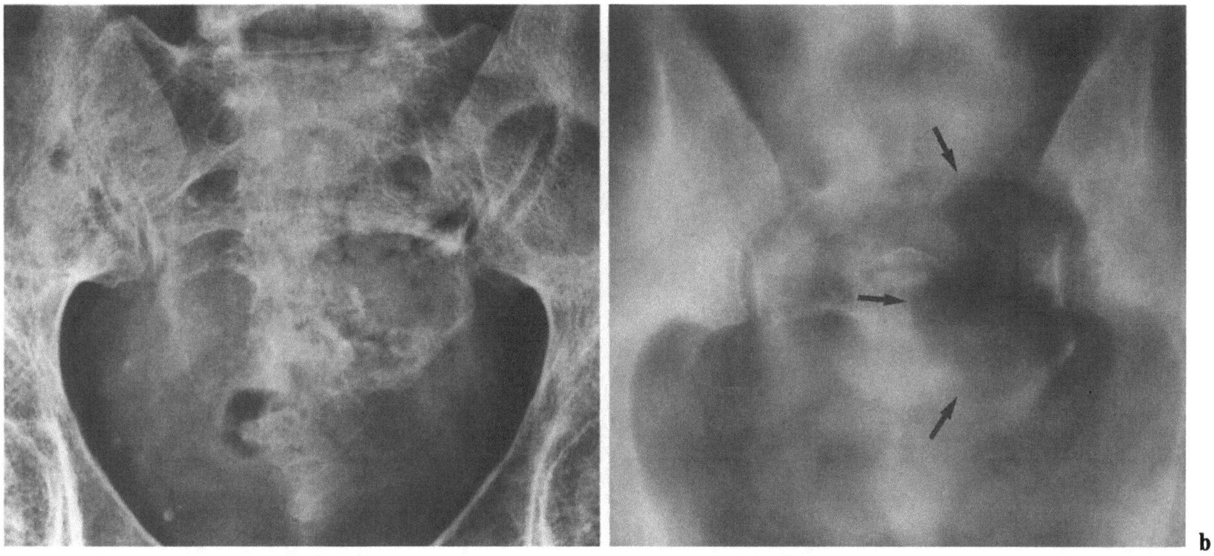

a b

Fig. 98 a, b. Tuberculous involvement of the sacrum. Chinese man, 38 years old. Other active tuberculous lesions were found in two ribs (*M. bovis*). Conventional radiography and tomography of the sacrum and sacroiliac joint: tuberculous bone cavity in the left wing of the sacrum without affection of the sacroiliac joint. Lytic well-defined lesion without marginal osteosclerosis (*arrows*)

◀ **Fig. 97 a, b.** Tuberculous arthritis of the sacroiliac joint. Woman, 67 years old. Other tuberculous focus in the cervical spine and previous tuberculous pleuritis. **a** High radioisotope uptake in the region of the right sacroiliac joint. **b** Active tuberculous sacroiliitis with destruction of the joint contours. Marginal osteosclerosis and probably a cortical sequestrum, suggestive of an older process

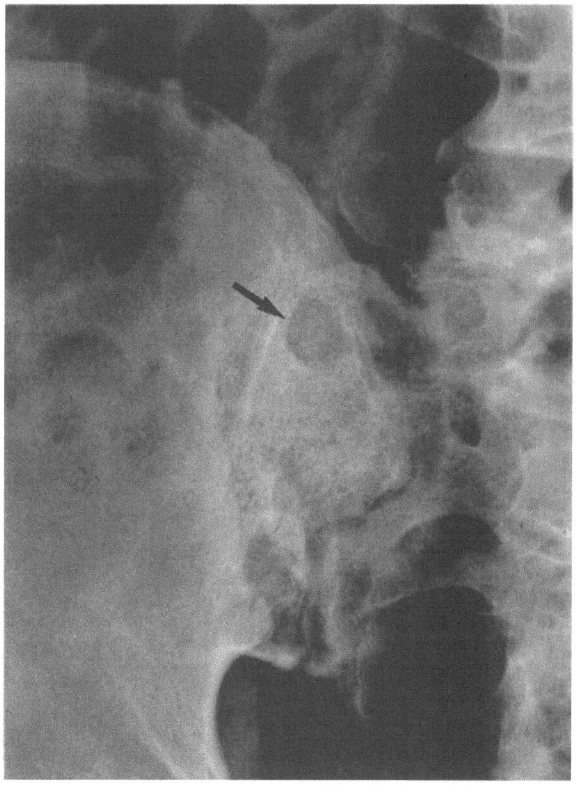

Fig. 99. Tuberculous involvement of the sacroiliac joint. Man, 70 years old. Previous tuberculous pleuritis and tuberculous gonitis. Some widening of the joint space, with irregular margins. Small osseous focus in the sacrum with slight marginal osteosclerosis and small sequestrum (*arrow*)

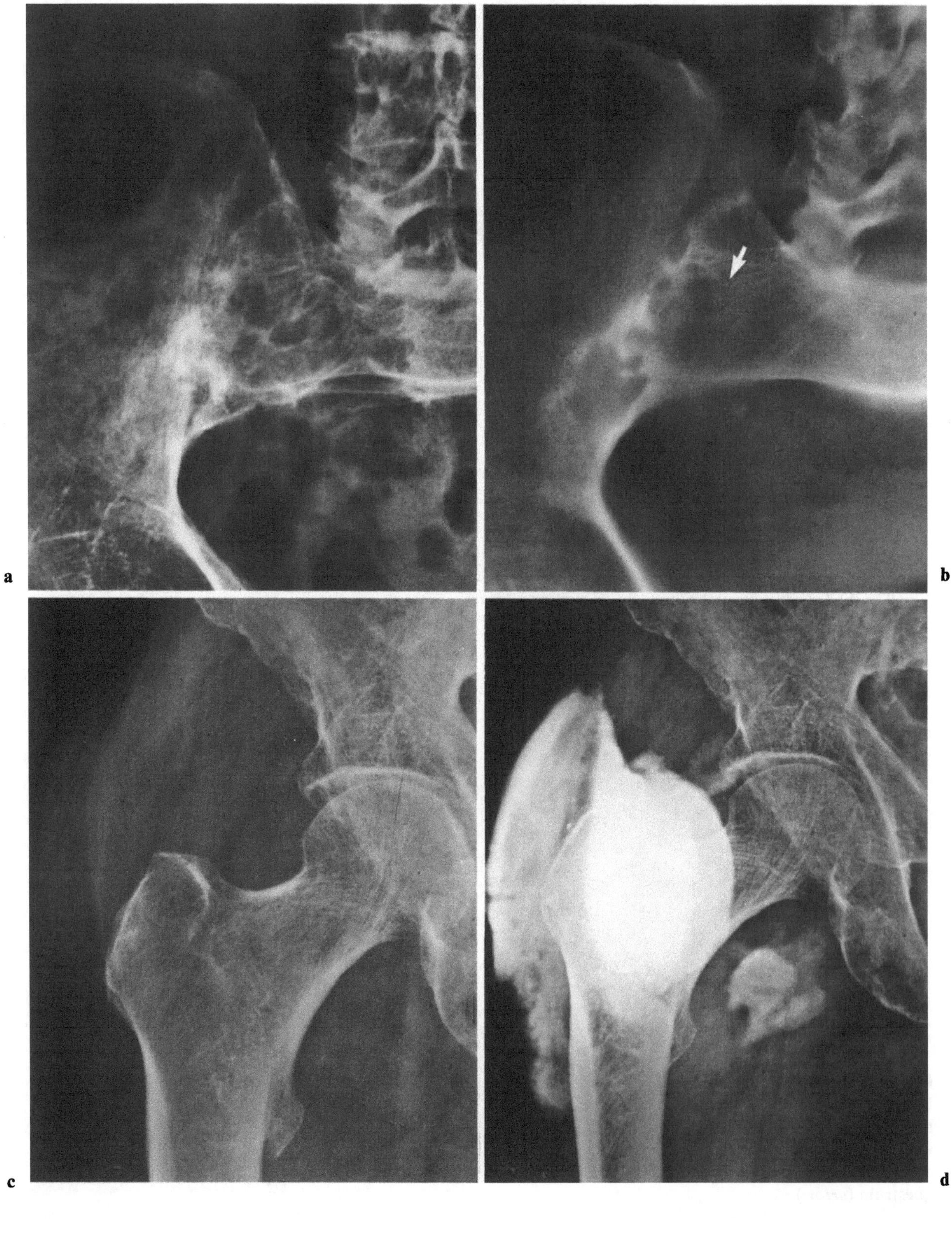
a
b
c
d

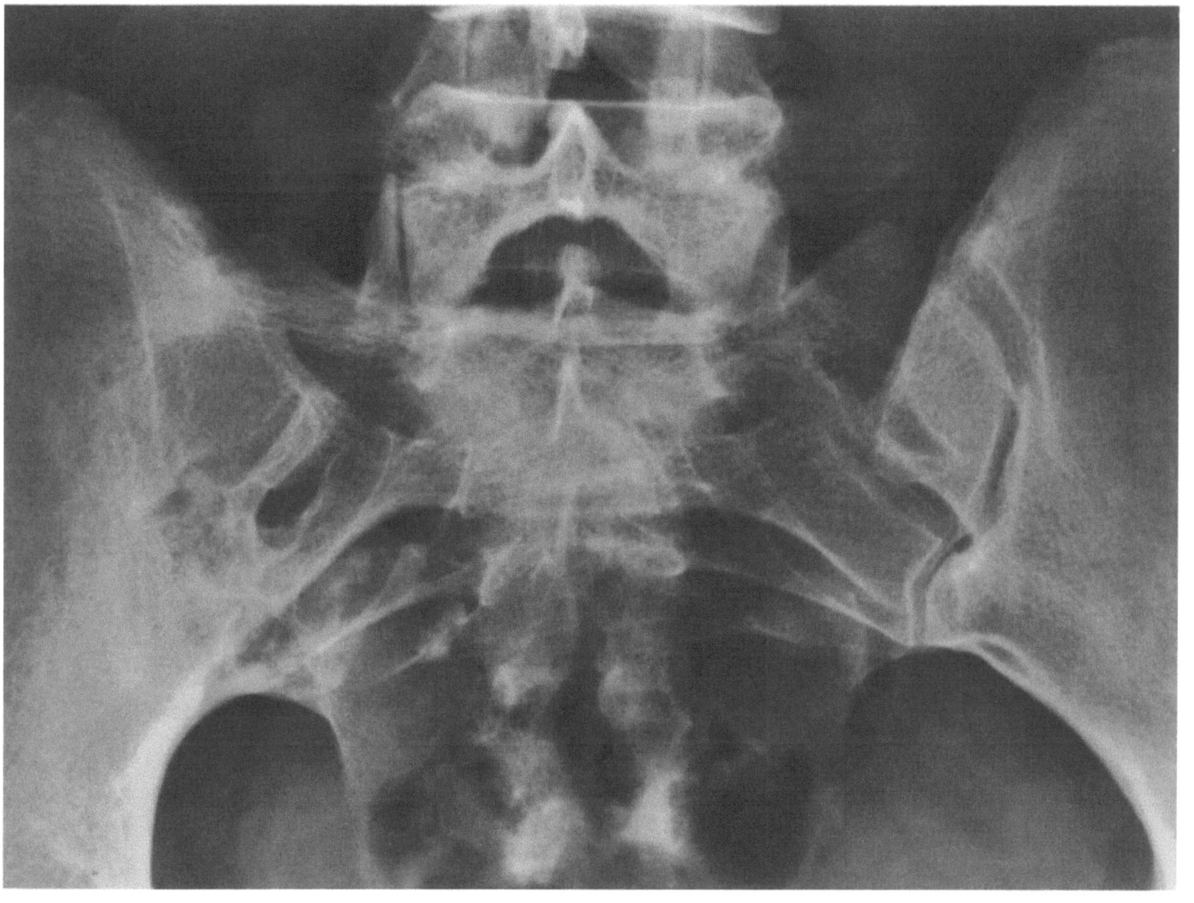

◀ **Fig. 100a–d.** Tuberculous involvement of the right sacroiliac joint and burrowing abscess. Man, 74 years old. **a, b** AP radiography and tomography present bony caverns adjacent to the right sacroiliac joint with at least one small sequestrum (*arrow*). The joint space is vanished. Marginal osteosclerosis. **c, d** Soft tissue swelling around the femoral neck caused by burrowing abscess. After puncture and injection of contrast medium, depiction of the abscess cavities (**d**)

Fig. 101. Healed tuberculous involvement of the sacroiliac joint. Woman, 37 years old. Previous pulmonary tuberculosis and multifocal tuberculous lesions of the spine and right kidney. Spontaneous bony fusion of the right sacroiliac joint with presacral calcification in the soft tissues

10 Tuberculous Osteomyelitis

In tuberculous osteomyelitis the disease is confined to an affected bone without involvement of an adjacent joint(s). In the tubular bones foci are localized in the epi/metaphysis or the diaphysis. Other manifestations of tuberculous osteomyelitis can be demonstrated in the flat bones (ribs, pelvic bones, skull, scapula) and at other sites, for example, in the greater trochanter. The frequency of tuberculous osteomyelitis has been reported at 3% [158] to 19% [109]. In our material the total incidence of tuberculous osteomyelitis of the greater trochanter, ribs, pelvic bones, sternum, and tubular bones together was 9%. Separate sections are devoted here to these localizations.

10.1 Long Tubular Bones

Tuberculous involvement of the small tubular bones of the hand and feet are discussed in Sects. 7.3 and 8.3.

In most cases the metaphyseal medulla of the long tubular bones are the sites where tuberculous bacilli settle. The tuberculous lesions may remain in the metaphyseal region or cross the growth plate and invade the epiphysis. Crossing of the growth plate is rarely found in pyogenic osteomyelitis but may be seen occasionally (Fig. 86). Checking the integrity of the joint is very important to make sure that the lesion is only tuberculous osteomyelitis and not an early stage of arthritis caused by perforation of the osseous focus into the adjacent joint [109].

Necrosis of bony tissue and caseation within the bone cavern causes abscess formation. Draining sinuses caused by rupture of tuberculous osteomyelitis may occur. In most series, cases of initial diaphyseal tuberculous osteomyelitis of the long tubular bones are rarely encountered, but sometimes the incidence proves to be rather high [102, 106, 109, 144]. In our material only two patients with this manifestation were found. Extensive periosteal bone formation may lead to a large expansion of the affected bone. As in other tuberculous skeletal lesions, multiple foci in the same individual may be present.

The characteristic radiologic presentation of tuberculous osteomyelitis is a slowly growing ill-defined skeletal lesion with bone destruction and only little formation of medullary or cortical bone [43, 172], however the radiologic aspects can vary widely.

10.1.1 Radiologic Findings (Figs. 102–106)

- Soft tissue swelling.
- Demineralization and osteoporosis.
- Bone cavity: This mostly metaphyseal cavity is either an ill-defined osseous lesion or a lesion with some marginal osteosclerosis [1, 2, 109, 172]. Tomography, CT, or MRI are often useful. The growth plate may be crossed by the tuberculous process (Figs. 67, 68, 78).
- Sequestra: As a necrotic sequela of spongiosal bone within a bone cavern, this is a quite characteristic phenomenon. Sequestration of cortical bone, however, presents a different radiologic finding, usually with huge periosteal bone formation. Examples of this are seen in patients with tuberculous dactylitis (Figs. 59–61).
- Destruction of the cortex: Fractures may occur.

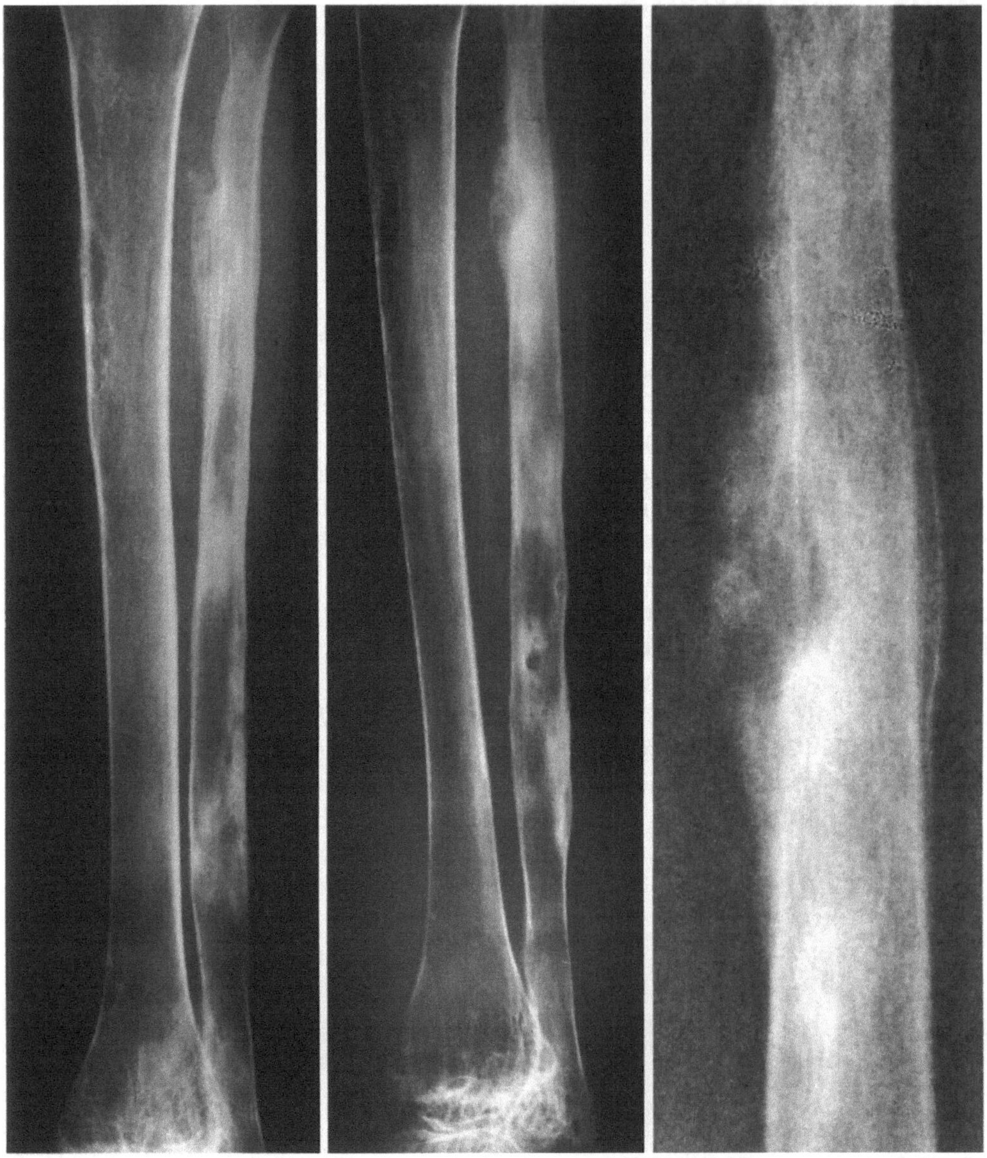

a–c

- Periosteal bone formation: Either slight or extensive periosteal bone formation may be found.
- Abscesses and sinuses.
- Disturbances in growth and ossification: These depend on affection of the growth plate(s).
- Osteosclerosis: Marginal osteosclerosis may be seen around a bone cavity. Usually osteosclerosis is predominant in the long-standing cases and during therapy.

Fig. 102a–c. Tuberculous osteomyelitis. Man, 17 years old. Previous tuberculous arthritis of the hip joint. After 2 years tuberculous affection of the right fibula. The diaphysis of the fibula is affected over a long distance. Focal osteosclerosis. Proximally in the fibula is an area of extensive osteosclerosis, cortical destruction, and periosteal bone reaction (*detail*, **c**). (By courtesy of Dr. J.A.M. Lemmens, Nijmegen, The Netherlands.)

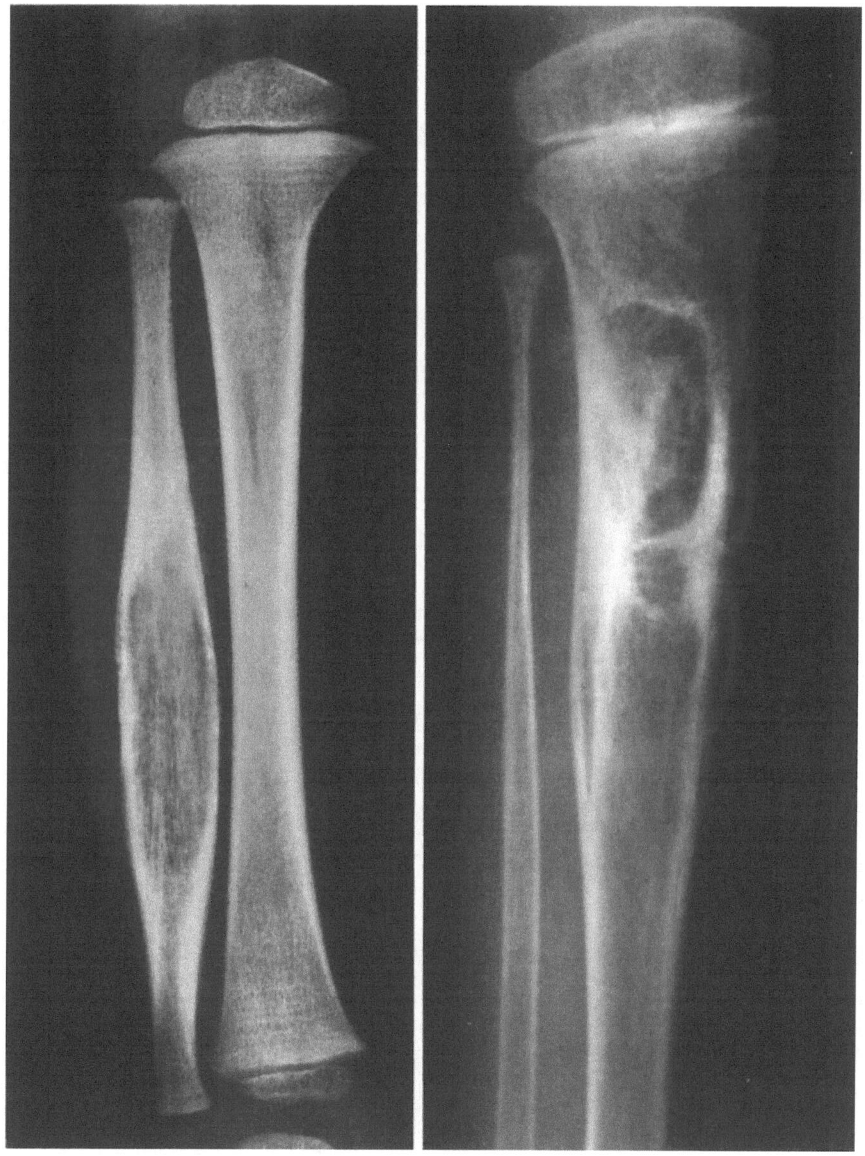

a b

10.1.2 Differential Diagnosis

- Pyogenic osteomyelitis.
- Primary bone tumor.
- Metastatic disease.
- Histiocytosis.
- Aggressive fibromatosis.

Fig. 103 a, b. Tuberculosis of the lower leg. **a** Tuberculous osteomyelitis of the fibula. The diaphysis of the fibula is largely expanded by periosteal bone formation. A cystlike tuberculous focus is clearly depicted. (By courtesy of Prof. B.J. Cremin, Cape Town, South Africa.) **b** Tuberculous osteomyelitis of the tibia. Osseous lesion with marginal osteosclerosis and periosteal bone formation. (By courtesy of Dr. W.P. Cockshott, Hamilton, Ont., Canada.)

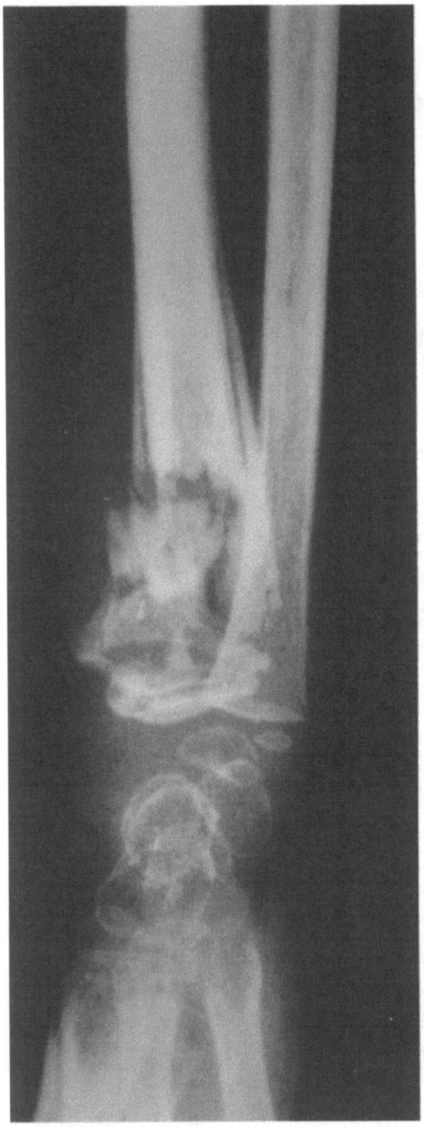

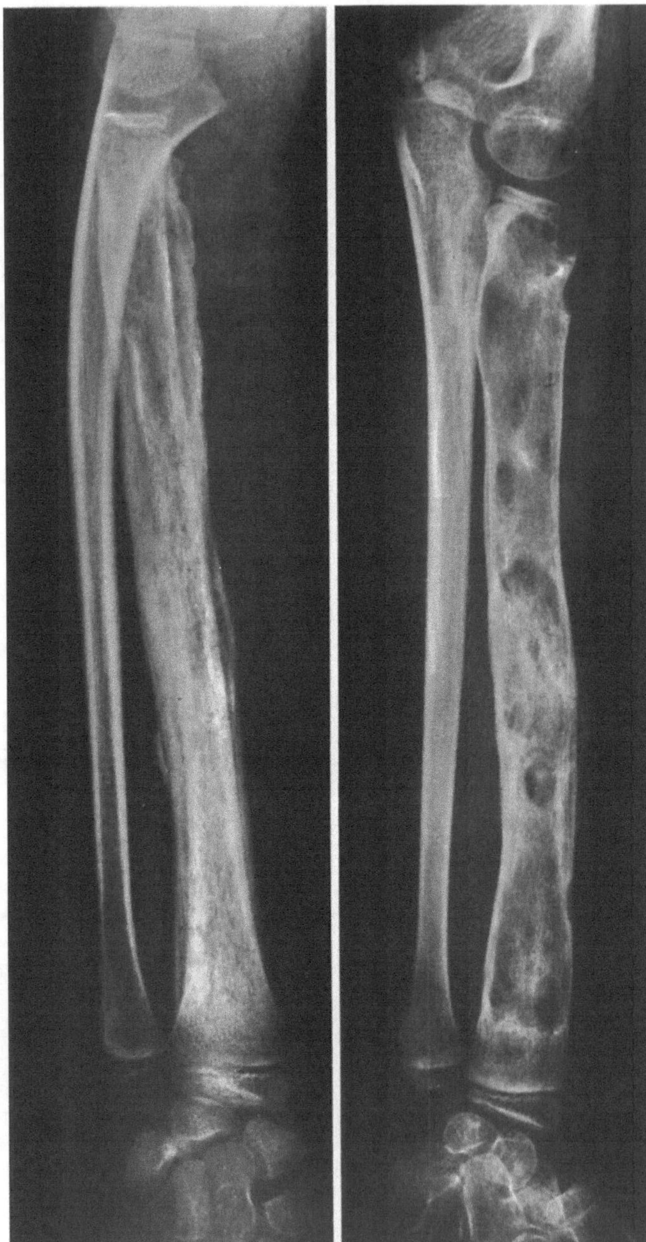

a b

Fig. 104. Tuberculous osteomyelitis of the radius in a child. The distal metaphysis of the radius presents a large osseous focus, probably with a large sequestrum. Cortex destruction and pathologic fractures have developed. (By courtesy of Prof. B.J. Cremin, Cape Town, South Africa.)

Fig. 105a, b. Tuberculous osteomyelitis of the radius. Child, 9 years old. (By courtesy of Prof. B.J. Cremin, Cape Town, South Africa.) **a** Affection of the whole diaphysis with extensive periosteal bone formation. The initial focus seems to be present in the middle of the radius. **b** After 5 months, chemotherapy: a pseudocystic appearance has developed, possibly with formation of a small sequestrum more distally in the radius. In the proximal metaphysis the radial contour presents a small area of destruction. As a whole, the width of the radius has increased

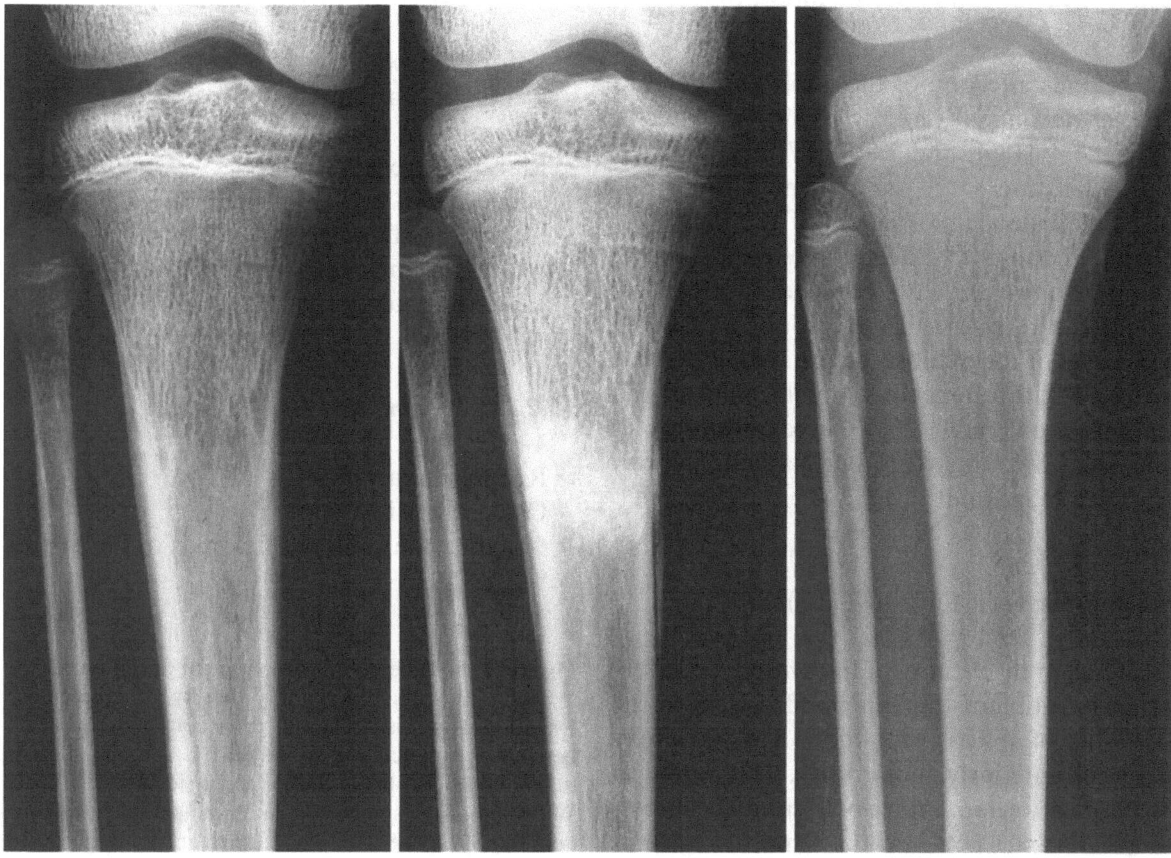

–c

Fig. 106a–c. Tuberculous osteomyelitis. Girl, 11 years old. Previous primary pulmonary tuberculosis. **a** Slight periosteal bone formation. **b** After immobilization and antituberculous chemotherapy: more prominent periosteal bone formation and osteosclerosis. **c** Complete restoration of the bony structures after one year

10.2 Pubis, Symphysis, Ischium, and Ilium

Tuberculous affection of the pubis and ischium is rather uncommon; rates of 0.3% [173], 0.5% [109], 0.7% [139], and 1.8% [67] are reported in the literature. Only one patient with an isolated tuberculous involvement of the ilium was encountered in our file. Examples of this manifestation, however, have been described in recent literature [145]. In our group of patients three cases of tuberculosis of the symphysis and two cases with tuberculous involvement of the ischium were found (1.2%). Three multifocal lesions were encountered in two patients (elbow, spine, sacroiliac joint).

10.2.1 Pubic Foci (Figs. 107–109)

Pubic foci in the vicinity of the symphysis rarely induce infection of this synchondrosis, with the possibility of abscess formation. Abscesses may be found anteriorly, posteriorly, and rarely in the perineal region. Anteriorly situated abscesses and/or extension into the femoral region is most common (Fig. 110). Radiologic findings vary with the degree of infection.

10.2.1.1 Active Disease

- Soft tissue swelling.
- Demineralization/osteoporosis.
- Widening of the symphysis.
- Marginal erosions.
- Sequestra.
- Marginal osteosclerosis.
- Abscesses and sinuses: CT is often of great value for detection of abscesses [173].

10.2.1.2 Healing and Healed Stages

- Remineralization.
- Osteosclerosis.
- Calcifications and ossifications in the soft tissue.

Fig. 107 a, b. Tuberculous involvement of the symphysis. ▶ Woman, 25 years old. Family history of tuberculosis. On admission, also bilateral cavernous pulmonary tuberculosis, tuberculous spondylitis L-2–L-3, and renal tuberculosis. Probably initial right-sided pubic focus. Widening of the symphysis, marginal osteosclerosis predominantly at the left side, and irregular margin in the lower half of the right pubic bone. Probably small sequestrum (*arrows*)

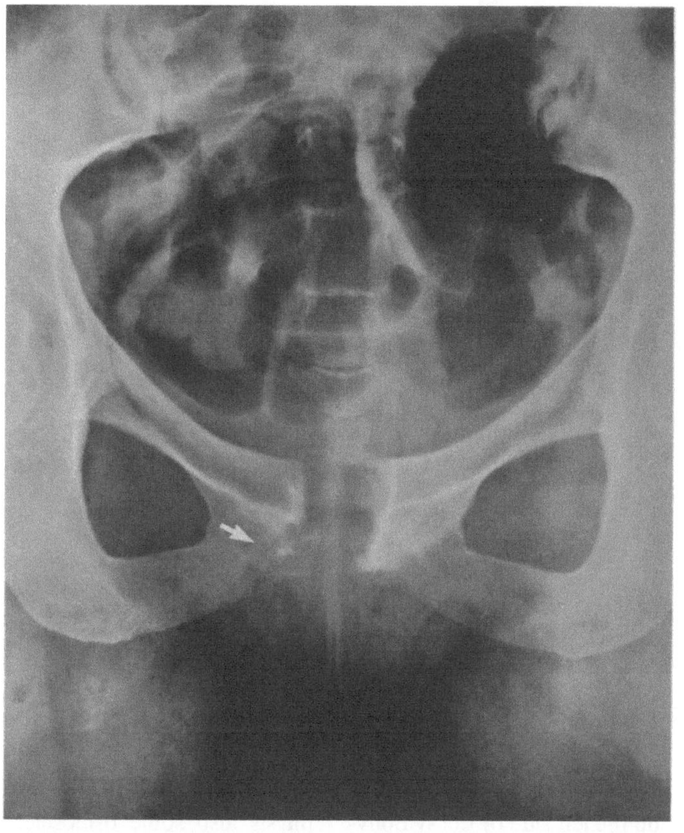

a

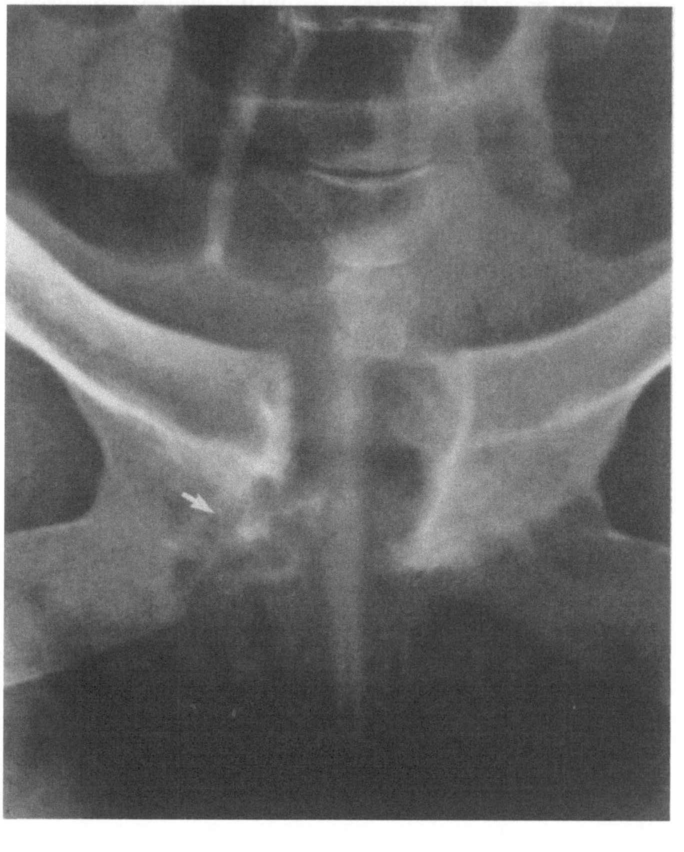

b

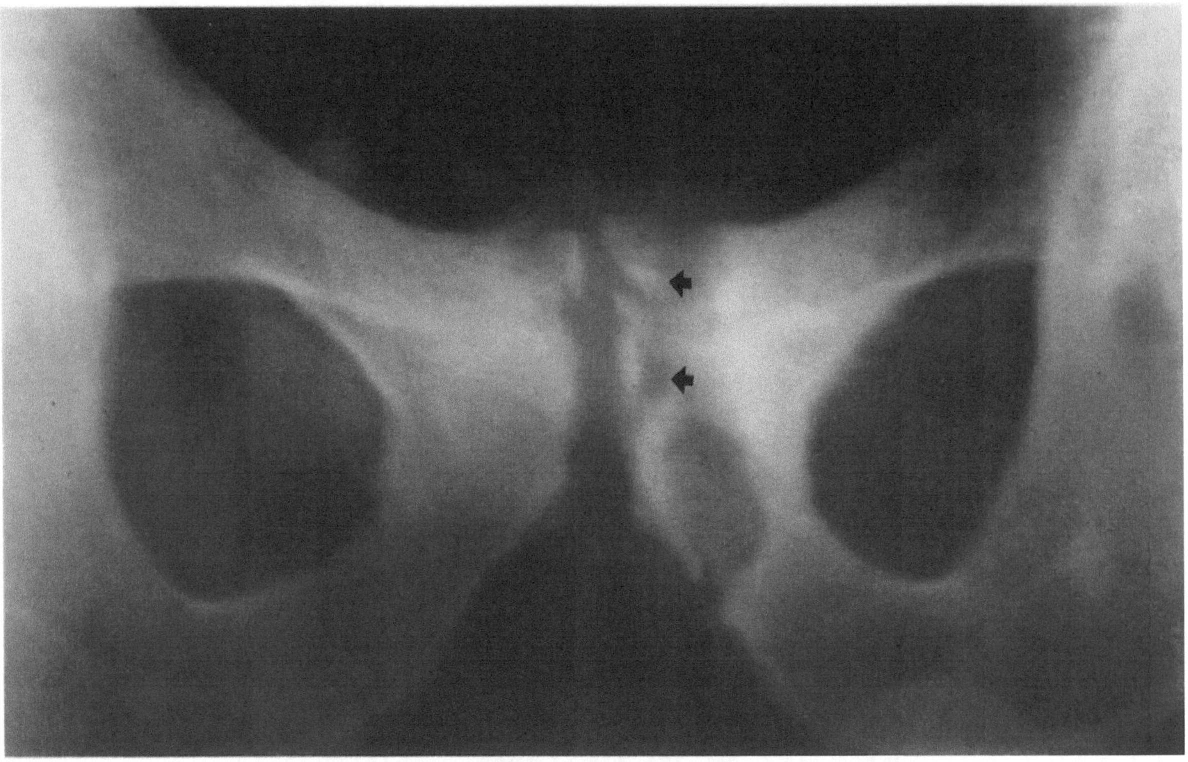

Fig. 108. Tuberculous involvement of the symphysis. Adult man. Bone caverns on the left side of the symphysis with marginal osteosclerosis and probably sequestra of cortical bone (*arrows*). On the right side of the symphysis also some osteosclerosis and marginal erosion cranially. Perifocal soft tissue swelling

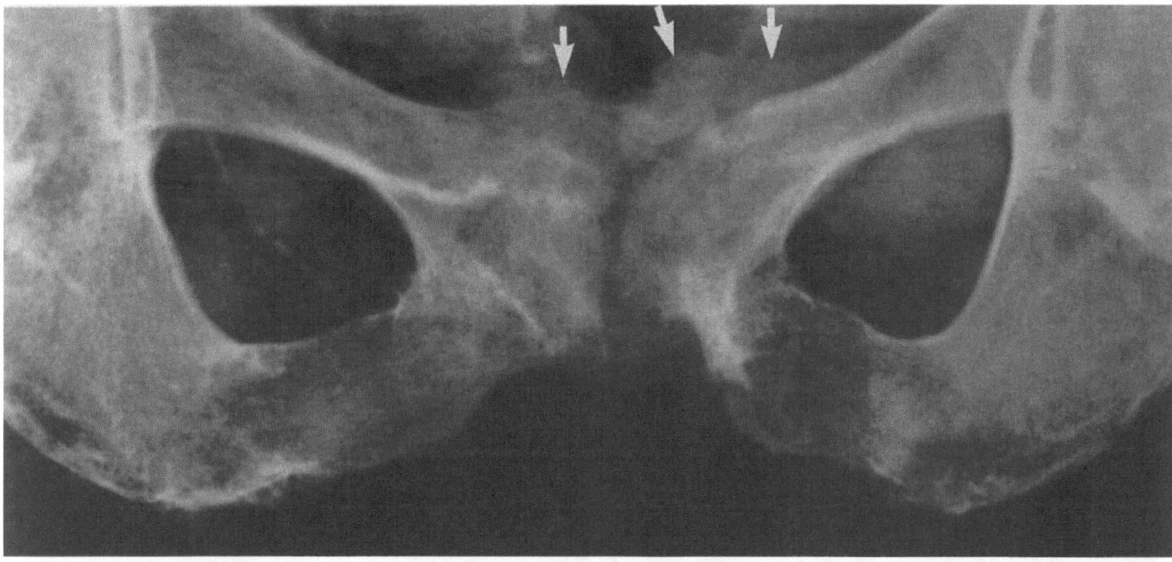

a

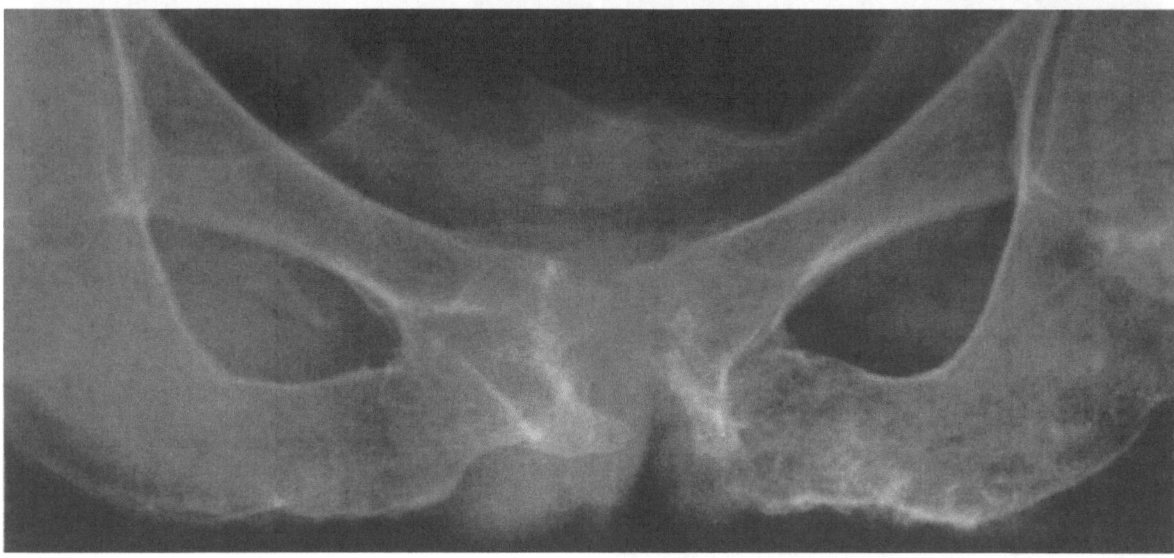

b

Fig. 109 a, b. Tuberculous involvement of the symphysis. Woman, 65 years old. No history of previous tuberculosis. Positive histologic findings of tuberculosis. **a** Severe demineralization of the pubic bone on both sides. Some widening of the symphysis, irregular bone contours, and some periosteal bone formation (*arrows*). **b** After 1 year: healing with remineralization and improved demarcation of the symphysis

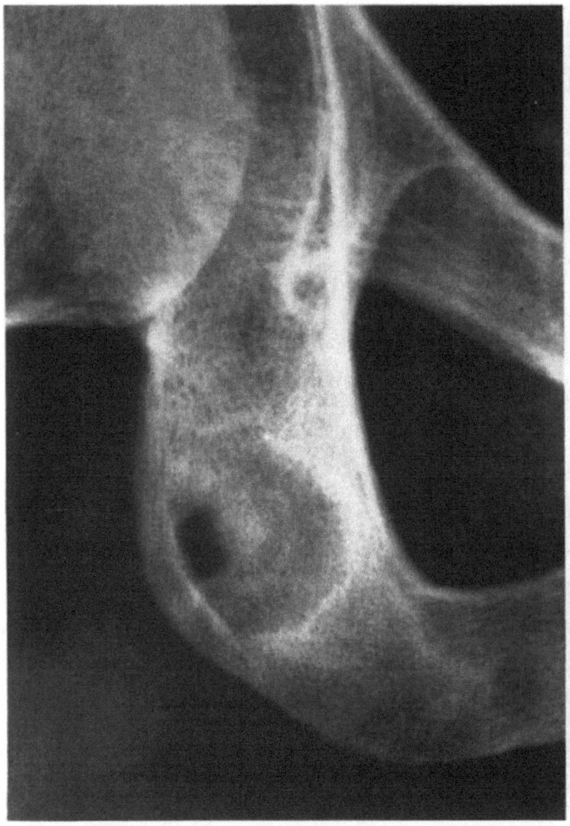

a

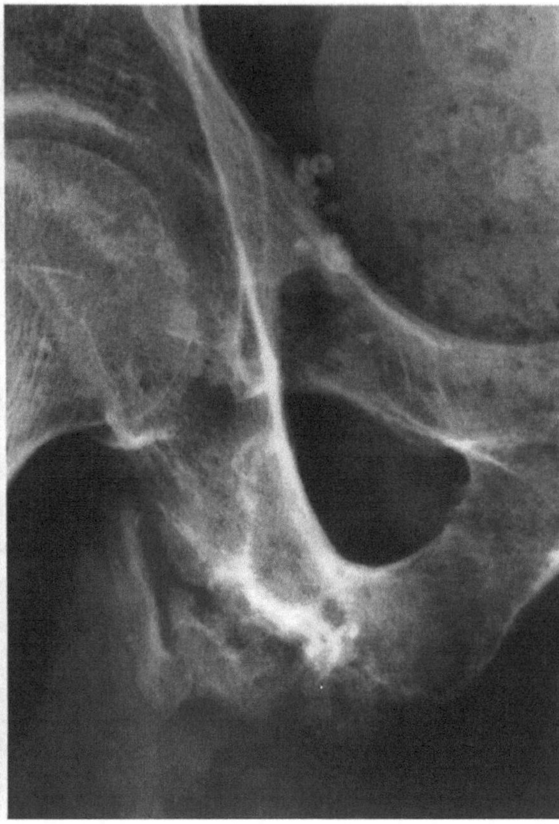

b

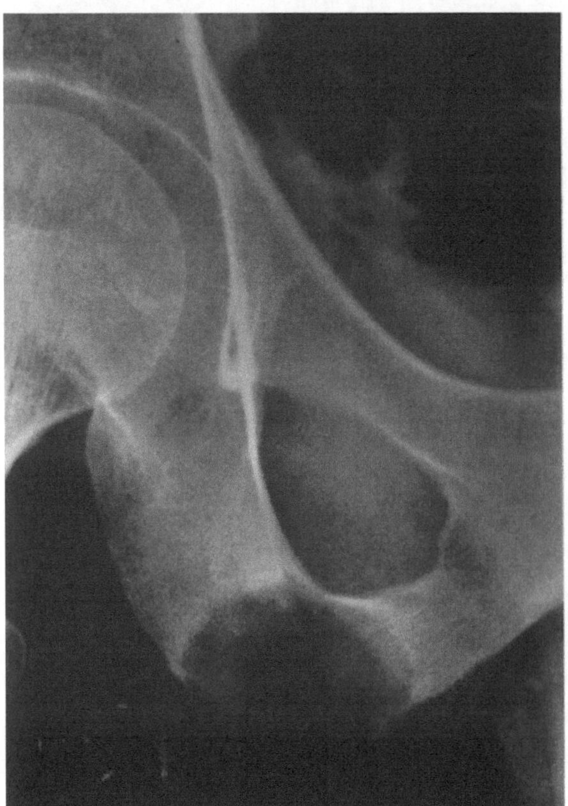

c

Fig. 110a–c. Two different patients with tuberculous involvement of the ischial tuberosity. **a** Man, 27 years old. Previous history of pulmonary tuberculosis and tuberculous arthritis of the left elbow (5 months after a local trauma). On admission, endogenous reactivation, also with positive sputum culture, tuberculous spondylitis T-10–L-1 and active tuberculous pleuritis. In the ischial tuberosity circumscribed cavern with marginal osteosclerosis. No affection of the hip joint. **b** Man, 71 years old. At the age of 51, draining sinus near the greater trochanter; "no diagnosis" at that time. Family history of tuberculosis. On admission, new draining sinus anteriorly and posteriorly. Positive culture for *M. tuberculosis*. The radiograph presents irregular contours of the ischial tuberosity and ossifications in the adjacent soft tissues. **c** Differential diagnosis: metastasis from bronchial carcinoma. Man, 41 years. Well-defined osteolytic defect without marginal osteosclerosis

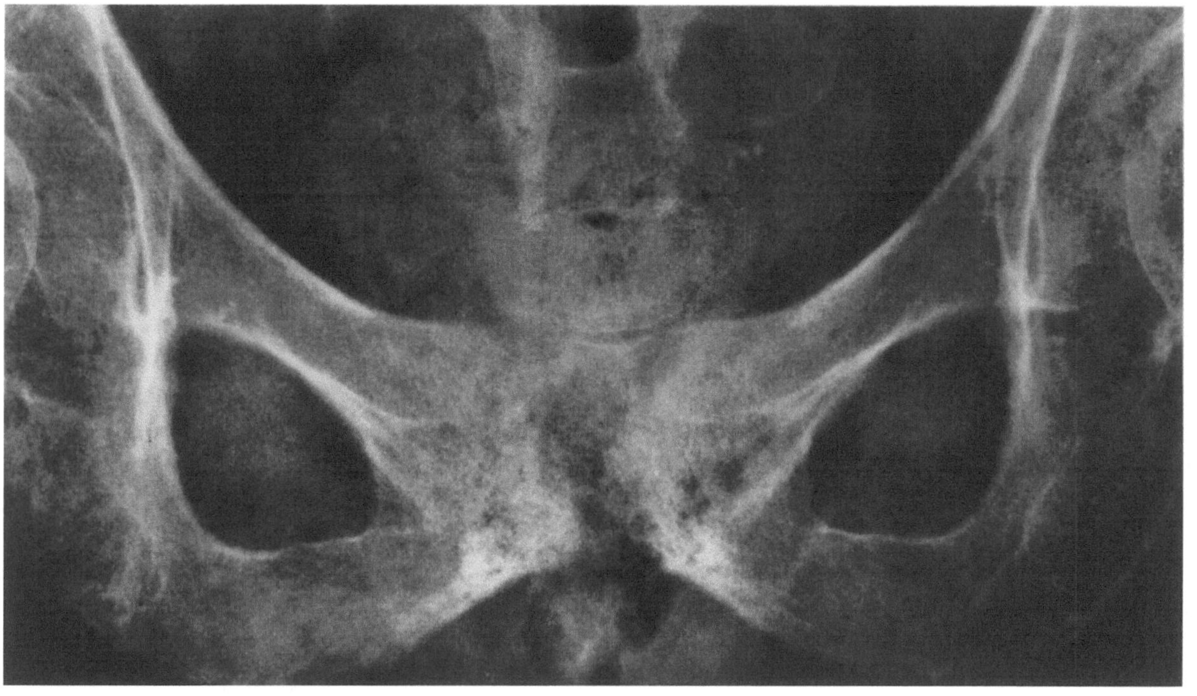

Fig. 111. Pyogenic affection of the symphysis. The radiologic findings are comparable to those of an acute stage of tuberculous involvement of the symphysis

10.2.1.3 Differential Diagnosis

- Pyogenic affection of the symphysis (Fig. 111).
- Symphysiolysis.

10.2.2 Ischial Foci (Fig. 110)

An ischial focus near the hip joint may infect the hip by perforation into the joint or infection of the synovial membrane. Ischial foci in the tuberosity usually do not extend to the hip. These present as osseous lesions with or without osteosclerotic margins and sequestra, depending on the time of onset and healing of this process. Secondary affection of the ischiogluteal bursa by an ischial tuberculous process may be found; otherwise the ischial tuberosity can be invaded by spread of the tuberculous infection from the adjacent affected bursa. In addition, long-standing traumatic bursitis has been described in patients sitting for a long time in a cross-legged position on a hard surface [26].

10.3 Ribs and Sternum

10.3.1 Ribs

Tuberculous affection of the ribs is rare. It may be present either as an initial rib lesion or secondary to tuberculous spondylitis or pleuritis [21, 64, 147]. In our hospital six examples of initial rib involvement have been found, and in three other patients the ribs were involved after tuberculous spondylitis (2%). Tuberculous osteomyelitis of the ribs is more common in patients from the tropics and is said to be the most common form of inflammatory lesions of the ribs in these patients. This is reported to be the most common site of bone tuberculosis in heroine addicts (we have seen this in one of our patients) and the second most common rib affection after metastatic disease [21, 57, 128, 165, 181]. One of the patients in our hospital presented other tuberculous lesions in another contralateral rib and in the sacrum. Multifocal lesions are described in the literature as common [47, 181]. Tuberculous rib involvement may be localized in the cartilage and/or in the osseous structures. In the former, only a soft tissue mass of the thoracic wall can be found without bone destruction.

10.3.1.1 Radiologic Findings (Figs. 112–114)

- Soft tissue swelling.
- Destruction of the rib with or without a pathologic fracture.
- Osseous focus: either ill-defined or well-defined.
- Periosteal bone formation: especially in non-white patients.
- Marginal osteosclerosis.
- Abscesses and sinuses.
- Residual deformity of the rib after healing.

10.3.1.2 Differential Diagnosis

- Myeloma.
- Metastatic disease.
- Primary bone tumor.
- Malignant lymphoma.
- Pyogenic osteomyelitis.
- Soft tissue tumors.

10.3.2 Sternum

Tuberculous infection of the sternum or the sternoclavicular joints is rare and is described at a rate of 1% or less [64, 109, 147]. In our material 14 patients (3%) with this manifestations were found. Four of these patients had multifocal osseous lesions (rib in one, spine in two, and mastoid in one). Infection of the sternum may be either hematogenous or secondary due to a tuberculous pleuritis. The osseous structures of the sternum are preferably affected, but extension to the manubriosternal synchondrosis or to the sternoclavicular joint is possible. The site of the sternum implies that abscesses may be difficult to detect. They may present themselves anterosternally or retrosternally or may spread into the sternocleidomastoid fascia [109]. They may also descend and perforate to the abdominal wall. In our patients at least three abscesses were found (anterosternally in one, upper abdomen in two). A sinus was present in one of these patients.

10.3.2.1 Radiologic Findings (Figs. 115, 116)

- Soft tissue swelling.
- Demineralization/osteoporosis.
- Osseous focus.
- Marginal erosions.
- Destruction of the manubriosternal synchondrosis.
- Abscesses and sinuses.
- Osteosclerosis.

10.3.2.2 Differential Diagnosis

- Pyogenic osteomyelitis.
- Myeloma.
- Metastatic disease.
- Primary bone tumor.

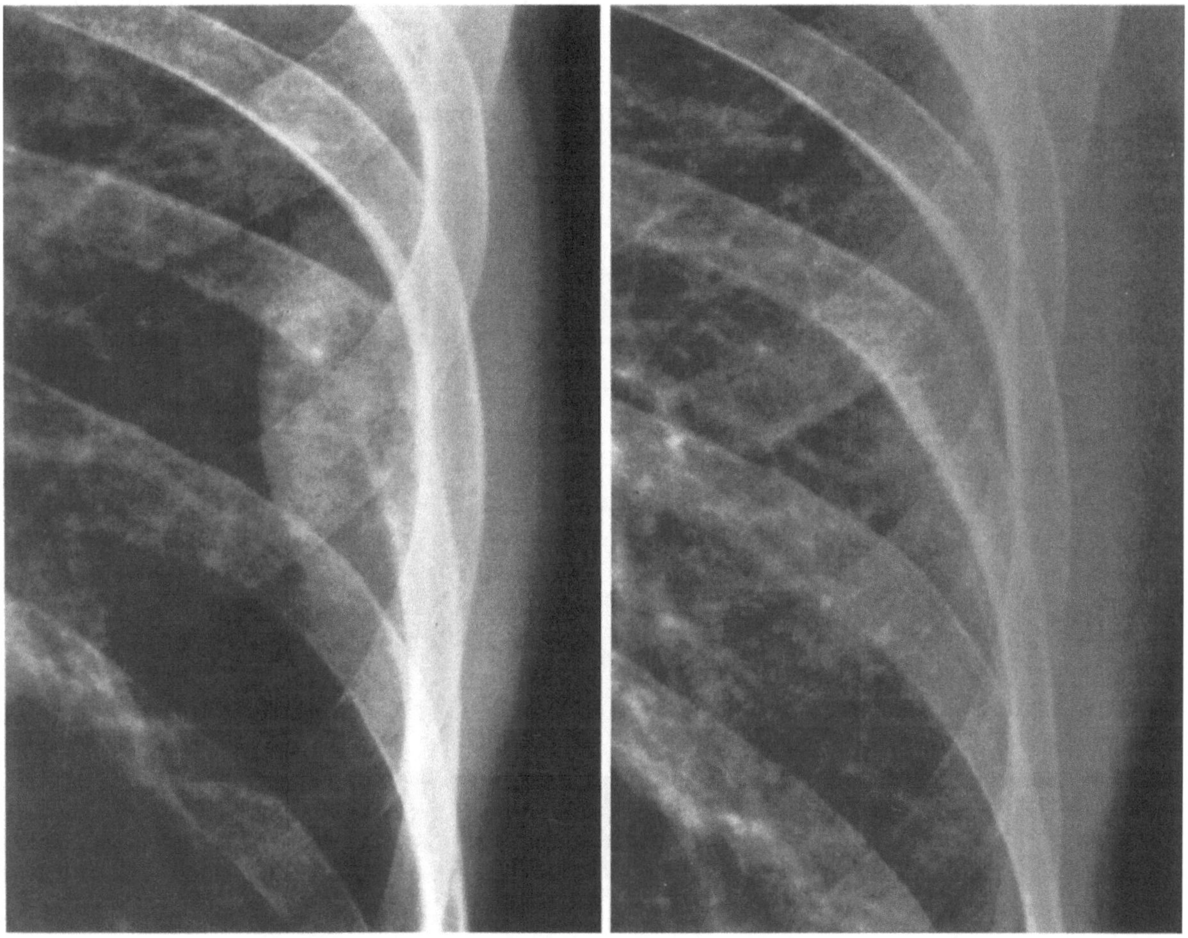

a b

Fig. 112 a, b. Tuberculous involvement of the rib. Same patient as in Fig. 98. **a** Osseous lesion in the eighth rib, with tuberculous abscess and positive culture for *M. bovis* by biopsy. Pathological fracture. **b** After 6 months, chemotherapy: healing of the tuberculous process with remineralization and consolidation of rib fracture. The abscess has vanished

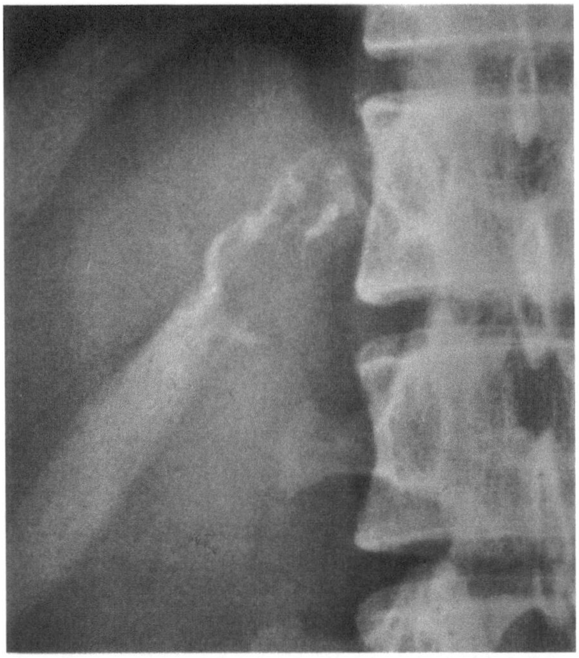

Fig. 113. Tuberculous involvement of the rib. Man, 43 years. No previous history of tuberculosis. On admission, pain during half a year on the right lower ribs posteriorly. Localized destruction of the 12th rib with cortex destruction and some osteosclerosis

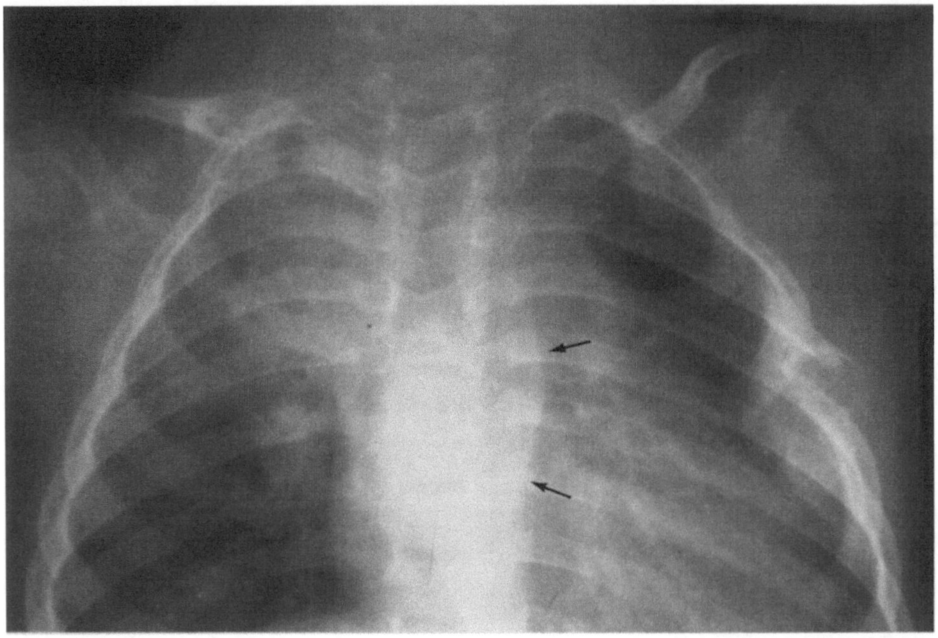

Fig. 114. Multifocal tuberculous affections. Tuberculous affections of the right clavicle, the upper lobe of the right lung, the thoracic spine, and the fourth left rib. Other foci were present in the humerus and the forearm. The rib lesion presents soft tissue swelling and a cystic appearance of the circumscribed tuberculous involvement. The right clavicle shows ballooning in the central part with intact contours. A paraspinal abscess as a consequence of tuberculous spondylitis is clearly detectable (*arrows*). (By courtesy of Dr. S.P. Bohrer, Winston-Salem, N.C., U.S.A.)

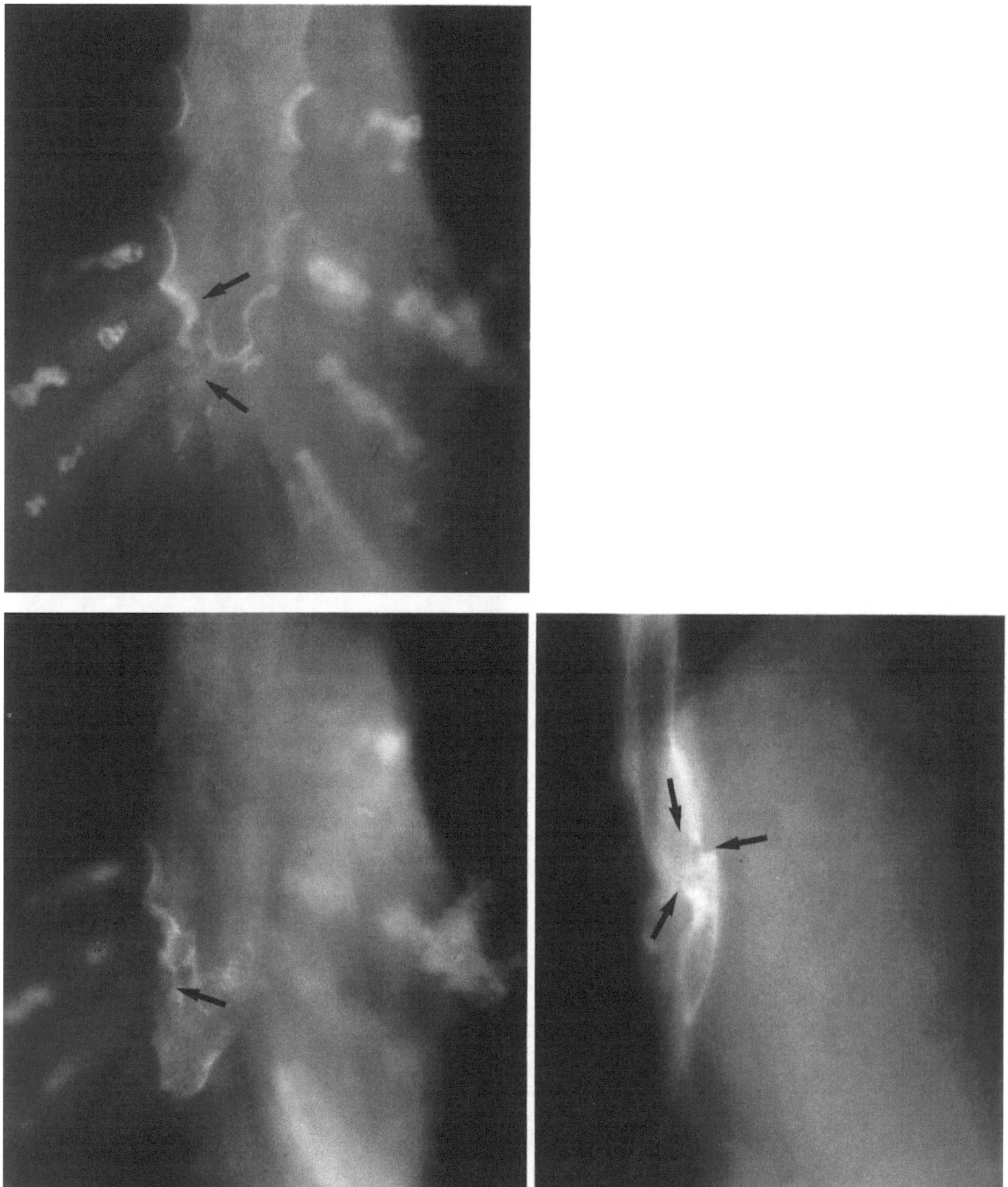

a

b

c

Fig. 115a–c. Tuberculous involvement of the sternum. Woman, 79 years old. Previous tuberculous pleuritis and tuberculous osteomyelitis of the greater trochanter and arthritis of the right elbow. On admission, draining sinus parasternally with positive culture for *M. tuberculosis*. Small osseous focus on the right posterior side of the sternum (*arrows*); a small bone cavern is present with cortical erosions and some osteosclerosis

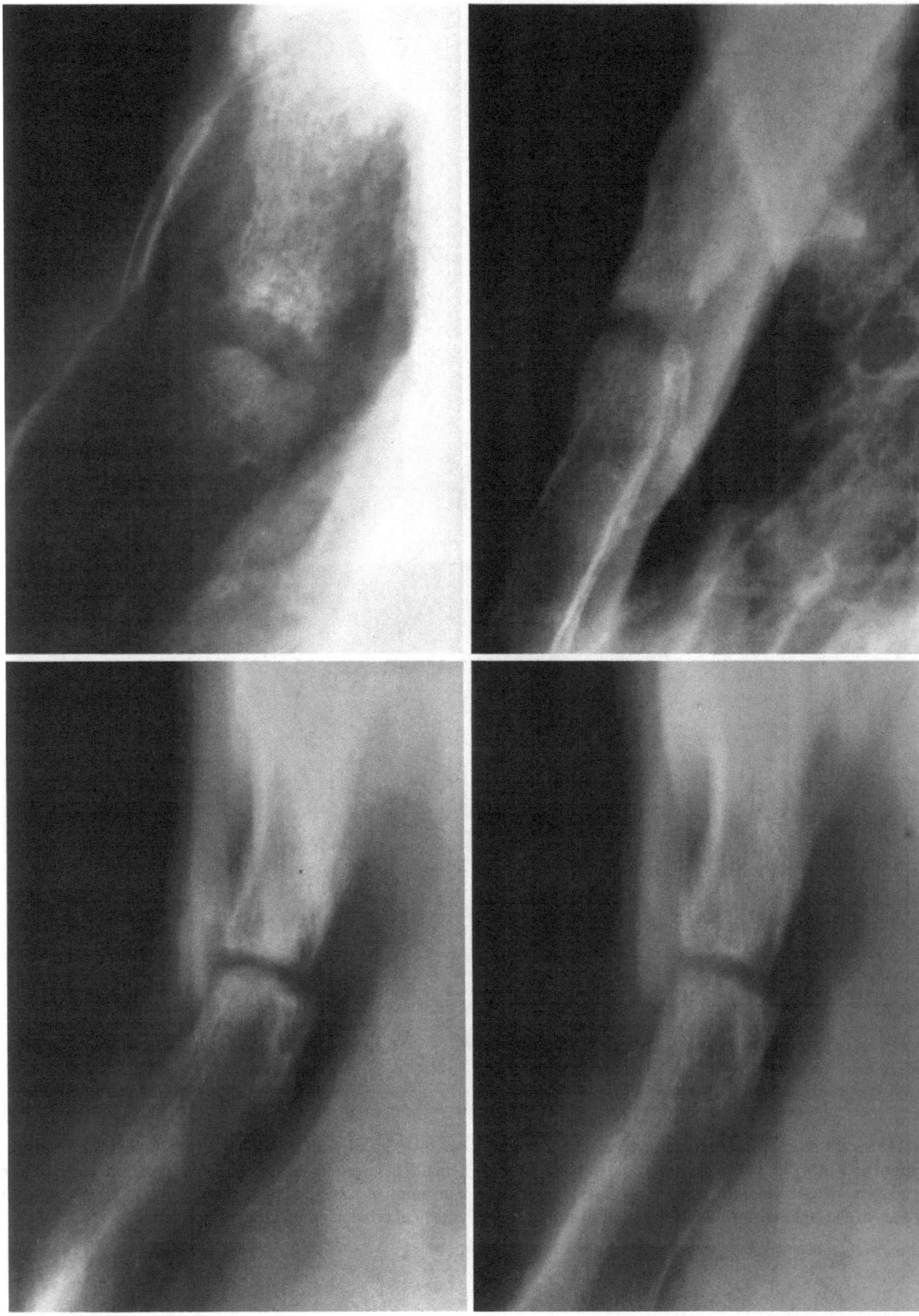

a b c d

◀ **Fig. 116a–d.** Tuberculosis of the sternum. Woman, 52 years old. At the age of 26, postpartum tuberculous pleuritis. Two years later, cavernous pulmonary tuberculosis; endogenous reactivation 10 years later. On admission, tuberculous involvement of the manubriosternal synchondrosis from a contiguous tuberculous empyema with draining sinus parasternally. **a** Demineralization and irregularity of the manubriosternal synchondrosis. **b** After 1 month: increased irregularity of the synchondrosis. **c** Ten months after **a**, during chemotherapy: narrowing of the synchondrosis with slight irregularity on the posterior border. Reconstruction of bone contours and some osteosclerosis. **d** Eight months after **c**: almost complete reconstruction of spongiosal bone. Residual irregularity around the synchondrosis

10.4 Greater Trochanter

Tuberculous osteomyelitis of the greater trochanter has been described in the literature at a rate of 0.2%–4% and seems to be the most frequent site of tuberculous osteomyelitis [103, 109, 112, 161]. We collected ten cases (2.2%) of this tuberculous manifestation, all in adult patients. In seven of these patients multifocal lesions were present: two in the sacroiliac joint, three in the hip, one in the knee, and one in the foot. The mode of infection is either initially as an osseous focus or secondary to a bursitis of the bursa lying between the gluteus medius muscle and the greater trochanter [103]. The osseous affection is mostly found in the craniolateral part of the trochanter, and, depending on the cause and duration of the tuberculous process, sequestra, osteosclerosis, and periosteal bone formation may be encountered. The bursa closely overlying the trochanter often presents bursitis, with thickening of the bursal wall and adherence to the bone. Abscess formation may occur. These abscesses have a tendency to progress to the region above the capsule. Spread of the tuberculous process to the hip joint may occur, leading to nonbacterial or tuberculous synovitis and some degree of joint destruction. This type of spread was seen in five of our patients (Figs. 65, 66). This affection of the soft tissues induces calcifications and ossifications adjacent to the trochanter.

10.4.1 Radiologic Findings (Figs. 117–121)

10.4.1.1 Osseous Focus

- Geode like cavities.
- Demineralization/osteoporosis.
- Sequestra.
- Marginal osteosclerosis.
- Cortical erosions.
- Periosteal bone formation.
- Abscesses and sinuses.

10.4.1.2 Healing and Healed Stages

- Osteosclerosis.
- Calcifications/ossifications in the soft tissues.

10.4.2 Differential Diagnosis

- Primary bone tumor.
- Metastatic disease.
- Pyogenic osteomyelitis.

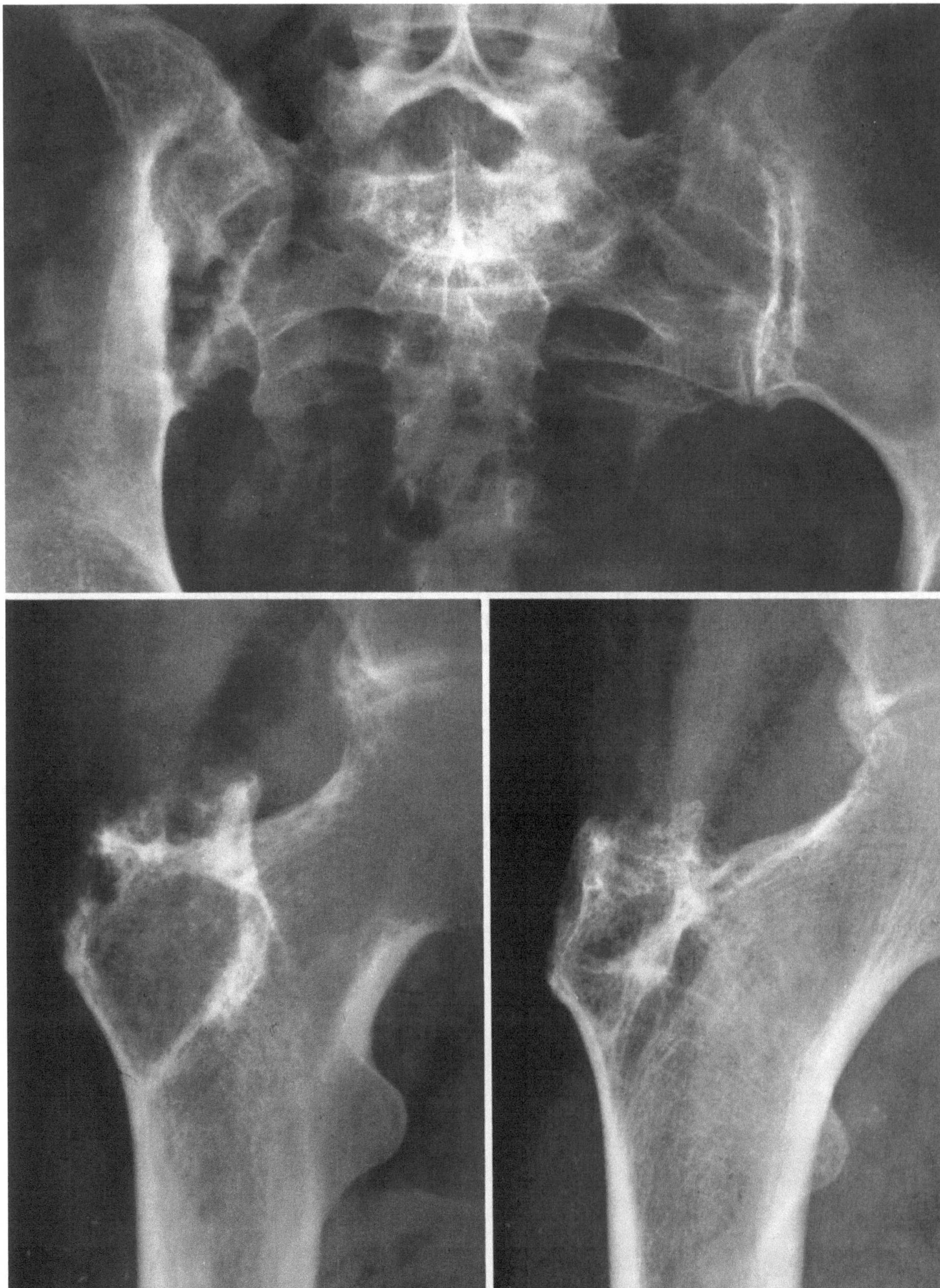

a

b

c

◀ **Fig. 117 a–c.** Multifocal skeletal tuberculosis. Woman, 61 years old. Previously bilateral tuberculous pleuritis and tuberculous involvement of the ischium. After 30 years involvement of the right sacroiliac joint. On admission, draining sinus over the right greater trochanter. **a** Unilateral sacroiliitis after exploration and excochleation. **b** Tuberculous affection of the greater trochanter with demineralization and cortical defects. **c** After 15 years: healed with remineralization and partial reconstruction of the contour of the greater trochanter

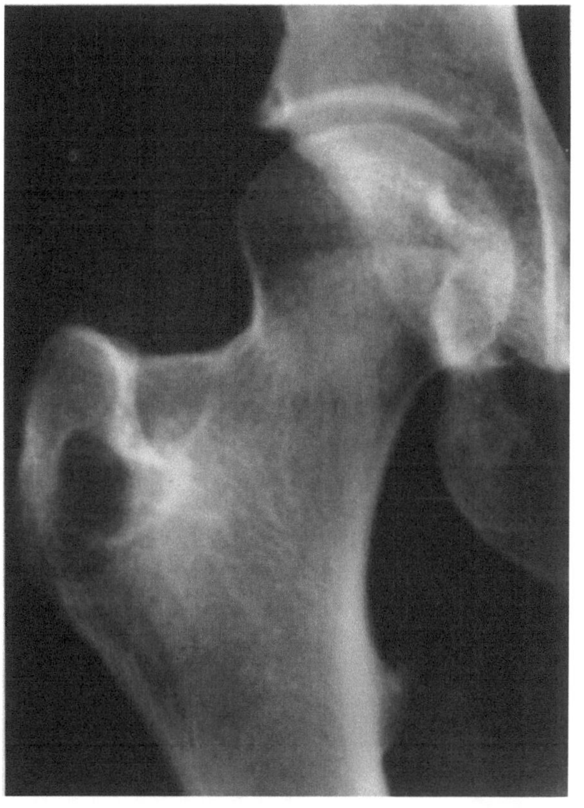

Fig. 118. Tuberculous affection of the greater trochanter. Adult woman. Osseous cavity and rather localized demineralization. Slight irregularity of the cortex. Positive culture for *M. tuberculosis*

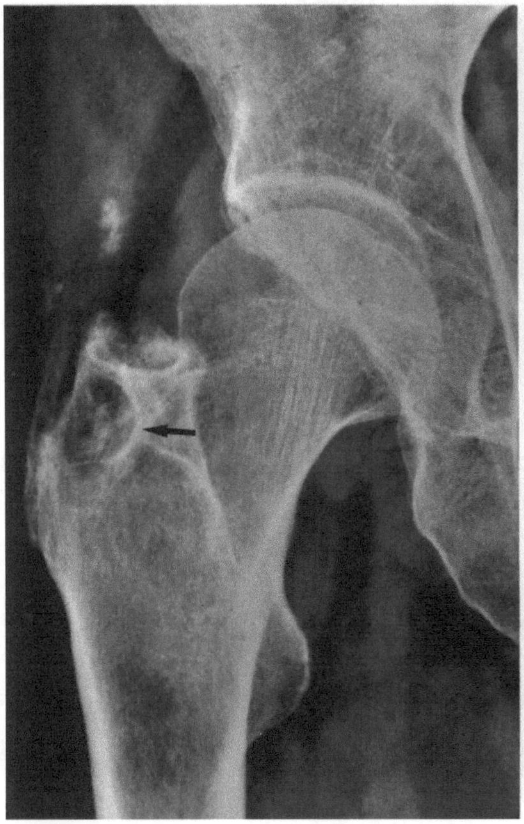
a

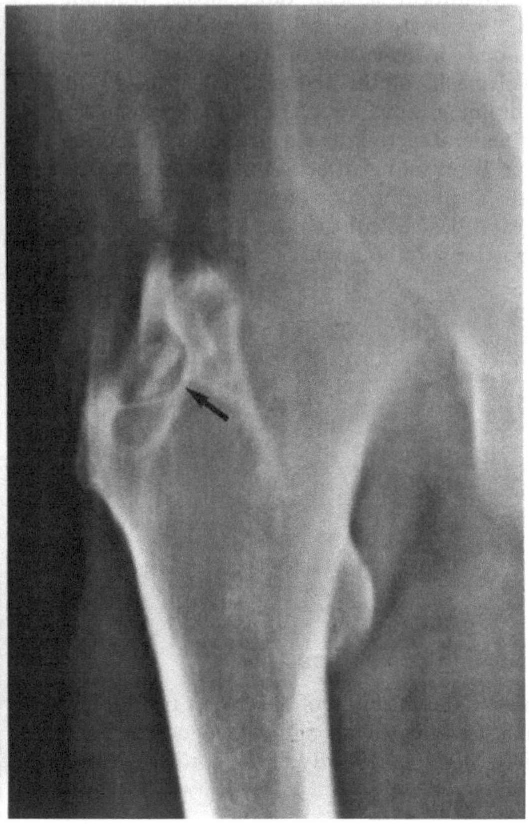
b

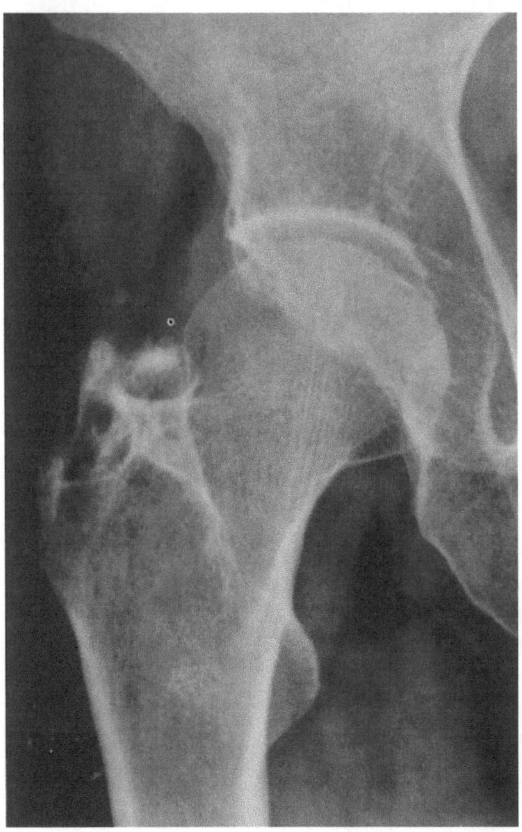
c

Fig. 119 a–c. Tuberculous affection of the greater trochanter. Woman, 65 years old. Previously left-sided pulmonary tuberculosis and tuberculous gonitis. On admission, detection of a reactivated osteomyelitis of the greater trochanter. **a**, **b** Bone cavity with marginal osteosclerosis and sequestrum (*arrows*). Marginal erosions. Calcifications and ossifications in the adjacent soft tissues, as a result of previous disease. **c** After 2 years: remineralization with residual bone defects. The sequestra seem to be incorporated in the bone structures. The calcifications are partly dissolved

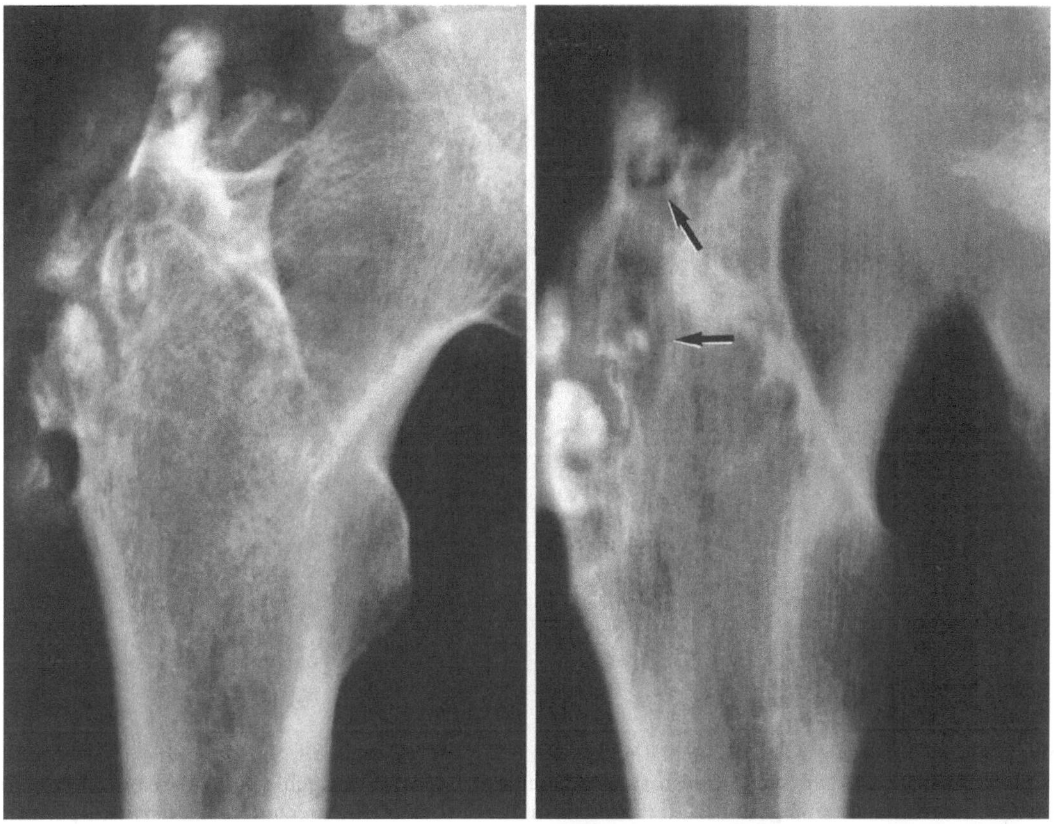

a b

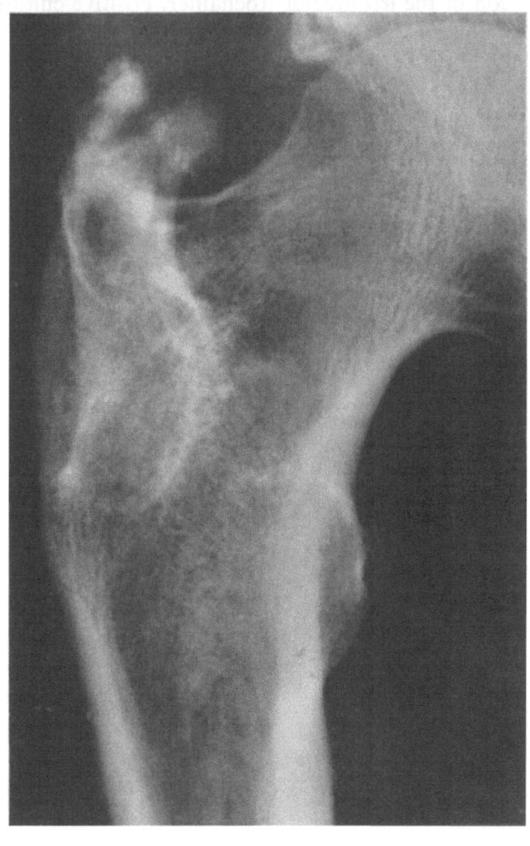

c

Fig. 120 a–c. Tuberculous affection of the greater trochanter. Woman, 64 years old. Previously right pulmonary tuberculosis and tuberculous involvement of the right kidney and right foot. On admission, tuberculous abscess of the right greater trochanter. **a**, **b** Bone cavities and marginal osteosclerosis with sequestra (*arrows*). Marginal erosions of the cortex. Calcifications in the soft tissues. **c** After 1 year, antituberculous therapy and surgery: remineralization and rather well-defined cortex

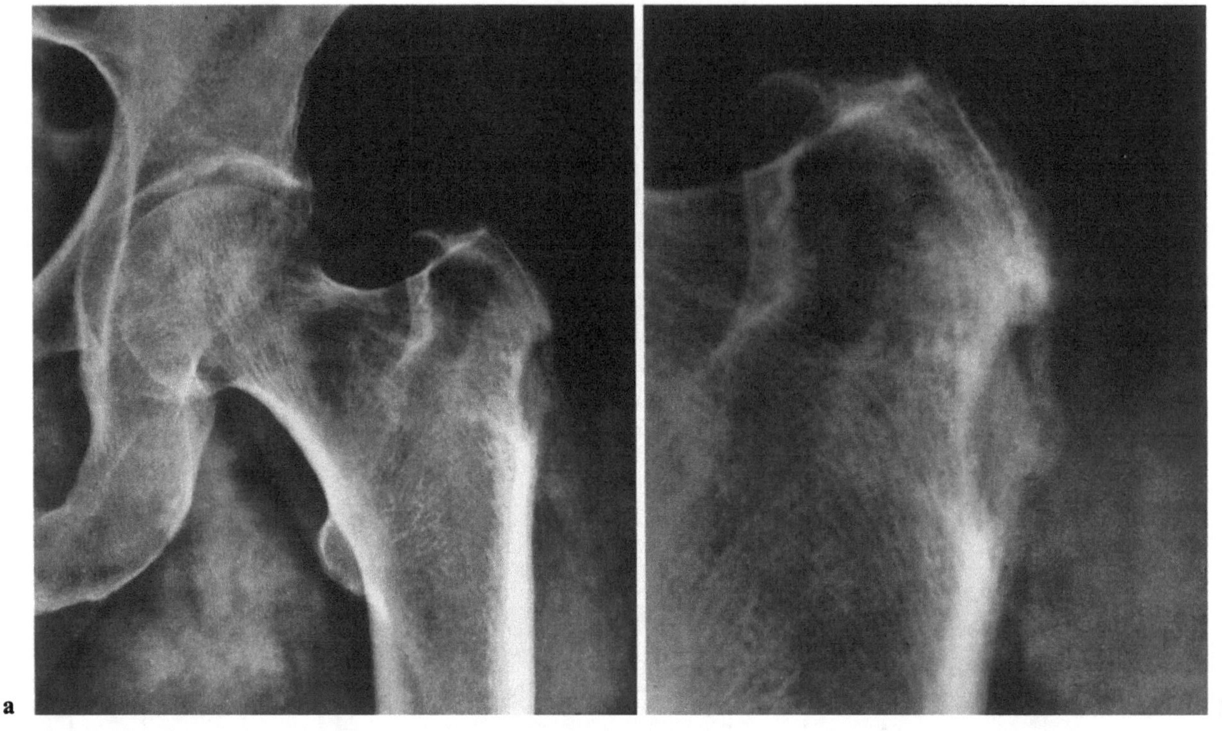

Fig. 121 a, b. Tuberculous affection of the greater trochanter. Woman, 68 years old. No history of tuberculosis. On admission, draining sinus after trauma in the region of the left greater trochanter. Positive culture of *M. tuberculosis*. Surgery and excision of the draining abscess and excochleation of the bone lesion. Irregular contour of the greater trochanter with periosteal bone formation

10.5 Cranium

Tuberculosis of the cranium is very rare. It may be found in the skullbones, facial bones, and bones of the skull base [10, 22, 23]. Infection of the cranial bones usually occurs by hematogenous spread of bacilli. Lymphogenous spread from affected cervical lymph nodes is also possible. In most cases of cranial tuberculosis, other lesions are found elsewhere in the body [23, 180]. The incidence of cranial tuberculosis has been reported at 0.1%–3.6% of patients with osseous tuberculosis [10, 38]. These bone lesions may be of initial osseous origin after hematogenous dissemination, or they may occur by spread of a tuberculous process from the subarachnoid space. Tuberculous meningitis or intracranial tuberculomas may lead to osseous involvement [27, 38, 180]. Most patients with cranial tuberculosis are children; there is an incidence of 50% below the age of 10 years and 75%–80% below the age of 20 [10]. In our material only three adult patients (0.7%) with cranial manifestations of tuberculosis were found.

10.5.1 Skull

A single frontal, parietal, or temporal spongiosal lesion is the most common manifestation of tuberculous affection of the skull. The internal as well as the external table of the vault may be destroyed, and subperiosteal and subcutaneous abscesses with sinuses may occur (Pott's puffy abscess). The dura usually prevents spread of the tuberculous process to the intracranial structures.

Typical radiologic findings of this type of tuberculosis are ill-defined and lytic lesions, with or without sequestra (Figs. 122, 123). Multiple skull lesions may coalesce and cross suture lines [10, 38]. Osteosclerosis caused by new bone formation has been described especially in association with secondary pyogenic infection, but otherwise this seems to be rare [22, 23, 147].

10.5.1.1 Differential Diagnosis

- Soft tissue tumors: lipoma, subaceous cyst, cephal hematoma.
- Histiocytosis X.
- Cholesteatoma.
- Myeloma.
- Metastatic disease.
- Growing fracture.
- Osteoporosis circumscripta.
- Hemangioma.

10.5.2 Facial Bones

Tuberculous involvement of the maxilla has been reported as the most frequent type of affection [90, 147]. In the mandible tuberculous lesions are usually localized in the angle and ramus. The radiologic aspect may be similar to that of nonspecific osteomyelitis with osteolysis and bone formation, but lesions with slow evolution seem to be more frequent. Abscesses, sequestra, and pathological fractures may occur [147]. In one of our patients a granulomatous tuberculous involvement of the left maxillary sinus was present originating in the maxilla.

10.5.3 Skull Base

Tuberculous osteitis of the skull base is very rare [119, 134, 180]. Radiographs usually present lytic destruction of the sphenoid bones with or without involvement of the orbits. Osteosclerosis is often absent [180]. In one of our patients tuberculous involvement of the left petrous bone was present, draining into the external auditory canal; the radiographs presented sclerosis of the mastoid with central osteolysis (Fig. 124).

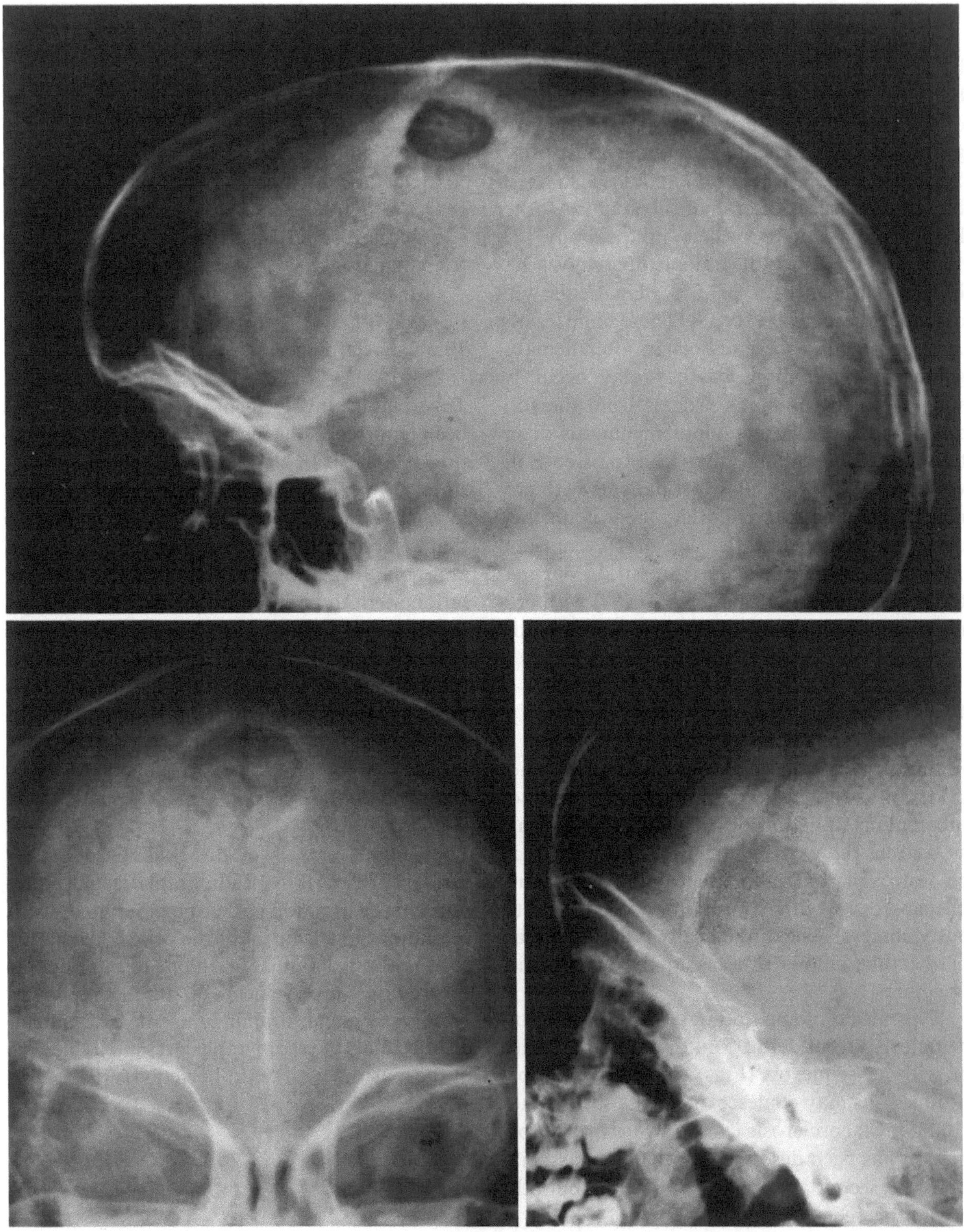

a

b

c

◀ **Fig. 122a–c.** Tuberculosis of the skull. Three different patients. (By courtesy of Prof. B.J. Cremin, Cape Town, South Africa.) **a** Circumscribed defect with significant marginal osteosclerosis and probably central reossification. **b, c** Rather well-defined defects with slight marginal osteosclerosis

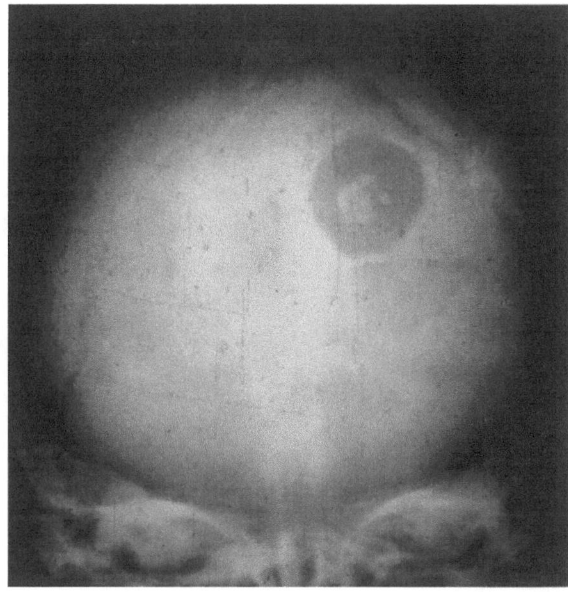

Fig. 123. Tuberculosis of the skull. Well-defined bone defect, marginal osteosclerosis, and sequestra (so-called bone sands). (By courtesy of Dr. W.P. Cockshott, Hamilton, Ont., Canada.)

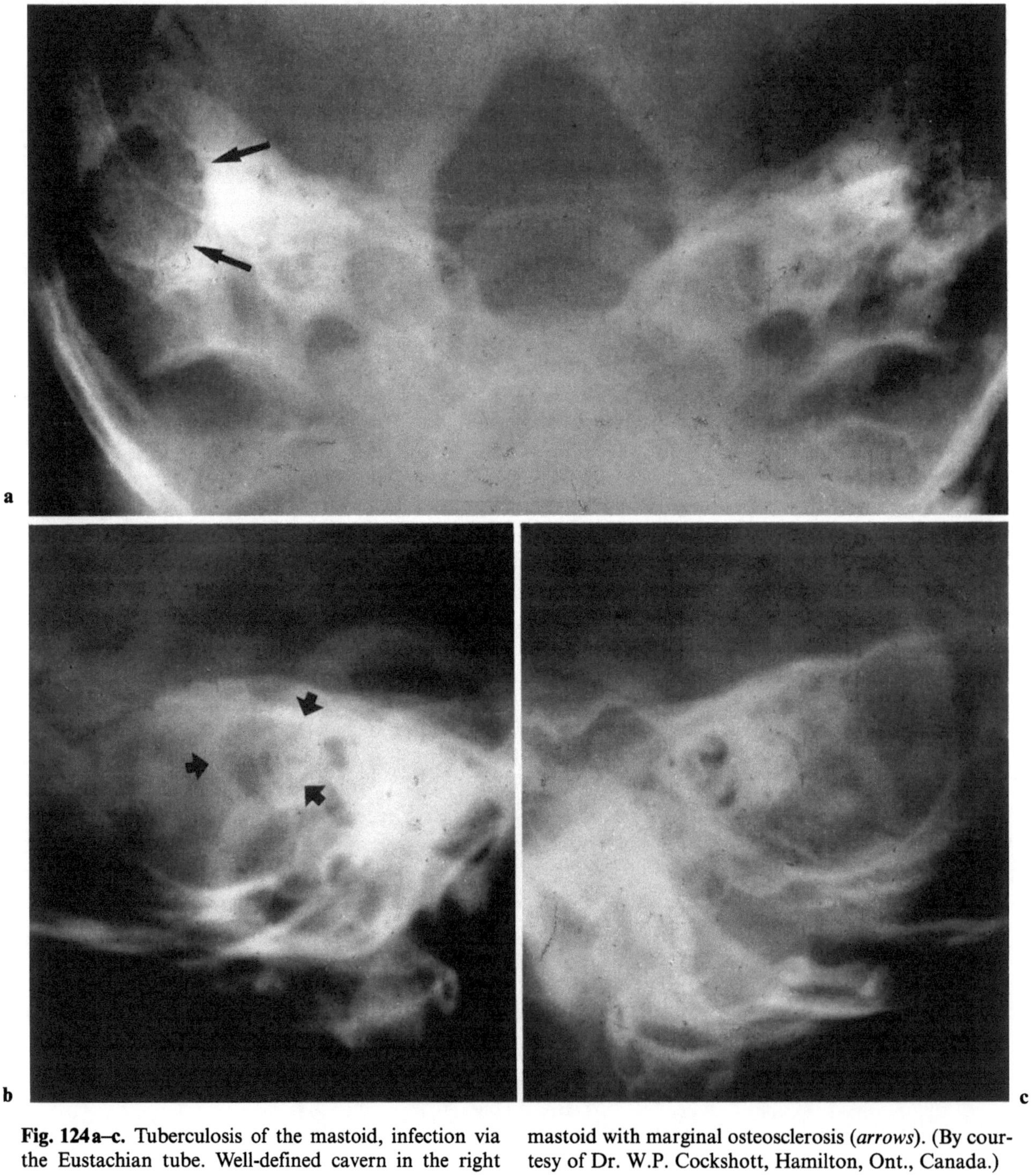

Fig. 124a–c. Tuberculosis of the mastoid, infection via the Eustachian tube. Well-defined cavern in the right mastoid with marginal osteosclerosis (*arrows*). (By courtesy of Dr. W.P. Cockshott, Hamilton, Ont., Canada.)

11 Therapy of Skeletal Tuberculosis

There is no single way of treating tuberculosis of bone and joints. Before antituberculous drugs could be used, it was known that children healed better than adolescents, adults healed slowly, and the elderly never achieved a final arrest. Nowadays even the outlook for the elderly is good, when adequate therapy is started in time. Still, the healing process in children remains faster than in adults and elderly persons.

Several aspects of therapy are dealt with briefly below: generalized therapeutic measures, immobilization, medicamentous therapy, surgical intervention, and rehabilitation.

The specific combination of therapeutic measures to be taken in a given case depends on extension and localization of the disease, the causative agent, and susceptibility to drugs. The only way to kill all mycobacteria is through the use of bactericidal drugs. According to Girdlestone [61], writing in 1940, the patient needs in the physician a combination of biologist, engineer, and surgical craftsman. One may add to this today a pharmacologist.

11.1 General Therapeutic Measures

Tuberculous disease of bone and joints is still a long-standing problem for the patient. Before the era of antituberculous drugs good nutrition and fresh air were considered to be most important; today the former is still considered valuable, although the value of the latter has become doubtful.

Certain general nursing matters are necessary with all patients. Optimal alimentation is important. The supine immobile patient must drink enough in order to avoid nephrolithiasis. Decubitus should be prevented, or treated as soon and as well as possible. Contractures must be prevented. The bedridden patient often has problems with his stool and must be laxated. For these patients anticoagulants are also recommended. Through enzyme induction in the liver, rifampicin accelerates the breakdown of many medicaments, including anticoagulants. The combination of anticoagulants and rifampicin needs close monitoring, both at the start and the first weeks after rifampicin is stopped.

Coexisting disease(s) should be treated accordingly. In case of a sinus, usually a late complication, prevention of secondary pyogenic infection is essential. Wounds must be taken care of with aseptic and antiseptic measures.

Psychological and social problems need attention. Repeated information on the course of the disease and on the treatment is most helpful to the patient in understanding his situation.

11.2 Immobilization

There is no common opinion about the value and duration of immobilization. In our opinion, immobilization is still an important measure in the treatment of tuberculosis of bone and joints. Antituberculous drugs, however, have considerably shortened the time necessary for healing. To give the patient the best opportunity for healing with the least extent of sequelae, immobilization should be part of the treatment. The capability of restoration in the original form, especially of vertebrae, is often astonishing. Destruction of joints, however, is usually permanent. Surgical intervention is often necessary.

When a patient with tuberculosis of bone and joints is treated on an ambulatory basis, one must accept the risk of further destruction of bony tissue and, especially in vertebral involvement, neurological complications. Destruction and necrosis may be advanced by weight load and activity. Even under modern medicamental treatment, demineralization and destruction in a tuberculous infection may proceed for some months. The bacilli are killed, but antigens (of bacilli dead or alive) may cause the hypersensitive reaction to continue (see Sect. 1.3.2), bringing tissue damage with caseation and formation of granulomas.

After operation immobilization is necessary to obtain reliable ossification. We prefer supine immobilization in the case of involvement of vertebrae or hips. Otherwise a brace is helpful. Circular caskets should be avoided because they do not allow one to follow the development of a cold abscess or sinus. Immobilization for a period of many weeks up to several months, of course, also has its disadvantages. Osteoporosis and muscle loss are important sequelae, especially in the elderly who are more prone to these phenomena. Static muscle contractions in the area where strict immobilization is necessary helps prevent muscle loss and osteoporosis.

11.3 Medicamentous Therapy

When Koch discovered the tubercle bacillus in 1882, the advent of efficient therapy seemed to be near at hand. However, it took until 1945 before the first antituberculous drug streptomycin was discovered [153]. With the antituberculous drugs today available, we aim at three goals [122]: (a) early bactericidal activity to prevent further spread of mycobacteria (bone and joint disease, however, is not contagious); (b) sterilizing activity to achieve definite cure; and (c) prevention of drug resistance through combination therapy.

Nowadays, the combination of isoniazid and rifampicin, suppleted by streptomycin and pyrazinamide during the first months (intensive phase), followed by isoniazid and rifampicin in the continuation phase, means that tuberculosis can be cured, thanks to the sterilizing capacity of these bactericidal drugs (first-line drugs). Ethambutol and thiacetazone are widely used second-line drugs. These are bacteriostatic, but in combination with first-line drugs they prevent drug resistance. Thiacetazone is much used in combination with isoniazid in Third World countries in the continuation phase (Table 2). If first-line drugs (isoniazid, rifampicin, pyrazinamide, streptomycin) cannot be used because of (multiple) drug resistance or intolerance or because of economic limitations (except for isoniazid, first-line drugs are not easily affordable in many developing countries), other drug combinations must be used. Short-course therapy, in which pyrazinamide also plays an essential role, is possible, however, only when isoniazid and rifampicin are used throughout the whole course.

Although they cause no sterilization, other combinations with second-line drugs are also sufficiently effective when given during a long enough period (±2 years in the case of bone disease). Patient compliance, however, is inversely proportional to the duration of therapy.

Table 2. Antituberculosis drugs in treatment of disease of bone and joints

Drug	Dosage
Isoniazid	4–8 mg/kg, 1–1.5 years
Rifampicin	10–15 mg/kg, 1–1.5 years
Pyrazinamide[a]	30–35 mg/kg (max. 2 g), 2–4 months
Streptomycin[b]	15–20 mg/kg (max. 1 g), 2 months
Ethambutol	25 mg/kg, the first 2 months; thereafter 15–20 mg/kg
Thiacetazone[c]	2 mg/kg (max. 150 mg)

Short-course therapy can only be given if isoniazid and rifampicin are given throughout the whole course. A 9 months therapy including these drugs may be sufficient in many cases.

[a] In case of *M. bovis*, pyrazinamide has no effect and can be replaced by ethambutol.
[b] Streptomycin can be replaced by ethambutol.
[c] When thiacetazone and isoniazid are given in the continuation phase, short-course therapy is not possible.

Thus, the combination of isoniazid and rifampicin is strongly recommended, in addition to pyrazinamide in the initial phase.

Drug therapy for tuberculosis is independent of localization and age. Multiple drug resistance, however, may influence the choice of drug combination and the duration of therapy. *M. bovis* is not sensitive to pyrazinamide because it lacks pyrazinamidase, which is necessary to convert pyrazinamide to the in vivo working compound pyrazinoic acid. Dosage is dependent solely on the patient's weight. In older treatment manuals, the dosage for children, especially that of isoniazid, is recommended to be higher than in adults because of greater distribution volume and total body clearance [3, 130, 131]. Recent studies have shown there to be no reason for this: in children and in adults dosage should be the same per kilogram body weight [118, 162].

In tuberculosis of bone and joints, cultures and a drug-resistance pattern are not always available. Yet good results can be obtained, even in those cases with resistant bacterial populations, when therapy is started with the four bactericidal drugs isoniazid, rifampicin, pyrazinamide, and streptomycin in the intensive phase and continued with isoniazid and rifampicin. Streptomycin may well be replaced by ethambutol in the intensive phase without influencing the final outcome [122].

There is no common opinion about the duration of antituberculous treatment in bone and joint disease. Studies by the British Medical Council in Third World countries have shown that short-course therapy (6–9 months) given under fully supervised conditions is very effective for pulmonary tuberculosis, and this is now accepted worldwide. Studies on short-course therapy for extrapulmonary tuberculosis are promising [46, 116]. The follow-up period varies from 3 to 10 years, which is relatively short for an infection of bone and joints. As disease may develop only decades after primary infection, diagnosis of a relapse might also take many years.

In most cases the bacterial load of an infection in bony tissue is low, but the penetration of drugs in an extensive cold abscess may be difficult. Dutt et al. [46] observed a good effect with short-course therapy (9 months) for extrapulmonary tuberculosis. Yet in 6 out of 47 patients (13%) with tuberculosis in bone and joints, treatment failed. These patients received additional drugs and/or surgery and were retreated for 1–1.5 years.

Since the introduction of rifampicin in 1968 the duration of treatment for bone and joint disease in the Netherlands has decreased from 2–3 years to 1–1.5 years. Since rifampicin has come to be used in the combination, we have seen neither failures or relapses nor an increase in bone lesions in the follow-up period after treatment is stopped. Short-course therapy (9 months) was introduced in 1978 for pulmonary tuberculosis and most other forms of extrapulmonary tuberculosis. Miliary tuberculosis and tuberculoud lymphadenitis are still treated for 1 year. Shortening of duration may be possible.

11.4 Surgical Therapy

Whether surgical therapy is necessary depends on localization and extension of the bone lesion(s) and/or (cold) abscess. Surgery has a threefold purpose: (a) removal of sick tissue (pus, sequestra, aseptic necrotic bone, and devitalized discs or cartilage), (b) restoration of stability, and (c) prevention of (further) deformities. Each of these three goals cannot always be achieved.

For the patient an operation often means (momentary) pain relief and the prevention of pain in the future, but sometimes also diminished function. Before antituberculous drugs became available, there was a high chance of reactivation of disease by surgery, and especially miliary tuberculosis was not uncommon after an operation was performed. When the first antituberculous drugs came into use, an operation was considered justified only when the patient had received drugs for several weeks in advance. Nowadays, with the use of bactericidal drugs, such as the combination of isoniazid, rifampicin, and pyrazinamide, there is no need to fear the (miliary) hematogenous spread of mycobacteria during operation. Yet one should always bear in mind that a tuberculous infection needs a special approach. Many operations need specially skilled and experienced orthopedic surgeons [114]. A brief summary is given below of how a tuberculous process in bone and joint disease may be handled surgically, discussing both the abscess and vertebral and joint involvement.

11.4.1 The Cold Abscess

Superficial lesions with a small abscess usually need no surgical intervention. However, even when it is relatively small, a cold abscess can, by its location, exert pressure on surrounding tissues and cause damage. This is especially the case in joint disease or progression of the bone lesions towards the vertebral canal. Immediate decompression may then prevent further destruction and (possibly) neurological complications. A puncture or drainage should preferably be carried out with the use of a closed system and with the help of negative pressure instead of gravity. We prefer repeated punctures over prolonged drainage because, properly performed, the chance of complications, especially that of secondary infection or sinus, is nil.

In order to prevent a sinus, the abscess should be approached from a higher level, i.e., cranially, but in the supine immobilized patient perhaps more from the anterior side. A long needle is used, going obliquely downwards through healthy skin and underlying tissues before entering the abscess wall. The skin should be shifted downwards before introducing the needle, so that after retraction the needle channel is bent upwards, against gravity; this method prevents pus coming down before closure of the channel [25]. The quantity of pus produced is sometimes tremendous. Drainage should not be prolonged for much more than 1 week in order to prevent a secondary pyogenic infection and/or a sinus. Local installment after puncture or drainage of isoniazid (100 mg) in combination with either kanamycin (250 mg) or rifamycin SV (250 mg) gives high concentrations in the abscess cavity. Not only tubercle bacilli may be killed, for both kanamycin and rifamycin have a bactericidal effect on a broad spectrum of gram-negative and gram-positive bacteria and thus prevent secondary infection [83]. After local installment of drugs drainage should be interrupted for about 2 h. If it is not possible to work under sterile conditions, one should avoid this mode of local treatment. The abscess wall is usually well vascularized, and the orally administered antituberculous drugs also penetrate into the abscess.

11.4.2 Surgery in Tuberculous Spondylitis

In tuberculous spondylitis adjacent vertebral bodies are usually involved. Destruction of arches or spinae is less common. In many cases the vertebrae fuse spontaneously with medication and additional conservative treatment. An abscess delays the healing process. Operation is to be considered before long, on the basis of destruction already present on admission and neurological complications. In the case of acute, increasing neurological symptoms immediate decompression is necessary. Since the problem is in the abscess, progressing from the focus in the vertebral body to the vertebral canal, the best way to remove diseased tissue is through the anterolateral approach. Laminectomy is an easier method for opening the vertebral canal and achieving decompression of the spinal cord. However, this usually increases instability, which may inhibit spinal fusion. Sometimes, nevertheless, there is no other choice. Although some correction is possible, collapsed vertebrae do not regain their original shape. In children the adjacent intervertebral discs may become asymmetrical, and the adjacent vertebrae may grow faster on the abdominal side, by which the kyphosis is (partly) compensated (Fig. 7d). Because of this compensation it is not crucial to measure the angle K that is described by Konstam and Bleskovsky to indicate the severity of kyphosis [89]; measurement of the angle between the upper and lower bone plates of the involved vertebrae is more suitable. Deformities in old lesions can often not be corrected. The fibrosis is extremely tough, and trying to change the situation can often do more harm than good.

Spondylodesis Anterior: Radical Operation. To enhance healing and restrict sequela a radical operation is advised [115, 116]. Radical operation consists of decompression by evacuation of the abscess and removal of all diseased tissue until a clean bleeding cavity remains. A mortise is made in the vertebrae and a strut graft of proper length to keep the vertebrae as much as possible in the normal position is introduced. The interval that remains between the vertebrae and the cavities in the corpora is filled with small bone chips [70–72]. It is very important to have the right length of strut graft. Only the destroyed vertebrae must fuse and regain stabilization. In the thoracic region a left-sided anterolateral approach is preferred because the vena cava is more vulnerable than the aorta. Parts of the rib that must be removed in order to reach the diseased area can be used as strut graft and bone chips. In the lumbar and cervical region bone from the tibia or pelvis can be used as such. In the higher lumbar region the lesions are approached by an incision as for nephrectomy. The fourth and fifth lumbar vertebrae can be reached via the abdominal wall, distal to the aortic bifurcation. The gross lesion is often more extensive than radiographs suggest. By leaving a drain behind in the affected focus and one in the abscess, it is possible to insert daily doses of antituberculous drugs. These drains must be inserted by separate means, not through the operation wound, and connected to a closed bottle. This mode of inserting drugs gives very high concentrations locally and may cause the attacking of mycobacteria that had perhaps remained, thereby preventing secondary infection [83, 84]. The drains are removed after 2–3 weeks.

Spondylodesis Posterior. If a radical operation by anterior approach is impossible for whatever reason, posterior fusion may be considered. This operation is easier to perform. The Albee method, whereby a bone graft is inserted into the split spinae, is suitable only over a short distance (2 or 3 vertebrae) and in the lower thoracic and lumbar region [5]. Long bone grafts tend to fracture. Better stability can be attained by inserting a bone graft over the arches, close to the vertebral body [68]. To obtain better fusion destruction of intervertebral joints is sometimes performed. The residual space can be filled with bone chips. The bone grafts need time to incorporate and obtain reliable fusion. Only thereafter is mobilization possible.

11.4.3 Surgery in Joint Tuberculosis

In the early onset phase a joint may be saved. Restoration of an already destroyed joint is not possible. In the case of a recently diseased joint it is very important to be aware of augmented pressure in the joint cavity, especially in the hip joint. Immediate decompression is necessary and may save the joint from further destruction.

The joint condyles and surfaces need time to regenerate (recalcify). Immobilization is important in this period and may, together with medicamentous treatment, lead to complete healing and normal function (Figs. 50, 68).

If the patient receives only antituberculous drugs and remains mobilized, the destruction continues; especially in the hip this may result in a completely destroyed joint within a few months. This happened, for example, to the patient in Fig. 65 before she was admitted. Unfamiliarity with treatment of bone and joint tuberculosis was disastrous, although the tubercle bacilli were adequately attacked.

Ankylosis after removal of all diseased tissue (pus, sequestra, aseptic necrotic bone, cartilage, and synovia) was until recently the first choice of treatment and is still a good solution in many cases (Figs. 125, 126). Nowadays, it is also possible to replace joints by a prosthesis (knee, hip). Whether this form of treatment is applicable, however, depends greatly on the extent of bone destruction and osteoporosis. The quality of remaining bone tissue must be sufficient to tolerate the implantation of a prosthesis. In the first place, however, the tuberculous disease must be adequately treated. Only after attaining a radiologically stable disease does a replacement ar-a 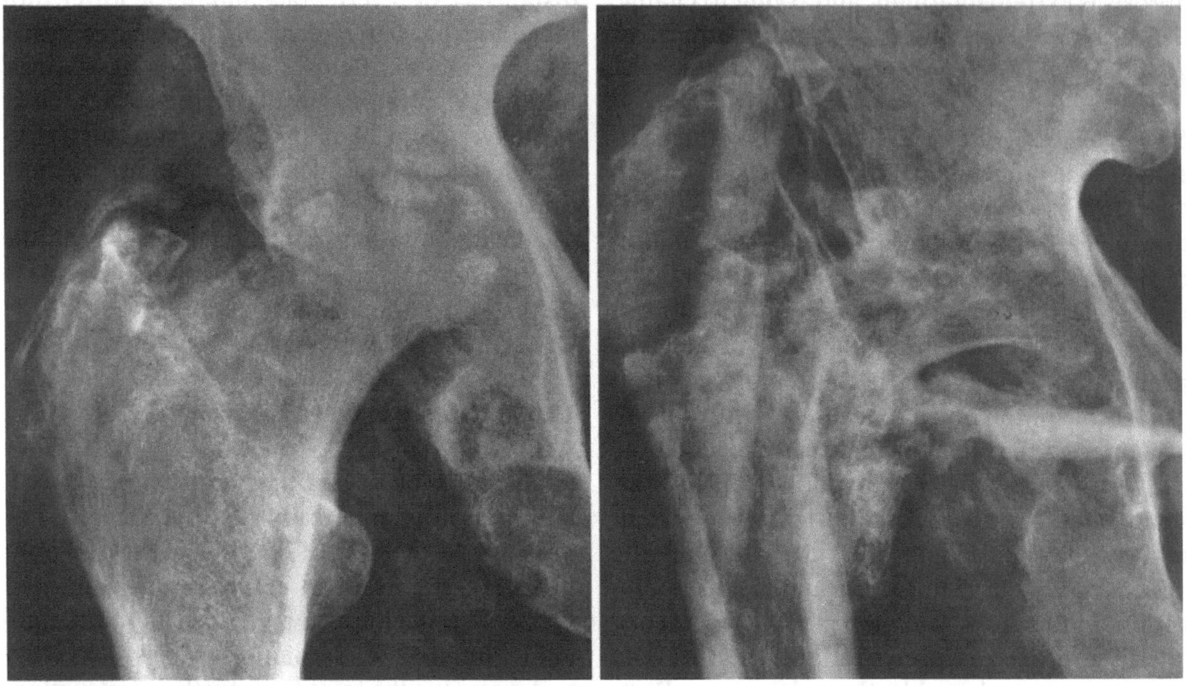 b

Fig. 125a, b. Tuberculosis of the hip. Man, 60 years old. Concomitant miliary tuberculosis and previous tuberculous affection of the right greater trochanter. **a** Old tuberculous affection of the greater trochanter. Ossifications in the overlying bursa. Severe involvement of the hip joint, with demineralization and destruction of femoral head and acetabulum. Narrowing of the joint space. The ischium also presents tuberculous foci. **b** Three years after **a**: situation after arthrodesis in a totally destroyed hip joint

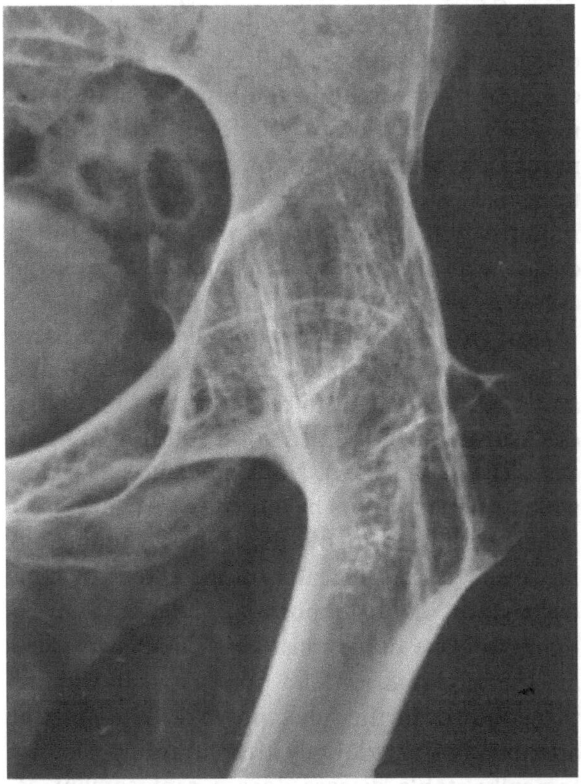

Fig. 126. Tuberculosis of the left hip. Man, 29 years old. Previous intermittent reactivation of tuberculosis in the left hip. Spontaneous bony fusion after immobilization in the prechemotherapy era. Seven years later, tuberculous meningitis

throplasty have a major chance of success [86, 100, 157]. Implantation of a prosthesis into a joint that was formerly infected with tuberculosis may result in a (local) flare up of tuberculosis if the surgeon is not aware of the patient's history of untreated tuberculosis and does not give (preventive) therapy [111, 125]

11.4.4 Other Locations of Osseous Tuberculosis

Tuberculosis in locations other than vertebrae and joints is treated in the same way: surgical débridement of all diseased tissue and possible local treatment with antituberculous drugs as long as wounds are open, together with oral therapy for about 1 year.

11.5 Rehabilitation

11.5.1 General Remarks

Rehabilitation is an important part of therapy in bone and joint disease. Pain and immobilization often result in muscle loss. Contractures and bone deformities give rise to abnormal function. In vertebral involvement with extension to the vertebral canal, neurological symptoms may result, and these may sometimes be permanent.

As long as the tuberculosis is still active, physiotherapy can do much harm. If the patient is forced to do exercises in this stage, the pain may worsen and diseased bony tissue collapse further, and a draining sinus may result, heal badly, or even relapse after drug therapy has started.

The healing stage, with restoration of bony tissue and resorption of the abscess, takes about 2 years after medicamentous treatment has started and continues until after the time at which the drugs are usually stopped. Aside from physiotherapy, the use of braces, adapted footwear, crutches, or cane are often necessary to restore or increase stability and optimal function.

The physical condition of the patient must be built up gradually. Progressive physical exercise is necessary to restore the strength and tone of the patient. Psychological and social problems need attention. Vocational guidance and occupational therapy is required when it is not possible for the patient to return to his previous employment.

Rehabilitation of a patient with bone and joint tuberculosis is a long process. One should not give up too early: with sufficient patience and perseverance from both patient and therapists, much can be achieved.

11.5.2 Rehabilitation in Tuberculous Spondylitis

If the disease is still active, pain may restrain the patient from much activity. The involved vertebrae should be given time to fuse. Therefore, immobilization is essential. Physiotherapy in this stage should consist of static muscle contractions in the area of the vertebral column. After a bony or fibrous fusion is established, the pain subsides or vanishes, and carefully supervised active exercises may be started.

After an operation with removal of diseased tissue and reimplantation of bone grafts or chips, the latter must be allowed time to incorporate in order to restore stability. In our experience, it is possible to start rehabilitation after 3–4 months of immobilization following an operation without threatening further collapse of vertebrae or relapse of sinuses.

However, this kind of treatment is not possible everywhere, due to lack of facilities, experienced orthopedic surgeons, physiotherapists, and/or funds. If the patient is treated on an ambulatory basis, the chance of further collapse of vertebrae and persisting neurological loss(es) is higher, but this must be accepted in many cases. As long as the vertebral column is unstable, a plaster-of-Paris jacket or the use of a collar in cervical involvement may relieve pain considerably [113a, 115]. If a stabilizing operation is not possible, and the vertebrae tend to dislocate and muscle strength remains insufficient, the use of a brace must be considered. Improvement, however, is possible still after 1–2 years.

In vertebral involvement the chance of back pain above and beneath the previously affected vertebrae is often seen many years after the disease and is mainly due to surmenage of adjacent intervertebral discs. Overweight and bearing of heavy loads should be avoided in patients with previous spondylitis.

11.5.3 Rehabilitation in Joint Disease

Static contractions of muscles that are inserted over the affected sites are advisable in the active stage of disease. In order to avoid contractures in adjacent joints, these may be passively exercised with full support of the physiotherapist in order to avoid weight bearing in the affected joint(s). After immobilization weight bearing, durance, and intensity of active exercises must gradually be augmented. It may take weeks or up to many months before optimal function is reestablished. Where there is permanent loss of function and/or shortening of extremities, e.g., in hip or knee involvement, other measures must be taken to improve function, such as adapted footwear, a brace, or the use of crutches or a cane in order to regain stability.

References

1. Abdelwahab IF, Present DA, Klein MJ (1986) Tuberculous pseudotumor of the proximal end on the right tibia without obvious synovial involvement. Case report. Skeletal Radiol 15:652–656
2. Abdelwahab IF, Present DA, Gould E, Klein MJ, Nelson J (1988) Tuberculosis of the distal metaphysis of the femur. Case report. Skeletal Radiol 17:199–202
3. Advenier C, Saint-Aubin A, Scheinmann P, Paupe J (1981) Pharmacocinétique de l'isoniazide chez l'enfant. Rev Fr Mal Respir 9:365–374
4. Al Arif LJ Goldstein RA, Affronti LF, Janicki BW (1979) HLA-BW 15 and tuberculosis in a North American black population. Am Rev Respir Dis 120:1275–1278
5. Albee FH (1930) The bone-graft operation for tuberculosis of the spine. Twenty years' experience. JAMA 94:1467–1476
6. American Thoracic Society (1981) Tuberculin skintest. Am Rev Respir Dis 124:356–363
7. Andersen JR, Ritchie AWS, Scobie WG (1979) Tuberculous osteitis of the talus. Tubercle 60:115–118
8. Babhulkar SS, Tayade WB, Babhulkar SK (1984) Atypical spinal tuberculosis. J Bone Joint Surg [Br] 66:239–242
9. Banacerraf B, Germain RN (1978) The immune response genes of the major histocompatibility complex. Immunol Rev 38:70–119
10. Barton CJ (1961) Tuberculosis of the vault of the skull. Br J Radiol 34:286–290
11. Bell D, Cockshott WP (1971) Tuberculosis of the vertebral pedicles. Radiology 99:43–48
12. Benkeddache Y, Gottesman H (1982) Skeletal tuberculosis of the wrist and hand: a study of 27 cases. J Hand Surg 7:593–600
13. Bergdahl S, Fellaender M, Robertson B (1976) BCG osteomyelitis. J Bone Joint Surg [Br] 58:212–216
14. Bjoerksten B, Boquist L (1980) Histopathological aspects of chronic recurrent multifocal osteomyelitis. J Bone Joint Surg [Br] 62:376–380
15. Blacklock JWS (1957) Injury as an aetiological factor in tuberculosis. Proc R Soc Med 50:61–64
16. Bleiker MA (1960) Specific and non specific tuberculin sensitivity in the Netherlands. van Gorkum, Assen
17. Blumensaat C (1932) Kortikale Kalkaneustuberkulose. Dtsch Z Chir 236:349–356
18. Bohrer SP (1969) Tuberculous synovitis with widening of the intercondylar notch of the distal femur. Br J Radiol 42:703–704
19. Bosworth DM, della Pietra A, Farrell RF (1950) Streptomycin in tuberculous bone and joint lesions with mixed infection and sinuses. J Bone Joint Surg [Am] 32:103–108
20. Brocher JEW (1946) Die Scheuermannsche Krankheit. Schwabe, Basel
21. Brown TS (1980) Tuberculosis of the ribs. Clin Radiol 31:681–684
22. Brown TS, Franklyn PP, Marikkar MSK (1980) Tuberculosis of the skull vault. Clin Radiol 31:313–315
23. Buehrer JHG, Van der Heyden AHM, Teertstra HJ, Van der Wolk DB, Weigel HM (1986) Tuberculose van de schedel. Ned Tijdschr Geneeskd 130:169–172
24. Burke HE (1947) The pathogenesis of Pott's disease. Trans Am Clin Climatol Assoc 59:122–137
25. Calve J (1935) La tuberculose ostéo-articulaire. Masson, Paris
26. Chafetz N, Genant HK, Hoaglund FT (1982) Ischioglutal tuberculous bursitis with progressive bony destruction. J Can Assoc Radiol 33:119–120
27. Chambers AA, Lukin RR, Tomsick TA (1979) Cranial and intracranial tuberculosis. Semin Roentgenol 14:319–324
28. Chaparas SD, MacVandiviere M, Melvin J, Koch G, Becker C (1985) Tuberculin test. Variability with the Mantoux procedure. Am Rev Respir Dis 132:175–177
29. Chapman M, Murray RO, Stoker DJ (1979) Tuberculosis of the bones and joints. Semin Roentgenol 14:266–282
30. Chaussee D (1981) Les infections articulaires chez l'adulte. Atteintes périférique et vertébrales à germes banals et à bacilles tuberculeux. Rev Rhum Mal Osteoartic 48:69–76
31. Chow SP, Yau A (1980) Tuberculosis of the knee: a long term follow-up. Int Orthop 4:87–92
32. Colombani S (1942) La tuberculosi del piede. Chir Organi Mov 27:390–393
33. Commission on Isoniazid Preventive Treatment (1985) Preventive treatment of tuberculosis. National Consensus Conference on Tuberculosis. Chest [Suppl] 87(2):128S–132S

34. Cortez LM, Pankey GA (1973) Mycobacterium marinum infections of the hand. Report of three cases and review of the literature. Am J Bone Joint Surg 55:363–370
35. Cremin BJ, Fisher RM, Levinsohn MW (1970) Multiple bone tuberculosis in the young. Br J Radiol 43:638–645
36. Cyrlak D, Pais MJ (1986) Chronic recurrent multifocal osteomyelitis. Skeletal Radiol 15:32–39
37. Dannenberg AM (1982) Pathogenesis of pulmonary tuberculosis. Am Rev Respir Dis 125(2)23:25–29
38. Danziger J, Bloch S, Cremin BJ, Goldblatt M (1976) Cranial and intracranial tuberculosis. S Afr Med J 50:1403–1405
39. David-Chaussé J, Dehais J, Effroy C (1984) L'ostéite vertébrale tuberculeuse centro-somatique. Rev Rhum Mal Osteoartic 51:123–129
40. Davidson PT, Horowitz I (1970) Skeletal tuberculosis. A review with patient presentations and discussion. Am J Med 48:77–84
41. Davies PDO, Humphries MJ, Byfield SP, Nunn AJ, Darbyshire JH, Citron KM, Fox W (1984) Bone and joint tuberculosis. A survey of notifications in England and Wales. J Bone Joint Surg [Br] 166:326–330
42. Davis JA, Bluestone R (1979) Case report 84. Skeletal Radiol 4:41–43
43. Day DL, Mikhail SH (1985) Topics in radiology: case of the month. JAMA 253:1593–1595
44. Dechairo DC, Kittredge D, Meyers A, Corrales J (1973) Septic arthritis due to Mycobacterium triviale. Am Rev Respir Dis 108:1224
45. Delilles S, Miller AE, Gudas J (1979) Tuberculous arthritis. J Am Pediatr Assoc 69:432–437
46. Dutt AK, Moers D, Stead WW (1986) Short course chemotherapy for extra pulmonary tuberculosis. Ann Intern Med 104:7–12
47. Echeverria J, Kaude JV (1978) Multifocal tuberculous osteomyelitis. Pediatr Radiol 7:238–240
48. Eckel H, Düe K (1985) Die Tuberkulose der kleinen Gelenke. ROFO 142:19–23
49. Editorial (1986) Rheumatoid arthritis and tuberculosis. Lancet 9:321–322
50. Editorial (1987) Depression stress and immunity. Lancet 27:1467–1468
51. Edwards LB, Palmer CE (1958) Epidemiological studies of tuberculin sensitivity. Am J Hyg 68:213
52. Ellis W (1974) Multiple bone lesions caused by avian-Battey mycobacteria. Report of a case. J Bone Joint Surg [Br] 56:323–326
53. Elting JJ, Southwick WO (1974) Acute infantile septic arthritis of the hip due to Mycobacterium triviale. A case report. J Bone Joint Surg [Br] 56:184–186
54. Enarson DA, Fuji M, Makielna EM, Grzybowski S (1979) Bone and joint tuberculosis, a continuing problem. Can Med Assoc J 120:139–145
55. Eng J, Aaneland T (1966) BCG-osteitis in a child. Scand J Respir Dis 47(3):182–186
56. Feldman F, Auerbach R, Johnston A (1971) Tuberculous dactylitis in the adult. AJR 112:460–479
57. Firooznia H, Seliger G, Abrams RA, Valensi V, Shamoun J (1973) Disseminated extrapulmonary tuberculosis in association with heroin addiction. Radiology 109:291–296
58. Forestier J (1929) L'aurothiope dans le rheumatisme chronique. Ann Med Interne (Paris) 53:323–327
59. Fraser RG, Paré JA (1970) Diagnosis of the diseases of the chest. Saunders, Philadelphia
60. Garber EK, Bluestone R (1981) Case report 138. Skeletal Radiol 6:75–76
61. Girdlestone GR (1940) Tuberculosis of bone and joint, preface. Oxford University Press, Oxford
62. Glynn LE (1962) Autoimmunity. J Bone Joint Surg [Br] 44:743
63. Göksan A, Yazicioglu Ö, Özger H, Tözün R, Türkmen M (1984) Die isolierte Knochentuberkulose am Talus. Z Orthop 122:657–658
64. Goldblatt M, Cremin BJ (1978) Osteo-articular tuberculosis: its presentation in coloured races. Clin Radiol 29:669–677
65. Gropper GR, Acker JD, Robertson JH (1982) Computed tomography in Pott's disease. Neurosurgery 10:506–508
66. Hartofilakidis-Garofalidi G (1969) Cystic tuberculosis of the patella. Report of three cases. Am J Bone Joint Surg 51:582–585
67. Hellstadius A (1934) Tuberculosis pubis. Acta Orthop Scand 5:148–151
68. Henle A, Huber E (1926) Die operative Versteifung der erkrankten Wirbelsäule durch Knochentransplantation. Ergeb Chir 19
69. Hermann G, Mendelson DS, Cohen BA, Train JS (1983) Role of computed tomography in the diagnosis of infectious spondylitis. J Comput Assist Tomogr 7:961–968
70. Hodgson AR, Stock FE (1956) Anterior spinal fusion: a preliminary communication on the radical treatment of Pott's disease and Pott's paraplegia. Br J Surg 44:266–275
71. Hodgson AR, Yan A (1969) Vordere operative Zugänge zur Wirbelsäule. II. Brustwirbelsäule. Thieme, Stuttgart (Actuelle Chirurgie, vol 4)
72. Hodgson AR, Yan A (1969) Vordere operative Zugänge zur Wirbelsäule. III. Lendenwirbelsäule. Sacrum. Thieme, Stuttgart (Actuelle Chirurgie, vol 5)
73. Hodgson AR, Wong W, Yau A (1969) X-ray appearances of tuberculosis of the spine. Thomas, Springfield
74. Holoshitz J, Klajman A, Drucker J, Lapidot Z, Yaretzky A, Frenkel A, van Eden W, Cohen JR (1986) T-lymphocytes of rheumatoid arthritis patients show augmented re-activity to a fraction of mycobacteria cross-reactive with cartilage. Lancet 9:305–309
75. Horsburg CR, Masom III UG, Fahri DC, Iseman MD (1985) Disseminated infection with Mycobacte-

ria avium-intracellulare. A report of 13 cases and a review of the literature. Medicine (Baltimore) 64(1):36–48
76. Hwang CH, Khan S, Ende N, Mangura BT, Reichman LB, Chou J (1985) The HLA, -B and DR phenotypes and tuberculosis. Am Rev Respir Dis 132:382–385
77. Isaacs AJ, Sturrock RD (1974) Poncet's disease – fact or fiction? A re-appraisal of tuberculous rheumatism. Tubercle 55:135–142
78. Jaffe HL (1972) Degenerative and inflammatory diseases of bones and joints. Lea and Febinger, Philadelphia
79. Johansson S (1926) Knochen und Gelenktuberculose in Kindesalter. Fischer, Jena
80. Johnstone JG (1938) Trauma in relation to tuberculosis of bones and joints. Tbc Assoc London 20:5
81. Kahan A, Feldmann Jl, Menkes CJ, Zenny JC, Vinh T (1983) Ostéo-condensation vertébrale plurifocale avec syndesmophytose d'origine tuberculeuse. Rev Rhum Mal Osteoartic 50:77–79
82. Kahan A, Amor B, Benhamou CL (1983) Rapidly progressive idiopathic chondrolysis simulating tuberculosis of the shoulder. J Rheumatol 10:291–293
83. Kastert J (1956) Traitement focal de la spondylite tuberculeuse, combinant l'opération chirurgicale et l'instillation locale d'antibiotiques. Rev Chir Orthop 42:207–210
84. Kastert J, Uehlinger E (1964) Skelettuberkulose. In: Hein J von, Kleinschmidt H, Uehlinger E (Hrsg) Formenkreis der extrapulmonalen Tuberkulose. Thieme, Stuttgart (Handbuch der Tuberkulose, vol 4)
85. Kelly PJ, Karlson AG, Weed LA (1967) Infection of synovial tissues by mycobacteria other than Mycobacterium tuberculosis. Am J Bone Joint Surg 49:1521–1530
86. Kim YY, Ko CU, Lee SW, Kwak B (1979) Replacement arthroplasty using Charnley prothesis in old tuberculosis of the hip. Int Orthop 3:81–88
87. Kisch E (1921) Diagnostik und Therapie der Knochen- und Gelenktuberkulose. Vogel, Leipzig
88. Kolodny A (1925) A contribution to the knowledge of pathogenesis of skeletal tuberculosis. J Bone Joint Surg [Br] 7:53–57
89. Konstam PG, Bleskovsky A (1962) The ambulant treatment of spinal tuberculosis. Br J Surg 50:26–38
90. Kremer W, Wiese O (1936) Tuberculosis de los huesos y articulaciones. Labor, Barcelona
91. Kumar K (1985) A clinical study classification of posterior spinal tuberculosis. Int Orthop 9:147–152
92. LaBerge JM, Brant-Zawadski M (1984) Evaluation of Pott's disease with computed tomography. Neuroradiology 26:429–434
93. La Fond EM (1958) An analysis of adult skeletal tuberculosis. J Bone Joint Surg [Am] 40:346–364
94. Lannelongue O (1894) La tuberculose chirurgicale. Gauthier-Villar, Paris
95. Lecklitner ML, Potter JL, Growcock G (1985) Computed tomography in acquired absence of thoracic pedicle. J Comput Assist Tomogr 9:395–397
96. Leibe H, Köhler H, Kessler P (1982) Osteo-articulare Tuberkulosis: Rückblick – gegenwärtiger Stand von Diagnostik und Therapie. Zentralbl Chir 107:322–342
97. Lévi-Valensin G, Bacques O, Guérin CL, Majer L, Hubault H, Bard M, de Sèze S (1976) L'ostéite tuberculeuse de l'africain transplanté. J Radiol Electrol Med Nucl 57:31–37
98. Liechti A (1948) Die Röntgendiagnostik der Wirbelsäule. Springer, Vienna
99. Lindemann K, Kuhlendahl H (1953) Die Erkrankungen der Wirbelsäule. Enke, Stuttgart
100. Linden A van der (1984) Osteoarticulaire tuberculose. Ned Tijdschr Geneeskd 128:108–113
101. Lurie MB (1964) Resistance to tuberculosis: experimental studies in native and acquired defense mechanisms. Harvard University Press, Cambridge, Mass
102. Lynder AF (1982) Tuberculosis of the greater trochanter: a report of eight cases. J Bone Joint Surg [Br] 64:185–188
103. Mabille JP, Collombier B, Magnet JL, Strauss J (1981) La trochantérite tuberculeuse. Son diagnostic radiologique. J Radiol 62:25–30
104. Madkour MM, Sharif HS, Aabed MY, Al-Fayez MA (1988) Osteoarticular brucellosis. AJR 150:1101–1105
105. Magnet JL, Thierry A, Couaillier JF, Tavernier C, Strauss J (1984) Ostéite tuberculeuse de l'atlas. Rev Rhum Mal Osteoartic 51:273–275
106. Manzella JP, Vanvoris LP, Hauska JF (1975) Isolated calcaneal tuberculous osteomyelitis: a case report. J Bone Joint Surg [Am] 61:946–947
107. Maritz NGJ, de Villiers JFK, van Castricum QS (1982) Computed tomography in tuberculosis of the spine. Comput Radiol 6:1–5
108. Marks J, Cook J, Pringle JAS (1975) Bone abscess due to Mycobacterium xenopi. Tubercle 56:157
109. Martini M (1988) Tuberculosis of the bones and joints. Springer, Berlin Heidelberg New York
110. Martini M, Ouahes M (1988) Bone and joint tuberculosis. A review of 652 cases. Orthopedics 11:861–866
111. McCullough CJ (1977) Tuberculosis as a late complication of total hip replacement. Acta Orthop Scand 48:508–510
112. McMurray B (1947) Tuberculosis of the greater trochanter. Br Med J 2:492–494
113. Meck JM, Collettis E, Parrot R, Le Gal J (1979) Aspects radiologiques de l'ostéite tuberculeuse chez l'africain immigré. Ann Radiol (Paris) 22:634–639
113a. Medical Research Council (1973) Working Party on Tuberculosis of the Spine: second report. A controlled trial of plaster-of-paris jackets in the management of ambulant outpatient treatment of tuberculosis of the spine in children on standard chemo-

therapy: a study in Pusan, Korea. Tubercle 54:261–282
114. Medical Research Council (1982) Working Party on Tuberculosis of the Spine: eighth report. A ten year assessment of a controlled trial comparing debridement and anterior spinal fusion in the management of tuberculosis of the spine in patients on standard chemotherapy in Hong Kong. J Bone Joint Surg [Br] 64:393–398
115. Medical Research Council (1985) Working Party on Tuberculosis of the Spine: ninth report. A 10-year assessment of controlled trials of inpatient and outpatient treatment and of plaster-of-paris jackets for tuberculosis of the spine in children on standard chemotherapy. Studies in Masan and Pusan, Korea. J Bone Joint Surg [Br] 67:103–110
116. Medical Research Council (1986) Working Party on Tuberculosis of the Spine: tenth report. A controlled trial of six-month and nine-month regimens of chemotherapy undergoing radical surgery for tuberculosis of the spine in Hong Kong. Tubercle 67:243–259
117. Menard V (1900) Etude pratique sur le mal de Pott. Masson, Paris
118. Micelli J, de Kantor JN, Sclavo L, Barbarelli G, Peluffo G, Broglia B, Albiero A (1981) Blood concentrations of isoniazid in children at doses of 5 or 10 mg/kg. Rev Fr Mal Respir 9:365–374
119. Miles J, Hughes B (1970) Tuberculous osteitis of the skull. Br J Surg 57:673–679
120. Miller KD, Moore ME (1983) Tuberculous arthritis of the shoulder: delayed diagnosis aided by arthrography. Clin Rheumatol 2:61–64
121. Mispar MS, Nuiz MA, Warni MA, Nazboo T, Chirui SK (1978) Regional lymph gland biopsy in tuberculous synovitis of the knee. Int Surg 63:25–27
122. Mitcheson DA (1985) The action of antituberculosis drugs in short-course therapy. Tubercle 66:219–225
122a. Morse D, Brothwell DR, Ucko PJ (1964) Tuberculosis in ancient Egypt. Am Rev Respir Dis 90:524–541
123. Mortensson W, Eklöf O, Jorulf H (1976) Radiologic aspects of BCG-osteomyelitis in children. Acta Radiol [Diagn] (Stockh) 17:845–855
124. Morvan G, Martini N, Massare C, Nahum H (1984) La tuberculose du rachis cervical. Rev Chir Orthop 70:76–80
125. Mouterde P, Deburge A (1978) Un cas d'infection tuberculeuse primitive sur prothèse totale de hanche. Rev Chir Orthop 64:171–174
126. Murray RO, Haddad F (1959) Hydatid disease of the spine. J Bone Joint Surg [Br] 41:499–506
127. Nathanson L, Cohen W (1941) A statistical and roentgen analysis of 200 cases of bone and joint tuberculosis. Radiology 36:550–567
128. Nicholson RA (1974) Twenty years of bone and joint tuberculosis in Bradford. J Bone Joint Surg [Br] 56:760–765
129. Obisesan AA, Lagundoye SB, Lawson EA (1977) Radiological features of tuberculosis of the spine in Ibadan, Nigeria. Afr J Med Sci 6:55–67
130. Ollivier A, Besson-Leaud M (1979) Principes d'emploi des medicaments antituberculeux chez l'enfant. Ann Pediatr (Paris) 26(3):141–147
131. Olson WA, Pruitt AW, Dayton PG (1981) Plasma concentrations of isoniazid in children with tuberculous infections. Pediatrics 67(6):876–878
132. Ottenhoff THM, Torres P, Terencio de las Aguas J, Fernandez R, van Eden W, de Vries RRP, Stanford JL (1986) Evidence for an HLA-DR4 associated immune response gene for Mycobacterium tuberculosis. Lancet 9:310–312
133. Pearson CM (1959) Development of arthritis in rat following injections of adjuvant. In: Schaeffer JH et al., Lo Grippi GA, Chase MW (eds) Mechanisms of hypersensitivity. Saunders, Philadelphia, p 647 (Henry Ford Symposium)
134. Pendergrass EP, Schaeffer JP, Hodes PJ (1956) The head and neck in roentgen diagnosis, 2nd edn. Blackwell, Oxford
135. Poncet A (1897) De la polyarthrite tuberculeuse déformante ou pseudorheumatisme chronique tuberculeux. Congr Fr Chir 1:732–739
136. Pott P (1779) Remarks on that kind of palsy of the lower limbs which is frequently found to accompany a curvature of the spine. Johnson, London
137. Probst FP, Björkstén B, Gustavson KH (1980) Radiological aspects of chronic recurrent multifocal osteomyelitis. J Bone Joint Surg [Br] 62:376–380
138. Psarras H, Faraj J, Gouliamos A, Kalovidouris A, Vlahos L, Pappavassiliou C (1985) Tuberculosis of the spine. Radiologe 25:339–341
139. Rebaudi F (1933) Tubercolosi dell'acetabolo. Arch Ital Chir 33:58–61
140. Reeder MM, Palmer PES (1981) Radiology of tropical diseases. Williams and Wilkins, Baltimore, pp 302–346
141. Reinhard W (1966) Die Tuberkulose der Knochen und Gelenke. Springer, Berlin Heidelberg New York
142. Resnick D, Niwayama G (1988) Diagnosis of bone and joint disorders. Saunders, Philadelphia
143. Rich AR (1951) The pathogenesis of tuberculosis. 2nd edn. Thomas, Springfield
144. Richter R, Krause FJ (1983) Primäre Diaphysentuberkulose der langen Röhrenknochen. ROFO 139:549–552
145. Richter R, Michels P (1982) Die isolierte Darmbeintuberculose und ihre Differentialdiagnose. ROFO 137:135–140
146. Robins RHC (1967) Tuberculosis of wrist and hand. Br J Surg 54:211–218
147. Sanchis-Olmos V (1948) Skeletal tuberculosis. Williams and Wilkins, Baltimore

148. Sandström S (1983) Multifocal sclerotic BCG spondylitis in a 13-years old girl. Pediatr Radiol 13(4):239–240
149. Deleted
150. Saphyakhajon P, Mukhopadhay D, Spiegel P, Grossman BJ (1977) Mycobacterium kansasii arthritis of the knee joint. Am J Dis Child 131:573
151. Satta F (1932) La tuberculose du poignet. Rev Orthop 19:609–613
152. Sbabaro MD (1985) Tuberculin test: a re-emphasis on clinical judgement. Am Rev Respir Dis 132:177–178
153. Schatz A, Waksman SA (1944) Effect of streptomycin and other antibiotic substances on Mycobacterium tuberculosis and related organisms. Proc Soc Exp Biol Med 57:244–248
154. Schinz HR (1952) Tuberkulose der Knochen und Gelenke. In: Schinz HR, Glauner R, Uehlinger E, Baensch WE (eds) Lehrbuch der Röntgendiagnostik. Thieme, Stuttgart, part 1, pp 525–584
155. Schonell ME, Crofton JW, Stuart AE, Wallace A (1968) Disseminated infection with Mycobacterium avium. I. Clinical features, treatment and pathology. Tubercle 49:12–30
156. Deleted
157. Sijbrandij S (1985) Een kwart eeuw heupgewrichts prothesen; terugblik, balans en toekomst-verwachtingen. Ned Tijdschr Geneeskd 129:1721–1725
158. Silva JF (1980) A review of patients with skeletal tuberculosis treated at the University Hospital Kuala Lumpur. Int Orthop 4:79–82
159. Simons B (1939) Röntgendiagnostik der Wirbelsäule. Fischer, Jena
160. Smyrnis P (1957) Hematogenous infection of closed fractures with mycobacterium tbc. J Bone Joint Surg [Am] 39:902–904
161. Sorrel E, Sorrel-Dejerine R (1932) Tuberculose osseuse et ostéo-articulaire. Masson, Paris
162. Steensma JT, Nossent G (1986) INH dosage in children. Bull Int Union Tuberc 61:109
163. Steindler A (1935) Sobre la tuberculosis de la muñeca. Rev Orthop Traumatol 4:223–228
164. Stutzer H (1985) Die Bedeutung verschmälerter Bandscheiben für die Diagnose der Wirbelsäulentuberculose. ROFO 143:595–596
165. Tatelman M, Drouillard EJP (1953) Tuberculosis of the ribs. AJR 70:923–935
166. Teertstra HJ, Taconis WK (1986) Veranderingen in het röntgenbeeld van tuberculose van het skelet. Ned Tijdschr Geneeskd 130:157–162
167. Trotsenburg L van (1977) Een destruerend wervelproces is gelukkig niet altijd maligne. Ned Tijdschr Geneeskd 121:1281–1284
168. Tuli SM (1975) Tuberculosis of the spine. American Publishing, New Delhi
169. Umerah BC (1977) Radiological patterns of spinal tuberculosis in the African. East Afr Med J 54:598–605
170. Urovitz EP (1982) Tuberculous dactylitis: a rare entity. Can J Surg 25:689–690
171. Valtancoli G (1924) Sul trattamento degli ascessi spondilitici prevertebrali del tratto medio dorsale del rachide. Chir Organi Mov 8:497–502
172. Versfeld GA, Salomon A (1982) A diagnostic approach to tuberculosis of bones and joints. J Bone Joint Surg [Br] 64:446–449
173. Vogelzang RL, Hendrix RW, Neiman HL (1983) Case report: computed tomography of tuberculous osteomyelitis of the pubis. J Comput Assist Tomogr 7:914–915
174. Warns EHJ (1979) Syllabus skelettuberculose. Koninklijke Nederlandse Centrale Vereniging tot Bestrijding der Tuberculose, 's-Gravenhage
175. Weaver P, Lifeso RM (1984) The radiological diagnosis of tuberculosis of the adult spine. Skeletal Radiol 12:178–186
176. Weir WRC, Muraleedharan MV (1983) Tuberculosis arising at the site of physical injury: eight case histories. J Infect 7:63–66
177. Whelan MA, Naidich DP, Post JD, Chase E (1983) Computed tomography of spinal tuberculosis. J Comput Assist Tomogr 7:25–30
178. Wilkinson MC (1967) A note on Poncet's tuberculous rheumatism. Tubercle 48:297–306
179. Williams CS, Riordan DC (1973) Mycobacterium marinum (atypical acid-fast bacillus) infections of the hand. A report of 6 cases. Am J Bone Joint Surg 55:1042–1050
180. Witcombe JB, Cremin BJ (1978) Tuberculous erosion of the sphenoid bone. Br J Radiol 51:347–350
181. Wolstein D, Rabinowitz JG, Twersky J (1974) Tuberculosis of the rib. J Can Assoc Radiol 25:307–309
182. Zeben W van, Wagenvoort MM (1980) Tuberculeuze ostitis door BCG. Ned Tijdschr Geneeskd 124:1765–1767

Subject Index

I. Fogelman, London (Ed.)

Bone Scanning in Clinical Practice

1987. XVIII, 260 pp. 217 figs. Hardcover
ISBN 3-540-16212-7

The technetium-99m-(99m Tc) – labelled diphosphonate bone scan remains the most frequently requested investigation in any nuclear medicine department because of its exquisite sensitivity for lesion detection. It has a wide, and apparently ever increasing, range of applications in clinical practice and the purpose of this book is to provide a comprehensive review of the use of bone scanning. In addition, important topics of current interest, such as single photon emission computed tomography, quantitation of bone uptake of diphosphonate and bone mineral measurements by photon absorptiometry, are included. The emphasis is on the clinical use of bone scanning. The book is extensively illustrated and provides a source of reference for all who are interested in the skeleton. It will be of value not only to nuclear medicine specialists, but also to those in the fields of orthopaedics, rheumatology, endocrinology and oncology.

Springer-Verlag Berlin
Heidelberg New York London
Paris Tokyo Hong Kong

Springer

MIX
Papier aus verantwortungsvollen Quellen
Paper from responsible sources
FSC® C105338

If you have any concerns about our products,
you can contact us on
ProductSafety@springernature.com

In case Publisher is established outside the EU,
the EU authorized representative is:
Springer Nature Customer Service Center GmbH
Europaplatz 3, 69115 Heidelberg, Germany

Printed by Libri Plureos GmbH
in Hamburg, Germany